INSULIN

RECEPTORS AND LIGANDS IN INTERCELLULAR COMMUNICATION

edited by
Bernhard Cinader

Institute of Immunology
University of Toronto
Toronto, Ontario, Canada

INSULIN

Its Receptor and Diabetes

edited by

Morley D. Hollenberg

Endocrine Research Group
Department of Pharmacology and Therapeutics
University of Calgary Faculty of Medicine
Calgary, Alberta, Canada

sponsored by

The Julia McFarlane Diabetes Research Unit
University of Calgary Faculty of Medicine
Calgary, Alberta, Canada

MARCEL DEKKER, INC.   New York and Basel

Library of Congress Cataloging in Publication Data
Main entry under title:

Insulin : its receptor and diabetes.

   (Receptors and ligands in intercellular
communication ; 6)
      Includes index.
      1. Insulin--Receptors. 2. Diabetes. I. Hollenberg,
Morley D., (date). II. Series: Receptors and
ligands in intercellular communication ; v. 6.
(DNLM: 1. Diabetes Mellitus--metabolism. 2. Receptors,
Insulin--physiology. W1 RE107LM v. 6 / WK 820 I583)
QP572.I5I5725 1985   616.4'62   85-25256
ISBN 0-8247-7383-7

MARCEL DEKKER, INC.
270 Madison Avenue, New York, New York 10016

Current printing (last digit):
10 9 8 7 6 5 4 3 2 1

PRINTED IN THE UNITED STATES OF AMERICA

Series Introduction

Cells communicate with one another to bring about orderly differentiation and regeneration. Receptor/ligand interaction can occur via secreted ligands; it can also occur between membranes of different cell types, i.e., via adhesion molecules which play a role in the structural development of organs, exemplified by neural cell adhesion and embryologic development under the influence of "master" cells. Communication during adult life maintains coordination and balance in the multicellular organism. The "words" of this communication are molecules, i.e., factors, which convey signals by combination with receptors. These signals can give rise to the production of other factors and thus to the "sentences" of the intercellular language; the resulting intercommunication is intense and continuous. In the immune system, macromolecules of the external world cause distortions of the internal conversation; the resulting change in the balance of molecular communication constitutes the immune response.

This series will be devoted to the study of biological language and will cover receptor-ligand interaction in health and disease. Special volumes will be dedicated to the development of drugs, modeled to fit receptors, to the understanding of the role of receptors in parasite-host interaction, and to receptor polymorphism, blockade, and activation.

Books are authored individually or consist of contributions from several investigators who have specialized in their topics. In each case, the preface will summarize the field for biologists who may not be specialists in the area covered in a particular book. This volume of our series summarizes an area in which biology, biochemistry, and clinical medicine interact intimately and rapidly to improve quality of life and survival. The volume surveys impressive recent progress in the analysis of chemical and biological properties of insulin receptors. It examines different organ systems which are directly affected by interaction of their insulin receptors with the hormone and deals with receptor-ligand interactions that relate, not only to diabetes, but also to other diseases.

Bernhard Cinader

Preface

There are few areas of clinical medicine to rival diabetes mellitus as a
disease entity that can so rapidly bring discoveries at the laboratory
bench to bear on the personal lives of such a widespread patient population. Perhaps in part as a result of the impact of diabetes on the
lives of so many individuals, research in areas related to diabetes is
not only progressing but is accelerating at an unprecedented rate.
Simply to keep track of the progress has become a full-time occupation
for those of us granted the luxury of digesting the piles of journal
articles facing us each week. For those with the time constraints imposed by dealing with patients on a day-to-day basis, the explosion
of information represents an intimidating challenge. The information
gap that I perceive developing between the practicing physician and
the biomedical research community is difficult to manage, either by the
"quick fix" of a lead article in a current medical journal or by an over-
loaded yearly "refresher course." This gap is widening not only for
today's physician at the bedside and for our future physicians in the
lecture halls, but also for many research scientists interested in following developments in the insulin receptor field. For instance, even
those researchers focused on a particular receptor system (e.g., for
steroid hormones) may be hard-pressed to keep track of developments
in other receptor systems (like the one for insulin).

The stimulus for this volume has come in part from a desire to address the issue of this widening knowledge gap; and to provide for
physicians, medical students (and their teachers), research graduate
students, and research scientists interested generally in receptor structure and function an in-depth profile of what I perceive to be today's
key areas related to insulin receptor research. A major focus of the
monograph is on areas related to the structure, biochemistry, and cell

biology of the receptor itself. Other areas deal with receptor-associated mechanisms thought to participate in insulin action and with some novel environments (e.g., central nervous system, immune system) in which the insulin receptor can play a role. Finally, the receptor is dealt with in the context of the disease entity, diabetes. An attempt has been made by all of the contributors to make the information accessible to a readership wider than simply the group working directly on insulin receptor biochemistry. The new insights concerning the insulin receptor itself and the mechanisms involved in insulin action represent a landmark not only in terms of diabetes per se, but also in terms of disease entities (e.g., cancer, birth defects) apart from diabetes. A synopsis of the menu offered, ranging from the discovery of insulin to the relationship of the insulin receptor to diabetes mellitus, is provided by the first chapter of this book.

I would like to take this opportunity to thank those who have given so generously of their time and energy to contribute to this volume and to acknowledge the support of the Julia McFarlane Diabetes Research Unit. I would also like to express my admiration and appreciation for all individuals who at this time are working so creatively on the complex areas of cell biology touched on by this volume. The collective effort of so many people not only makes a monograph like this one possible but also makes this a particularly exciting time to do research on topics related to diabetes.

Morley D. Hollenberg

Contents

Contributors

Paulos Berhanu, M.D., Department of Medicine, University of Colorado Health Sciences Center, Denver, Colorado

Michael Bliss, Ph.D., Department of History, University of Toronto, Toronto, Ontario, Canada

J. Harold Helderman, M.D., Department of Internal Medicine, The University of Texas Health Science Center at Dallas and The Southwestern Medical School, Dallas, Texas

Morley D. Hollenberg, D. Phil., M.D., Department of Pharmacology and Therapeutics, University of Calgary Faculty of Medicine, Calgary, Alberta, Canada

Steven Jacobs, M.D., Department of Molecular Biology, The Wellcome Research Laboratories, Research Triangle Park, North Carolina

Leonard Jarett, M.D., Department of Pathology and Laboratory Medicine, University of Pennsylvania School of Medicine, Philadelphia, Pennsylvania

Frederick L. Kiechle, M.D., Ph.D., Department of Clinical Pathology, William Beaumont Hospital, Royal Oak, Michigan

M. Daniel Lane, Ph.D., Department of Biological Chemistry, The Johns Hopkins University School of Medicine, Baltimore, Maryland

Jerrold M. Olefsky, M.D., Department of Medicine, University of California School of Medicine, San Diego, La Jolla, California

Barry I. Posner, M.D., Department of Medicine, McGill University Clinic and Royal Victoria Hospital, Montreal, Quebec, Canada

Robert M. Smith, B.A., Department of Pathology and Laboratory Medicine, University of Pennsylvania School of Medicine, Philadelphia, Pennsylvania

Mark van Houten, M.D., Ph.D.,* Department of Medicine, McGill University Clinic and Royal Victoria Hospital, Montreal, Quebec, Canada

Cecil C. Yip, Ph.D., Banting and Best Department of Medical Research, University of Toronto, Toronto, Ontario, Canada

Kenneth Zierler, M.D., Departments of Physiology and Medicine, The Johns Hopkins University School of Medicine, Baltimore, Maryland

Present affiliation: Department of Neurology, University of California at Los Angeles, School of Medicine, Los Angeles, California

INSULIN

1

Insulin, Its Receptor and Diabetes: An Overview

MORLEY D. HOLLENBERG *University of Calgary Faculty of Medicine, Calgary, Alberta, Canada*

I. TO THOSE WHO HAVE BEEN WAITING SINCE THE DISCOVERY OF INSULIN: AN OPTIMISTIC PROGRESS REPORT

In the field of diabetes-related research, it will be difficult to re-capture the kind of excitement that surrounded the discovery of insulin, and it may be impossible to match the dramatic impression made both on the lay public and on the scientific community by the administration of insulin to diabetic subjects such as Leonard Thompson. Bliss has artfully recreated for us in his recent book the true scenario surrounding insulin's discovery, and in his chapter in this treatise (Chapter 2), he summarizes events as they "really happened." Doubtless, many believed euphorically that the discovery of insulin represented the key "breakthrough" that would lead quickly to a "cure" for diabetes. Yet here we are now, over 60 years after the discovery of insulin, all of us much sobered by the enormous amount of effort that has yet to yield a full understanding of the complex disease entity—diabetes. Clearly, insulin does, in terms of diabetes-related research, represent a rosetta stone of sorts. Nonetheless, despite our optimism based on the accelerated rate of the discovery of new clues in this rapidly advancing area of research, we have yet to crack the code. There is, however, just cause for our cautious optimism. As will be evident from the work described in this book, we now have a much broader grasp than ever before of the clinical heterogeneity, cell biology, and cellular chemistry related to diabetes. It is now clear to the lay public as well as to the scientific community that no "single big breakthrough" will lead to the total understanding of the disease; rather, many discoveries both apparently big and small

will contribute to our understanding. It is also clear that to talk in
terms of finding "the cure" for diabetes may be misleading. One may
rather talk optimistically about an understanding of the disease entity
that will permit a rational approach to the total management of all diabetics. Thus, the heady excitement that initially surrounded the
discovery of insulin has, largely because of progress made over the
past decade, been replaced by a new kind of cautious enthusiasm that
has served as a major stimulus for this book. It is our goal in this
book to provide the reader with a perspective on today's focus on what
are considered by many to be key areas of diabetes-related research
and to summarize some of the exciting advances that have been recently made in those areas. As will be apparent from many of the
chapters, the discoveries relating to insulin and its receptor bear on
a much wider area of pathophysiology than that of diabetes alone. For
instance, the newly discovered enzymatic activity of the insulin receptor (tyrosine kinase) relates directly to analogous enzymes produced by so-called oncogenes. This relationship between the receptor
and oncogene products, predicted on the basis of the receptor's enzymatic activity, has been elegantly substantiated by the discovery
of the sequence homology between the β-subunit of the receptor and
the sequence of tyrosine kinases encoded by sarcoma viruses. Thus,
unexpectedly, the information relating to the action of insulin is now
providing a most useful paradigm for the action of a variety of "insulinlike" growth factors and oncogene products that may play a critical
role in normal and abnormal cell growth. It is hoped that the topics
dealt with in this book will provide some insight not only with respect
to the pathophysiology of diabetes, but also with regard to areas of
research that relate to disease entities (e.g., cancer and birth defects) apart from diabetes.

II. FOR THE INTENDED READERSHIP: SOME COMMENTARY

There have been and will continue to be detailed monographs published
on various aspects of insulin-related research. Yet, it is often difficult if not impossible to gain from such monographs a grasp as to
where research on insulin receptor mechanisms has been; where it is
now; and where it is hoped we will go in the future. This kind of
perspective is, of course, important to those working on a day-to-day
basis in the laboratory on diabetes-related research and on the mechanism of insulin action. However, this kind of perspective is also important to a much wider audience. The perspective is of value to physicians who regularly treat diabetics and who may be too occupied with
the demands of patient care to follow the complex details of the progress
in diabetes-related research; and the perspective is important for
medical students and research graduate students who represent the

most precious source of new insights relating to diabetes. Finally, the perspective is of value to the ever increasing sector of the lay public, who in their university education may study advanced cell biology.

Clearly, no single treatise can hope to satisfy the needs of all of the audience outlined above. Nonetheless, an attempt has been made in this volume to try and include topics that represent, on a broad front, the texture of many areas of diabetes-related research, and to make the information accessible at least in part to a wide readership. Contributors to the book have been asked to paint their pictures in broad strokes, without the necessity of documenting each comment (as is usually required in research-oriented literature) with multiple references in the bibliography. Some contributors have kept the reference material used to a minimum by selecting only key references and review articles; other bibliographies are more lengthy. However, all chapters have provided a core of reference material (references and bibliographies) that may help medical students and graduate students delve further into the subject matter without having to consult innumerable references. Thus, it is hoped the reader will have a more-or-less uncluttered access to the overall perspective provided by the various contributors, as well as a key to additional reference material that will further substantiate the claims made in each chapter. It is hoped that contributors may be forgiven by their colleagues for not citing all of the pertinent references, as is usually done in research monographs.

To facilitate the accessibility of the text for some individuals, attempts have been made to describe some concepts in a manner that to a number of readers may appear oversimplified; to the cognicenti, apologies are offered. For instance, in order to understand the effects of insulin on membrane polarization, it is essential, as briefly outlined in Chapter 8, that the reader understand what a membrane potential is and how it is measured. Unfortunately, a number of topics dealt with in the text are necessarily of a complexity that does not lend itself to simple models. Hopefully, the technical aspects of such portions of this book will not obscure the general picture that the authors have tried to convey. In the final analysis, it must be admitted that some of the chapters may be far too technical for a general readership. It is expected, nonetheless, that many chapters will provide information in a form which will balance the technical portions of this treatise. On the whole, it is hoped that all of the chapters will be accessible at least in part to medical students (and their instructors), advanced graduate students and to practicing physicians. It is hoped that, with some effort on the part of the reader, that at least parts of the book and much of the book's perspective may be accessible to a wider readership, as described above.

III. ABOUT THE TOPICS SELECTED FOR THIS BOOK

The disease entity, diabetes, is now inextricably linked in many minds
with the hormone, insulin. Yet, except for the minority of diabetic
patients who like Leonard Thompson are critically dependent on insulin
supplementation for survival, insulin per se does not appear to represent the major disease-related causative factor. Rather, in the majority of diabetics, who are not dependent on insulin for survival, the
defect would appear to lie somewhere in the complex chain of reactions
whereby insulin activates its target cells. Yet, despite the discovery
of insulin over 60 years ago, as outlined in Chapter 2, we still do not
know the mechanism of action of insulin. As pointed out at the turn
of the century by Paul Ehrlich and J. N. Langley, in order to act,
substances such as insulin must first bind to a highly specialized component of the cell called the "receptive substance" (Langley's term)
or, more commonly, the receptor. The receptor performs the critical
function of detecting the presence of insulin among the millions of
molecules present in the extracellular milieu and transmitting to the
cell the activation signal mediated by insulin. Thus, apart from work
directed at elucidating the detailed amino acid sequence and three-
dimensional structure of insulin, much interest has focused on determining the regions of the insulin molecule that are responsible for receptor binding. This topic is dealt with in Chapter 3. As work on
the mechanism of insulin action has progressed, the emphasis has begun to shift away from the detailed chemistry of insulin itself to the
details of the structure and function of the insulin receptor. Excitement has been generated over the past decade by progress dealing
with the isolation and characterization of the insulin receptor. Methods
that have led to the isolation and characterization of the receptor are
largely outlined in Chapter 4, and molecular models of the insulin receptor are described in Chapters 3 and 4. Work outlined in Chapters
3 and 4 has paved the way for the isolation of the receptor gene and
for the elucidation of the sequences of the receptor subunits. Somewhat surprisingly, the structure of the insulin receptor has turned
out to have its parallel in the structure of receptors for other insulinlike polypeptides, as described in Chapter 5. Work with the receptor
has now progressed to the point where its biosynthesis and turnover
can be monitored (Chapter 12) and where its presence and mobile
characteristics can be measured in a variety of intact cell and subcellular membrane preparations (Chapters 6 and 7). Strikingly, techniques that permit the counting of individual receptors within groups
reveal interesting differences between various cell types in terms of
insulin receptor topography (Chapter 7). In all, as summarized in
Chapters 3 to 7, work over the past decade has yielded a most interesting picture of the receptor as a dynamic (both in terms of cell surface mobility and turnover) intrinsic membrane glycoprotein that

possesses a novel enzymatic activity. The enzymatic (kinase) activity enables the receptor to transfer a phosphate moiety from adenosine triphosphate (ATP) to a specific amino acid residue (tyrosine). The phosphate can be transferred from ATP to a tyrosine residue in the receptor β-chain and possibly to other proteins that interact with the receptor. This enzymatic activity can now be understood in terms of the β-chain sequence that exhibits homologies with other tyrosine kinases. The availability of the receptor sequence provides for new vistas in our understanding of the overall function of the receptor.

Now that detailed information has been obtained about the receptor, substantial effort is being directed toward determining the immediate postbinding events leading to cell activation. As outlined in Chapter 8, one of the earliest events that has been detected subsequent to receptor binding is a change in membrane polarization. Whether or not the hyperpolarization caused by insulin in skeletal muscle, myocardium, and adipose tissue can be related to the kinase activity of the receptor remains to be determined. In more general terms, Chapter 9 discusses a number of membrane-localized reactions that may form the basis of insulin's action on intracellular enzyme systems. Specifically, Chapter 9 points to the newly discovered tyrosine kinase activity of the receptor and focuses on the exciting new evidence that the binding of insulin to its receptor in membrane preparations releases low molecular weight compounds (1000 to 2000 M.W.) that can regulate enzyme activities such as pyruvate dehydrogenase in a manner that mimics insulin action. It has been suggested that these low molecular weight compounds represent mediators of insulin action that originate in the plasma membrane. In the very near future, one can look forward to the chemical identification of these putative insulin mediators and to new insights concerning the mechanism of insulin action.

In addition to the book's focus on the way insulin acts, Chapters 10 and 11 are included as a reminder of how widespread is insulin's spectrum of target tissues. Traditionally, insulin has been thought of as a hormone that regulates metabolic events primarily in muscle, liver, and adipose tissue. Now, however, it is clear that cells as diverse as lymphocytes, fibroblasts, and lens cells can all bind and respond to insulin. In particular, as alluded to in Chapters 10 and 11, the effects of insulin on the central nervous system (Chapter 10) and on the immune system (Chapter 11) must be considered in terms of the pathogenesis of diabetes. The biosynthetic dynamics of the insulin receptor are illustrated by the receptor induction and receptor changes that can occur in the lymphocyte, as outlined in Chapter 11. The biochemistry of the biosynthesis and turnover of the receptor is dealt with at some length in Chapter 12.

Finally, one may ask: How do the discoveries concerning receptor structure and function relate to our understanding of the pathogenesis

of diabetes? It is the wish to solve the puzzle of diabetes that has
served as a major stimulus for much of the work described in this
treatise. This difficult question is addressed in Chapter 13. Thus,
in summary, in the first nine chapters of this book, the reader is
taken on a trip from the discovery of insulin to an in depth look at
its receptor, which is now known to represent a critical link in the
activation of cells by insulin, and from there the reader is led to a
consideration of the biochemical mechanisms related to insulin action.
Three chapters (Chapters 10 to 12) then point out the widespread
nature of insulin's action and illustrate the biosynthetic dynamics of
the receptor. The final considerations (Chapter 13) return to the
initial motivating questions that led to insulin' discovery: what causes
diabetes? In all, this treatise illustrates the exemplary multidisciplin-
ary cooperative effort by many individuals to understand the nature
of diabetes. The acrimony and interpersonal jealousies surrounding
the discovery of insulin seem to have dissipated somewhat. Thus,
recent progress has benefited greatly from rewardingly supportive
(although sometimes competitive) interactions between many individuals
working in this exciting field. Hopefully, this treatise will provide
some perspective for all and a stimulus for many to continue their
search to discover the cause of diabetes.

2

The Discovery of Insulin: How It Really Happened

MICHAEL BLISS *University of Toronto, Toronto, Ontario, Canada*

Everyone involved with the discovery of insulin at the University of Toronto in 1921-1922 was aware that there had been "trouble" involving conflicting claims of credit. To many outsiders, it seemed clear that insulin had been discovered by Dr. Frederick G. Banting, a private practitioner who had conceived an idea, been given research facilities at the University of Toronto, and then carried the idea to a triumphant conclusion. Banting himself said that the help of his student assistant, Charles Best, was indispensable. Scientists familiar with the work and reputation of the professor of physiology in whose lab Banting worked, J J. R. Macleod, were impressed by Macleod's brilliant lectures and articles outlining the many steps that had to be taken in the research before it was clear that a discovery had been made. Macleod always took care to credit a fourth member of the team, J. B. Collip, with vital research accomplishments.

To the friends of Macleod, the award of the 1923 Nobel Prize in physiology or medicine to Banting and Macleod for the discovery of insulin seemed a fair division of credit. Banting considered it manifestly unfair, immediately announcing that he was dividing his share of the prize money with his research associate, Charles H. Best. A few days later Macleod announced the division of his money with J. B. Collip. For most of the 60 years since that award, there has been recurrent speculation about what must have really happened in Toronto, and possibly in Stockholm, to have caused such lack of clarity about how and by whom insulin had been discovered. Not simply because of the alphabetical precedence and assonance of their names, Banting and Best seem to have garnered most of history's laurels as the true discoverers of insulin. Macleod's name has faded into a half-light infused with suspicions of sinister machinations to appropriate credit. Collip's name in connection with insulin is usually forgotten.

The most recent trend in historical writing about the discovery of insulin has been to draw attention to the precursors of the Toronto group. Many other scientists, it now appears, were working with occasionally effective extracts of pancreas in the months and years before the publications of Banting, Best, and the other Toronto researchers. A German physician, G. L. Zuelzer, had treated human diabetics with his pancreatic extract as early as 1906, bringing one of them out of diabetic coma. An American graduate student, E. L. Scott, announced in his 1911 Master of Arts thesis that he had discovered the internal secretion of the pancreas, but apparently acquiesced in his thesis supervisor's determination to tone down the claim, thereby losing priority of publication. In the summer of 1921, just as Banting and Best were beginning their work in Toronto, a Roumanian physiologist, N. C. Paulesco, published several short papers describing his work with a pancreatic extract that repeatedly lowered the blood and urinary sugar in diabetic dogs as well as relieving their acidosis. Paulesco has been given much attention in recent years as having deserved far more credit for the discovery of insulin than anyone (outside of Roumania) ever gave him. "Banting and Best are commonly believed to have been the first to have succeeded in isolating insulin," concludes one of the revisionist medical historians. "They have been hailed as its 'discoverers.' Their work, however, may more accurately be construed as confirmation of Paulesco's findings" (Murray, 1969; Bliss, 1982).

The passage of time, the opening of documents for scholarly research and a determined application of standard methods of historical scholarship, have made it possible to outline, for the first time, how, why, and by whom the discovery of insulin was made. This chapter is a greatly condensed summary of a much more intricate history narrated in my 1982 book, *The Discovery of Insulin* (Bliss, 1982). It should be noticed that many of the facts established in that book and this paper are derived from a detailed recreation of Banting and Best's research; this was made possible by the location in archives of their complete notebooks.

The hypothesis that an internal secretion of the pancreas controls carbohydrate metabolism had been widely held from the discovery in 1889 by von Mering and Minkowski that total pancreactectomy induces severe diabetes. A large number of researchers during the next 30 years—as many as 400, J. J. R. Macleod once estimated—attempted to administer pancreas or pancreatic extracts to diabetic subjects in the hope that the internal secretion would be thereby supplied and the diabetes relieved. Although it was possible to prepare pancreatic extracts that, on occasion, reduced the glycosuria and/or hyperglycemia created by diabetes, it was not clear that the favorable results could be obtained consistently or in the absence of the toxic effects commonly accompanying administration of such extracts. Zuelzer's pancreatic extract, for example, was judged so toxic as to be unsafe to administer even to severely ill diabetics. Scott could neither eliminate the toxic effects of his extract nor repeat its early favorable impact on sugar content. As many others before him had done, not the least because of the expense and difficulty of sustained research using dogs, Scott abandoned the work (Bliss, 1982).

Frederick G. Banting graduated in medicine from the University of Toronto in 1916. After war service and a hospital residence in surgery, he began practicing medicine in London, Ontario, in 1920. On the evening of October 30, Banting read an article in a medical journal describing a rare case in which a pancreatic stone had blocked the main pancreatic duct. It had appeared to cause the acinar cells of the pancreas to atrophy, while the cells known as the islets of Langerhans had not. Banting had been mustering his knowledge of the pancreas to give a talk to medical students at a local university the next day. He could not sleep that night.

> About two in the morning after the lecture and the article had been chasing each other through my mind for some time, the idea occurred to me that by the experimental ligation of the duct and the subsequent degeneration of a portion of the pancreas, that one might obtain the internal secretion free from the external secretion. I got up and wrote down the idea (Banting, 1940).

The idea he wrote down was as follows:

> Diabetus
>
> Ligate pancreatic ducts of dogs. Keep dogs alive till acini degenerate leaving Islets.
>
> Try to isolate the internal secretion of these to relieve glycosurea (Banting, 1920-1921).

A few days later, Banting discussed his idea with the Professor of Physiology at the University of Toronto, J. J. R. Macleod. Macleod was an internationally known expert on carbohydrate metabolism. "I found that Dr. Banting had only a superficial text-book knowledge of the work that had been done on the effects of pancreatic extracts in diabetes," Macleod wrote of this meeting 2 years later, "and that he had very little practical familiarity with the methods by which such a problem could be investigated in the laboratory" (Macleod, 1978). He advised Banting that the research necessary to test his idea would be arduous, unlikely to succeed, and time consuming. He concluded, however, that the idea was worth testing, if only to produce negative results, and that he would make facilities available if Banting was determined to pursue the idea. After considerable hesitation during the winter of 1920-1921, during which he pondered such alternatives as service in the Indian army and a job with an oil-drilling expedition into Canada's Northwest Teritories, Banting decided to spend a month or two in Toronto that summer seeing what might come of his idea. When he arrived in Toronto in May, Macleod introduced him to Charles H. Best, a graduating student in the Honour Physiology and Biochemistry course, who would serve the first stint as his research assistant. (Another student, Clark Noble, had lost a coin toss with Best and was to come in later. Noble decided, however, to let Best do the whole job, a mistake he regretted for the rest of his life.)

Banting and Best began work on May 17, 1921, under Macleod's direction. The early weeks were spent experimenting with the technique of pancreatectomy, as well as ligating the pancreatic ducts of several dogs. It was assumed that the acinar cells of the ligated pancreases in these dogs would atrophy, leaving the islet tissue healthy. It had long been hypothesized that the islet cells produced the elusive internal secretion.

Banting's notebooks contain two important entries apparently outlining the intended plan of work:

June 9
suggestion

Have depancreatised dog $\bar{c}$ pedicle
graft into it remnant of degenerated pancreas
later remove pedicle
then remove graft

-Prof. McLeod-

1　put remnant free in peritoneum;
2　put remnant subcutaneously.
3　emulsions.
　　whole remnant in one shot
4　repeated smaller shots.
5　50 gms glucose to totally diabetic dog
　　60 gms glucose with whole gland remnant.

June 14. Dr. McLeod's parting instructions
have dogs diabetic $\bar{c}$ DN ratio constant for
3 days. meat diet.

(1)　intraperitoneal graft
(2)　subcutaneous graft
(3)　whole remnant intravenous injection.
(4)　divided aq. 2 h intravenous
(5)　subcutaneous injection.

microscopic sections of remnant before and after transplant
(Banting 1920−1921).

While open to differing interpretations, these notes provide clear evidence of two facts: (1) That some kind of grafting technique involving the degenerated pancreas was an integral part of the research plan. This realization may explain the absence of the word "extract" in Banting's original idea and is less surprising than it first appears when we reflect that Banting was a surgeon in an era before the rejection phenomenon had been fully understood. (2) That J. J. R. Macleod was in Toronto and actively involved in planning the research during the first month of the experiments. This contrasts with a widely held view that Macleod set Banting and Best to work on their first experiment and then left town for his holidays.

Banting and Best abandoned the grafting proposal, perhaps because they realized it would be difficult and time consuming, perhaps because they had experienced serious wastage of dogs in the summer heat and because of their fairly primitive techniques. On July 30, they removed the apparently atrophied pancreas from one of their duct-ligated dogs, sliced it up in ice-cold Ringer's solution, macerated the pancreas particles, filtered the solution, and allowed the filtrate to warm before injection. "We followed your directions in preparing the extract," Best wrote to Macleod a few days later. (Best, 1921).

They injected 4 ml of the extract into the vein of a depancreatized dog that was showing a blood sugar of 0.20%. One hour after injection, the blood sugar had fallen to 0.12%. Subsequent readings and the movement of the blood sugar after administration of sugar appear inconclusive, but were interpreted as being favorable. The dog died that night. A second dog appeared to awaken from coma under the influence of extract on August 1, but died so quickly that the experiment was never reported. Injections of extract given to a third dog between August 4 and 7 seemed more conclusive in their good effect in reducing its blood sugar; extracts of other organs were ineffective. On August 11, Banting and Best depancreatized two dogs; one was given extract, the other left untreated. The control dog died of severe diabetes on August 15; the dog that was given injections of the extract of degenerated pancreas lived almost 3 weeks, dying only when no more extract was available. It was unfortunate that Banting and Best misread the result of an experiment injecting an extract of whole pancreas into this dog on August 17; their notebooks and publication show that the extract was effective; assuming it could not be effective, they dismissed it as lacking potency (Banting and Best, 1921, 1922a).

Banting and Best were tinkering with other methods of administering and obtaining the extract when Macleod returned from Scotland in

September. He urged them to eliminate the possibility of diurnal variation or a dilution phenomenon as explanations of their extract's potency. They did so, taking more care to control the time of injection and making hemoglobin estimations. After a good deal of background reading (during which their mistranslation of Paulesco's recent article caused them to conclude that his results were much more negative than was actually the case), Banting apparently decided to attempt his original idea of tissue grafting. Macleod seems to have intervened, urging the pair to repeat and buttress their summer's experiments. They tried, got mixed results, and stopped again (Bliss, 1982).

In mid-November, Banting and Best drafted a report of the research project. It was published in February, 1922, in the *Journal of Laboratory and Clinical Medicine*, under the bold title, "The Internal Secretion of the Pancreas." The key sentences of the paper were a bold summary and claim:

> In the course of our experiments we have administered over seventy-five doses of extract from degenerated pancreatic tissue to ten different diabetic animals. Since the extract has always produced a reduction of the percentage [of] sugar of the blood and of the sugar excreted in the urine, we feel justified in stating that this extract contains the internal secretion of the pancreas (Banting and Best, 1922a).

Careful analysis of Banting's notebooks does not support their contention. As inexperienced enthusiasts, deeply committed to a preconception, they had always put the most favorable interpretations upon their results. My interpretation of their first seventy-five injections of extract (which is also bound to be somewhat subjective) is that they had produced 42 favorable results, 22 unfavorable ones, and 11 inconclusive observations. They took little account of the clinical conditions of their animals and did not test for the most common toxic effect that other researchers had observed with pancreatic extracts—that they caused the dogs to show fever.

A second stage of the work began in mid-November when, on the advice of another member of the department and under Macleod's direction, Banting and Best began a longevity experiment to see if their extract could prolong the life of a diabetic dog well beyond the usual term of a few days or weeks. The first dog used in the experiment died suddenly after 2 weeks from what was interpreted as an anaphylacticlike reaction to the extract. A second dog, No. 33, was started on the longevity experiment.

In the meantime, Banting and Best had discovered that extract made from fetal calf pancreas was just as effective as extract of degenerated, duct-ligated pancreas. A few days later they tried Macleod's suggestion that they use alcohol as an extractive (rather than Ringer's solution). When it worked, using fetal pancreas, they immediately tried using fresh whole pancreas extracted with alcohol. When that worked, they had solved the principal problem involved in producing extract, and the experiments could go forward rapidly and in several directions. In the group's haste to go forward, little thought was given to the physiological implication of the discovery that extract of whole pancreas was effective (a discovery that Banting and Best could have made as early as August 17, had they correctly interpreted their own results). The hypothesis with which Banting had started the work, that duct ligation and atrophy were necessary to eliminate the external secretion, was in fact incorrect. As was known at the time, the proteolytic external secretion, trypsin, exists in an inactive state in the pancreas. It was the immediate chilling of the extirpated pancreas, not any duct ligation procedure that nullified the possibility of autolytic activity at that stage (Pratt, 1954).

The advance in ability to produce extract coincided with Macleod's decision to accede to Banting's request that J. B. Collip join the team. Collip was a trained biochemist who had received his Ph.D. in Toronto in 1916. He normally taught at the University of Alberta, but was in Toronto that autumn to work with Macleod as part of a sabbatical year of research. Collip had happened to sit in on one of Banting and Macleod's early discussions and had expressed an interest in the work. He began experiments with pancreatic extract about December 12, 1921.

Collip immediately began making extract from whole beef pancreas. Following a suggestion Macleod had made at a group discussion, Collip began working with rabbits, finding right away that the extract lowered the blood sugar of normal rabbits. This observation immediately gave the group a quick, easy way of testing the potency of their extract.

Macleod also assigned to Collip the task of determining the extract's effect on the glycogen-forming capacity of the liver, an experiment that would provide solid evidence as to whether or not the extract did more than reduce glycosuria and hyperglycemia. On December 22, Collip observed that the extract enabled the liver of a diabetic dog to form glycogen, a most encouraging result. At the same time, Collip made the first observation that the extract caused the ketone bodies to disappear from a diabetic dog's urine. During that week, Collip was also making slight improvements in Banting and Best's method of producing extract. (They evaporated all the alcohol from the pancreas—alcohol solution, using a warm air current. Collip used a laboratory vacuum still and found it better not to evaporate to dryness.)

Banting and Best, on their part, had a frustrating few days attempting to produce extract in larger quantities. Their insulin notebook for 1921 ends with seven successive failures in the week before Christmas as they attempted to reduce the blood sugar of diabetic dogs, normal dogs, and normal rabbits. They also attempted to reduce the sugar circulating in the system of a diabetic human, a classmate of Banting's named Joseph Gilchrist, and must have been disappointed when extract that had worked on dogs failed to have any beneficial effect on Gilchrist. At that time they did not know that oral administration would never work. The Gilchrist test appears to have been informal and impromptu; Macleod probably did not know about it.

On December 31, 1921, Banting presented a paper about his and Best's work to the American Physiological Society conference at Yale University in New Haven. Entitled, "The Beneficial Influence of Certain Pancreatic Extracts on Pancreatic Diabetes," it was a version of the paper written in November and due for publication in February. Rumors of interesting experiments in Toronto had caused a large attendance of distinguished diabetologists. They questioned Banting closely about his findings. As the inexperienced and shy Banting later admitted, the experience was a personal ordeal (Banting, 1940). It must have been made worse by the fact that his and Best's experiments had not been particularly well done, making it difficult or impossible to answer some of the questions that must have been asked. There were no temperature readings on the dogs, few autopsies to show that total pancreatectomies had in fact been done, poor recording of the DN (dextrose to nitrogen) ratio, which was a standard measurement of the diabetic condition in depancreatized dogs, and other shortcomings. As Macleod wrote 9 months later, "It was evident that he [Banting] had not succeeded in convincing all of his audience that the results obtained proved the presence of an internal secretion of the pancreas—the primary object of the work—any more definitely than had those of previous investigators."

Macleod, who was serving as chairman of the session, joined the discussion to defend the work as best he could. Elliott Joslin later recalled the general reaction to the session as being "little praise or congratulation, and a moderate amount of friendly but serious criticism of the work." There seems to have been a general impression that the Toronto group might be onto something, but further reports would be necessary.

Frederick Banting came home from New Haven in a state of severe emotional turmoil. His personal failure at New Haven, combined with his and Best's problems in the laboratory before Christmas, reinforced a temperamental insecurity to the point where he became nearly paranoic in his belief that Macleod and Collip were appropriating his idea and his extract. Banting had not related well to Macleod at any stage of the work, had had a major quarrel with him about research facilities in September, and now misunderstood Macleod's motives in inserting himself into the New Haven discussion. He was worried by Collip's success, alarmed that Macleod had assigned to Collip the task of purifying the extract for clinical trials, and was then given a final shock when he learned that his lack of qualifications to treat diabetics (he had never treated any) barred him from the hospital appointment necessary for him to participate directly in the clinical testing.

In his determination not to be cast aside, Banting managed to persuade Macleod that he and Best ought to have the opportunity to make the first extract tested on a human. Macleod consented. Best made extract using the method worked out in December (one which incorporated Collip's modifications), and determined it was potent on a dog. On January 11, 1922, 15 ml of the extract were injected into the buttocks of a 14-year-old diabetic, Leonard Thompson, at Toronto General Hospital.

Although Banting and Best were not directly involved in the test on Thompson, they were among the coauthors of the paper describing its results. Thompson's blood sugar dropped from 0.440 to 0.320. The excretion of glucose in his urine fell from 91.5 gm in 3625 ml over 24 hr to 84 gm in 4060 ml. Tests for ketones continued to be strongly positive. "No clinical benefit was evidenced." A sterile abscess developed at the site of one of the injections (Banting, et al., 1922a). The modest improvements in Thompson's blood sugar and glycosuria were judged to be outweighed by the reaction the injection had caused. No further extract was given. The clinical test of Banting and Best's extract had failed. As Banting himself wrote in 1929, "These results were not as encouraging as those obtained by Zuelzer in 1908."

In the meantime, Collip had continued his efforts to remove impurities from the extract. One of his important findings as he began to produce more powerful extract was that it could cause a violent and sometimes fatal reaction in the test rabbits. When he found that administration of glucose was an almost instant antidote to the reaction, Collip realized he was seeing a hypoglycemic effect caused when the extract reduced the blood sugar well below normal levels.

Collip's notebooks do not survive. He appears to have worked long hours and with many trials and failures in attempting to remove impurities from the extract. He could get fats and salts out of the solutions by applying reasonably standard methods. The more difficult job of removing contaminating proteins from the solution while retaining the active principle involved endless tinkering with concentration of alcohol and degrees of acidity, trying to find a state in which the proteins would be soluble and the active principle insoluble, or vice versa. We will never know all the steps Collip took, all the twists and turns of the path he followed during those January experiments. Late one night, probably that of the sixteenth, he discovered that he could "trap" the active principle by first producing a concentration of alcohol in which most of its protein contaminants were not soluble, and then raising the concentration to just over the 90% level. At that point the active principle itself would precipitate out of the solution. "I experienced then and there all alone in the top story of the old Pathology Building

perhaps the greatest thrill which has ever been given me to realize,"
Collip wrote many years later (Bliss, 1982).

Tests of Collip's extract began on Leonard Thompson on January 23.
The injections were spectacularly successful in eliminating his ketonuria,
virtually eliminating his glycosuria, and lowering his blood sugar to
normal. The Toronto group then knew that they had made a very big
discovery. After further clinical testing, as well as such important
buttressing experiments as measurement of the extract's impact on the
respiratory quotient, the Toronto team presented a thorough summary
paper, "The Effect Produced on Diabetes by Extracts of Pancreas,"
at the Association of American Physicians meeting in Washington, D.C.
on May 3, 1922 (Banting, et al., 1922b). In this paper, they finally
gave a name to "this extract which we propose to call insulin." At
the time of naming they did not know that E. A. Schafer had proposed
"insuline" in 1916 as the name for the hypothetical internal secretion.
Schafer did not know that J. de Meyer had made the same suggestion
in 1909. The response to the Washington presentation was a standing
vote of appreciation to honor what Frederick M. Allen, the world's
leading diabetologist, said in the discussion was "one of the greatest
achievements of modern medicine."

Having misread Paulesco's work, Banting and Best had not known
that they had a competitor anywhere near success. On February 25,
Paulesco first tested his extract on a human. Because his aqueous
extract had caused toxic side effects in dogs when injected intra-
venously, Paulesco decided to administer it to humans by rectum.
Paulesco's extract was ineffective, of course, in these clinical trials,
and appears never to have been used successfully to treat humans.
Paulesco's work had been hampered by limited resources, primitive
techniques (particularly for obtaining blood sugars), and theoretical
misconceptions (most notably that which influenced him in his claim
to have reduced a diabetic animal's blood sugar to 0.000) (Paulesco,
1923b).

Banting and Best did not discover insulin. Their experiments,
initiated to test a physiologically incorrect hypothesis (that it was
the presence of the external secretion in the pancreas that destroyed
the internal secretion), led to the production of crude pancreatic extracts that were often effective in reducing hyperglycemia and glycosuria. Almost anyone who set his mind to it could produce such an
extract, and many had, including Zuelzer, Scott, and Paulesco. An
argument later advanced by Banting and Best to the effect that the
longevity experiment on their dog No. 33 proved that they had discovered an antidiabetic agent flounders on the fact that the autopsy
on dog No. 33, killed 70 days after pancreactectomy, disclosed a small
pancreatic remant, sufficient to cast doubt on whether or not the dog
had been completely diabetic (Banting and Best, 1922b). The records
of the longevity experiment were also extremely spotty, and it had

extended past the time when Collip's purification indicated that the group had discovered insulin.

Banting and Best had produced findings attractive enough to convince themselves and Macleod that the work should continue and be extended. Enough of their extracts were potent that the Toronto researchers decided they must contain an internal secretion. In December and January, the Toronto team isolated the internal secretion. The discovery of insulin was complete when either (a) a nontoxic preparation of the extract reduced the cardinal symptons of diabetes in a human being (i.e., on January 23, 1922) or (b) the Toronto group presented convincing evidence of insulin's existence to the Association of American Physicians on May 3, 1922. Insulin was discovered at the University of Toronto as the result of collaboration among a number of researchers, directed by J. J. R. Macleod, who expanded upon and carried to triumphant success a project initiated by Banting with the help of Best. The single most important technical achievement was that made by Collip in the purification of the extract. Among other factors making possible this brilliant success, we should include the then vast resources of the University of Toronto (in a very real way it can be said that Toronto had more man-hours, money, and dogs to invest in the problem than most of the predecessors had had) and the fact that advances in the technology of blood sugar measurement had made it possible after about 1916 to perform the crucial experiments with much greater reliability and sophistication.

The Nobel Committee of the Caroline Institute carried out a reasonably thorough investigation of the discovery. It was impressed by the advice, direction, and management Macleod had supplied at every stage in a very impressive total orchestration of a discovery. A four-way division of the prize was forbidden by statute. A three-way division would have been to Banting, Macleod, and Collip. All things considered, the formal award to Macleod and Banting and then the informal division of the money among Banting, Best, Macleod, and Collip, was a fair distribution of honor. Unfortunately, the profound personal antagonism that developed among members of the discovery team meant that first Banting and then Best carried out long and successful campaigns to ignore or discredit the work of their collaborators. Collip was correct in his frequent statements in later years that what had really happened during the discovery of insulin would not be disclosed until all the discoverers had died.

REFERENCES

Banting, F. G. (1920-1921). Unpublished notebook, Academy of
    Medicine, Toronto.
Banting, F. G. (1929). *Edinburgh Med. J.*, 1.

Banting, F. G. (1940). Unpublished manuscript, "The Story of
    Insulin," Banting Papers, University of Toronto.
Banting, F. G. and Best, C. H. (1921). Unpublished insulin note-
    books, Banting Papers, University of Toronto.
Banting, F. G., and Best, C. H. (1922a), *J. Lab. Clin. Med.*,
    VII:256.
Banting, F. G , and Best, C. H. (1922b), *J. Lab. Clin. Med.*,
    VIII:3.
Banting, F. G., Best, C. H., Collip, J. B., Campbell, W. R., and
    Fletcher, A. A. (1922a). *Can. Med. Assoc. J.*, 2:141.
Banting, F. G., Best, C. H., Collip, J. B., Campbell, W. R., and
    Fletcher, A. A., Macleod, J. J. R., and Nobel, E. C. (1922b).
    Trans. Assoc. Am. Phys., 1.
Best, C. H. (1921). Unpublished letter to J. J. R. Macleod, Aug. 9,
    1921, Banting Papers, University of Toronto.
Bliss, M. (1982). *The Discovery of Insulin*. University of Chicago
    Press, Chicago.
Macleod, J. J. R. (1978). *Bull. Hist. Med.*, 52(3):295.
Murray, I. (1971). *J. Hist. Med. XXVI*:2, 150.
Paulesco, N. C. (1923a). *Arch. Intern. Physiol.*, 21:71.
Paulesco, N. C. (1923b). *Arch. Intern. Physiol.*, 21:215.
Pratt, J. H. (1954). *J. Hist. Med.*, 9:281.

BIBLIOGRAPHY

Banting, F. G., and Best, C. H. (1922). The internal secretion of
    the pancreas. *J. Lab. Clin. Med. VII*:256-271.
Banting, F. G., Best, C. H., Collip, J. B., Campbell, W. R., and
    Fletcher, A. A. (1922). Pancreatic extracts in the treatment of
    diabetes mellitus. Preliminary report. *Can. Med. Assoc. J.*,
    141:94-98.
Banting, F. G., Best, C. H., Collip, J. B., Campbell, W. R.,
    Fletcher, A. A., Macleod, J. J. R., and Noble, E. C. (1922).
    The effect produced on diabetes by extracts of pancreas. *Trans.
    Assoc. Am. Physic.*, 1-11.
Bliss, M. (1982). *The Discovery of Insulin*. University of Chicago
    Press, Chicago.
Bliss, M. (1982). Banting's Best's, and Collip's accounts of the
    discovery of insulin, *Bull. Hist. Med.*, 56:554-568.
Collip, J. B. (1923). History of the discovery of insulin, *North-
    west Med.*, 22:267-273.
International Diabetes Federation, Report of the special committee set
    up to present a written summary of work leading up to the dis-
    covery of insulin. *News Bull. Intern. Diabetes Fed.*, 16(2):
    29-40.

Macleod, J. J. R. (1978). History of the researches leading to the discovery of insulin, September 1922. *Bull. Hist. Med.* 52(3): 295-312.

Murray, I. (1969). The search for insulin. *Scot. Med. J.*, *14*: 286-295.

Pavel, I. (1976). *The Priority of N. C. Paulesco in the Discovery of Insulin*. Bucharest.

Pratt, J. H. (1954). A reappraisal of researches leading to the discovery of insulin, *J. Hist. Med.*, *9*: 281-289.

3

Insulin Structure: Receptor Binding and Probing Structure with Photoreactive Derivatives

CECIL C. YIP *University of Toronto, Toronto, Ontario, Canada*

I. INTRODUCTION

Insulin-induced biological responses are the results of the specific
interaction between insulin and its target cells. The specificity of
the interaction resides in both insulin itself and its cellular receptor.
The potency or intrinsic activity of insulin is dependent on its structural integrity. A decrease in the cellular response to insulin can,
therefore, arise from either a structural abnormality of the hormone
or from some unknown defects of the insulin receptor, for instance,
a decrease in receptor number. A comparison of biological potency
of insulins from different animal species has provided telling information on the structure--function relationship in this hormone. Direct
chemical modifications together with semisynthesis of insulin analogues
have further advanced our understanding of the structural requirements in this hormone. Physical analyses, such as x-ray crystallography and circular dichroism, have made it possible to visualize the
structure of insulin in three dimensions. Results from these studies
have led to the conclusion that the structure of the insulin molecule
contains a special region or domain that interacts with the receptor.
While much has been learned about insulin in these respects, information on the structure of its receptor has only begun to accumulate.
The interaction between insulin and its receptor, as is generally the
case with polypeptide hormones, takes place primarily on the cell surface. Although insulin receptors have been detected in subcellular
organelles, such as the nuclei, the function of these intracellular insulin receptors is not clear. The study of the structure—function
relationship in the insulin receptor has been hampered by the

reversibility of the hormone—receptor interaction and by the small quantity of insulin receptors in target tissues.

In this chapter, I will review the structure—function requirement for insulin and illustrate how such information has been used to study the insulin receptor. In particular, I will review our own studies of the insulin receptor using two specifically designed photoreactive insulin derivatives. The results of these studies have led us to postulate a model of the insulin receptor being composed of disulfide-linked subunits and capable of undergoing reduction and oxidation to give rise to three interconvertible redox forms.

II. STRUCTURE—FUNCTION REQUIREMENTS

The structure—function relationship in insulin has been studied using two different approaches: comparing insulins from different animal species and altering the activity of insulin by chemical modifications of the hormone. In this section, I will summarize some of the important findings and the current view on the relationship between structure and function. In particular, I will focus my discussion on the overall structure of insulin and on specific regions of the hormone that have been studied extensively.

A. The Dual-Chain Structure of Insulin

One of the characteristic structural features of insulin is that it is composed of two polypeptide chains linked by two disulfide bridges (Fig. 1). The shorter chain, called the A chain because of its relative acidic nature, has 21 amino acid residues and an internal disulfide bridge. There are 29-31 amino acids, depending on the animal species, in the less acidic B chain. This dual-chain structure and the positions of the two interchain and the one intrachain disulfide bridges are invariant in all the different species of insulin that have been isolated and characterized (Hunt, 1969). The conservation of these structural features in insulins from the most primitive vertebrate alive, the cyclostome North Atlantic hagfish, through fish, birds, and rodents to human is evidence of their functional role. The functional requirement for the integrity of this basic molecular structure is further illustrated by a complete loss of biological potency when the interchain disulfide bridges are broken by reduction (Dixon and Wardlaw, 1960).

Within this dual-chain structural framework, the amino acid sequences of the A and B chains are highly conserved as well. For example, the amino acid sequence of hagfish insulin differs from that of port insulin by 18 residues (Peterson et al., 1975) whereas pork insulin itself differs from human insulin by only one amino acid at

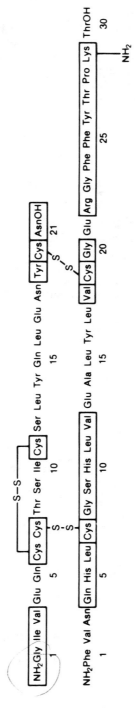

Figure 1 Amino acid sequence of human insulin. The highly conserved amino acid residues are outlined.

the carboxyl terminus of the B chain. Among all naturally occurring insulins that have been studied covering an evolutionary time span of about 400 million years, the maximum difference in amino acid sequence between them is about 40% or about 20 replacements or substitutions of amino acid residues. This can be translated to a rate of mutation of about 4 PAM (accepted point mutations per 100 residues per 100 million years), comparing to a rate of 60 PAM for growth hormones (McLaughlin and Dayhoff, 1969). However, as shown in Table 1, the biological potencies of naturally occurring insulins when assayed in a mammalian system, such as the rat fat cells, differ greatly when compared with pork or beef insulin. Thus, regions or sequences in insulin, other than those that have been highly conserved in evolution, must also play a role in the functional requirement of the molecule.

B. The Amino-Terminal Regions

In addition to the invariant positions of the six cysteine residues (Fig. 1), one of the striking features of insulin is the complete conservation of the amino-terminal A1 glycine of the A chain. Chemical modifications of this amino terminus have demonstrated its functional role in binding of insulin to its receptor and its biological activity. An extension of this terminal region by neutral and bulky nonflexible groups causes a parallel loss in both biological activity and receptor binding activity; the bigger the extension, the greater is the loss of

Table 1 Biological Activity of Insulin from Different Species

Insulin	Activity (%)	Reference
Bovine or pork	100	
Guinea pig	5-10	Zimmerman et al. (1974)
Coypu	10	Horuk et al. (1979)
Casiragua	10	Horuk et al. (1979)
Chinchilla	29	Horuk et al. (1979)
Porcupine	4	Horuk et al. (1980)
Chicken or turkey	150-190	Simon et al. (1974)
Atlantic hagfish	5	Emdin et al. (1977)
Codfish	50	Grant and Reid (1968)
Toadfish	30	Humbel and Renold (1963)
Angler fish	100	Humbel and Crestfield (1965)

activity. The positive charge on this terminal residue seems to play an important role in binding to the insulin receptor, since insulin derivatives with positively charged bulky groups have a higher receptor binding activity relative to their biological activity (Pullen et al., 1976).

In contrast to the highly conserved A-chain amino terminal, the amino terminus of the B chain is less invariant among the insulins. The amino-terminal residue B1 phenylalanine is conserved in all known mammalian insulins, but is replaced in bony fish, hagfish, and avian (chicken and turkey) insulins by other amino acids. While deletion or shortening of this region of the B chain results in little change of biological activity, suggesting that this region is functionally not essential, there is strong evidence in support of its functional importance. It is, therefore, significant to note that in insulins with higher biological activity relative to pork or beef insulin, such as chicken and turkey insulins, this terminal residue is replaced by a neutral amino acid, alanine, whereas in insulins with lower biological activity, such as the hagfish insulin, it is replaced by a basic amino acid, arginine. While there is hardly any difference in biological potency among the mammalian insulins, insulins of the hystricomorph rodents, including guinea pig, casiragua, and coypu, exhibit less than 10% of the potency of pork insulin (Moody et al., 1974; Zimmerman et al., 1974). Although there are substitutions and deletions in the hydrophobic carboxyl-terminal region of the B chain in these hystricomorph insulins, a basic amino acid, either arginine or lysine, has replaced either the B4 glutamine or B5 histidine at the amino-terminal end of the B chain. The functional role of the amino-terminal region of the B chain, as manifested particularly by this apparent deleterious effect of positively charged basic amino acid replacement, is further supported by the observation that an extension of the B-chain amino terminus by the addition of an arginine or lysine results in a significant parallel loss of both receptor binding and biological activity and that elongations of this N-terminal end by neutral residues have little effect (Yeung et al., 1979). Extensions by bulky hydrophobic residues also cause a loss of biological activity (Geiger et al., 1980).

C. The Carboxyl-Terminal Regions

Other invariant and thus likely functional important sequences in the insulin molecule are found in its A-chain and B-chain carboxyl-terminal regions. In the A chain, the terminal tripeptide sequence (positions 19-21) Tyr-Cys-Asn is totally conserved in all known, naturally occurring insulins. Monoiodination of the A19 tyrosine leads to a loss of receptor-binding activity and biological potency (Gliemann et al., 1979). Removal of the A-chain terminal asparagine residue by carboxypeptidase digestion results in a loss of more than

90% of insulin activity (Carpenter, 1966). This loss of activity has
been attributed to the destruction of a salt bridge between this terminal asparagine and the B 22 arginine in the carboxyl-terminal region
of the B chain. The importance of this salt bridge in fulfilling the
functional requirements may also explain the low activity of hystricomorph insulins, in which the B 22 arginine residue is replaced by
aspartic acid. On the other hand, it is of interest to note that when
the A 21 asparagine in guinea pig (a hystricomorph) insulin is removed,
there is a further tenfold reduction of activity (Yip and Moule, 1976).
Thus the A-chain carboxyl-terminal residue itself may also interact
directly with the receptor.

The carboxyl-terminal region of the B chain is characterized by
its invariant sequence of hydrophobic amino acids of Phe-Phe-Tyr at
positions 24-26. Highly purified desoctapeptide insulin, obtained by
tryptic digestion to remove the carboxyl-terminal sequence containing
this hydrophobic core, is practically devoid of activity (Kikuchi et al.,
1980). The functional importance of these hydrophobic residues is
substantiated further by a recent finding that in a variant of human
insulin with greatly reduced activity, isolated from the pancreas of a
diabetic patient, the phenylalanine residue at either position 24 or 25
is replaced by a leucine (Olefsky et al., 1980). This observation has
been confirmed by studies using semisynthetic insulin analogues containing leucine at these two positions (Gattner et al., 1980).

D. The Functional Domain in Insulin

At first glance, the structure—function requirements in insulin as discussed appear to be located in different parts of the insulin molecule.
However, it is clearly evident from the tertiary structure, as determined by x-ray crystallography, that there is a structural domain consisting of the amino-terminal A1 glycine, the A-chain carboxyl-terminal
sequence Tyr-Cys-Asn at positions 19-21, and the carboxyl-terminal
region of the B chain. The amino acid residues in this putative receptor-
binding domain of the insulin molecule are outlined in Figure 2. In
fact, this structural domain contains the region involved in the formation of insulin dimers. In this context, it is interesting to note that the
poorly active hystricomorph insulins, in contrast to other mammalian
insulins, are unable to form dimers. These considerations have led
to the hypothesis (Pullen et al., 1976) that the receptor-binding domain of insulin includes the hydrophobic region involved in dimerization as well as other exposed polar residues peripheral to this region.
These polar residues would include the A1 glycine, A21 asparagine,
and B 22 arginine for which the functional importance has been discussed.

As shown in Table 1, the potency of naturally occurring insulins
varies greatly. Among those insulins with low potency, such as those
of the hystricomorphs and the hagfish, the receptor-binding domain,

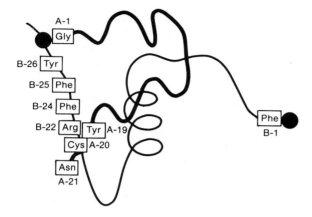

Figure 2 Schematic representation of the three-dimensional folding of the A and B chains of insulin. The A chain is represented by the heavy line, the B chain by the thin line. Adapted from Blundell et al. (1972).

as postulated and discussed above, is nevertheless conserved. Furthermore, it is also significant that, in spite of these great differences in potency, the three-dimensional structures of these native insulins are nearly identical to each other, as revealed by high-resolution x-ray crystallography and by other spectroscopic methods. An appropriate three-dimensional structure alone is, therefore, apparently insufficient to fulfill all the functional requirements in insulin; other factors, such as charge and hydrophobicity of specific regions, are also required for the full expression of insulin activity through their interactions with the insulin receptor. These interactions with the insulin receptor should be viewed as a dynamic, rather than static, process, involving conformational changes of both the insulin molecule and its receptor. The formation of the insulin-receptor complex is then a result of an induced fit or allosteric interaction between these two entities. In this context, it is significant to note that insulin derivatives, cross-linked between A1 glycine and B29 lysine and exhibiting little conformational change from native insulin, have greatly reduced biological potencies (Dodson et al., 1980b). The cross-linking may have prevented such essential dynamic allosteric interactions. In insulin, other structural regions outside of the postulated receptor-binding domain, but exhibiting functional requirements, may play a role in this allosteric interaction. Results from the x-ray crystallographic study of insulin polymers suggest that the amino-terminal sequence of B1-B8 of the B chain is capable of a great deal of conformational movement (Dodson et al., 1980a). Indeed, as already discussed, insulins modified at the amino terminus of the B chain have altered receptor-binding activity and biological potency. Therefore, it is likely that the functional importance of this area of the insulin molecule may be attributed to its participation in the allosteric interaction with the receptor.

III. PROBING THE STRUCTURE OF THE RECEPTOR WITH PHOTOREACTIVE INSULIN DERIVATIVES

In contrast to insulin, little is known about the structure-function aspect of the insulin receptor. Experiments using insulin linked to insoluble substances such as cellulose and polydextran, demonstrated that insulin may not need to enter the cell to elicit biological responses. Binding studies using radioiodinated insulin and subcellular fractions have established that the plasma membrane fraction contains the bulk of the insulin-binding activity. Autoradiographic electron microscopy, using radioiodinated insulin also demonstrates the initial localization of radioactive insulin on the cell surface (see Chapter 7). These observations have established that the insulin receptor is localized on the cell membrane. Treatments of the cell membrane by enzymes, salts, detergents, and chemical modifications using reagents such as sulfhydryl reagents to react with specific functional groups have led to the conclusions that the insulin receptor is probably a glycoprotein partially buried in the membrane bilayer and that sulfhydryl groups may be involved in the cellular response to insulin. One direct approach to studying the receptor is through its isolation and purification. This approach has been successful in establishing the glycoprotein nature of the insulin receptor and in showing that there may well be other membrane factors or components affecting the insulin-binding behavior of the receptor. The details of this approach are dealt with in Chapter 4.

In addition to the relative low abundance of receptors, one other hurdle in the structure-function analysis of the insulin receptor is the reversibility of the binding reaction. Ideally the receptor should be studied in situ with little or no disturbance of its environment. With this in mind, we have taken the direct approach of photoaffinity labeling of the insulin receptor, using light-sensitive derivatives of insulin that, upon activation, can form irreversible covalent bonds with the receptor in situ, so that the receptor can then be extracted and identified.

A. Designing the Photoreactive Insulin Probe

Compared to other reagents that cross-link proteins, photoreactive cross-linking reagents have certain distinct advantages. The reagents

remain inert and unreactive until the appropriate time when they are
activated by light. Chemical cross-linkers require specific reactive
groups, such as amino groups in the case of disuccinimidyl suberate,
appropriately spaced on the proteins for successful cross-linking.
Photoaffinity linkers, on the other hand, do not require specific reactive groups to be present for cross-linking to occur. The most
commonly used photoreactive reagents belong to the aryl azide family.
As outlined in Figure 3, upon exposure to light, the azido group of
the reagent generates a very reactive nitrene intermediate that is
capable of breaking and forming covalent bonds through extraction
of electrons from a neighboring component, such as a protein to which
the photoreactive probe is bound. However, there are a number of
nonproductive side reactions resulting in a low efficiency of cross-
linking. One major difficulty in the use of photolabeling technique in
biological studies is the synthesis of an appropriate probe that retains
the biological properties of the original compound.

In designing a photoreactive insulin probe, we have chosen to prepare the aryl azide derivative of insulin. There are three reactive
amino groups (the amino termini of the A and B chains and the B29
lysine ε-amino group) in insulin available for derivatization. These
amino groups can be derivatized by reacting with an activated ester
of an aryl azide, in this case the succinimide ester of 4-azidobenzoate.
Based on what is known about the structure-function requirements in
insulin as discussed in the previous sections, we decided to prepare
two different photoreactive insulins. One would have the aryl azide

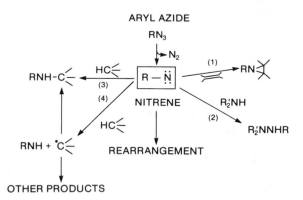

Figure 3 Schematic outline of the reactions of the reactive intermediate
nitrene generated from the photolysis of an aryl azide. As an example,
reactions 1, 2, and 3 will lead to covalent-linked products, while there
are side reactions that do not result in the formation of covalent bonds.

azidobenzoyl group added to the B29 lysine to yield $N^{\epsilon B29}$-monoazido-
benzoyl insulin (B29-MABI). The other one would have the azido
group at the B1 phenylalanine to yield $N^{\alpha B1}$-monoazidobenzoyl insulin
(B1-MABI). In the case of B29-MABI, the photoreactive group is
therefore located within the receptor-binding domain of insulin. In
contrast, the photoreactive group in B1-MABI is in that region of insulin that may participate in the allosteric interaction between the
hormone and its receptor. The locations of these two photoreactive
groups on the insulin molecule are shown as black circles in Figure 2.

We use two different strategies to synthesize the two different
photoprobes of insulin. In the case of B29-MABI (Yip et al., 1980),
insulin is reacted with the ester under conditions that favor derivatization of the B29 lysine, although a mixture of mono-, di-, and tri-
substituted insulins is obtained. The B29-MABI derivative is purified
by ion-exchange chromatography on carboxymethyl (CM)-cellulose.
To prepare B1-MABI (Yeung et al., 1980), insulin is reacted with Boc-
azide (*t*-butyloxycarbonyl azide) to give di-Boc insulin. The remaining
amino group of B1 phenylalanine of this di-Boc insulin is then reacted
with the ester. Removal of the Boc groups after this reaction gives B1-
MABI, which is purified by chromatography on CM-cellulose. Both
azidobenzoyl insulins are fully characterized with respect to the site of
derivatization, purity, covalent bond formation when photolyzed, and
biological activity. B1-MABI and B29-MABI retained 75% and 65% of biological potency, respectively. Both probes are found to be able to form
covalent bonds with the H and L chains of anti-insulin immunoglobulin
but not with preimmune immunoglobulin. This covalent linking to the
anti-insulin immunoglobulin chains is specifically blocked by insulin.
These observations demonstrate that the two photoreactive insulins
probes are suitable for use to study the insulin receptor.

B. The Insulin Receptor as Revealed by Photoaffinity
   Labeling

We have chosen fat cells to study the insulin receptor because they
are highly sensitive to insulin and because their binding of insulin has
been studied most extensively. The procedure is relatively simple.
Fat cells are isolated from the epididymal fat pads of the rat by digestion with the enzyme collagenase. The fat cells are then incubated
with either one of the two photoreactive insulin probes that have been
made radioactive by iodination with radioactive iodine. Incubation is
usually carried out at room temperature in the dark for 40-60 min.
The cells are then exposed for 20-30 sec to a light source from a high-
pressure mercury lamp. A plasma membrane fraction is then prepared
from the cells. The membrane fraction is then made soluble using an
ionic detergent, sodium dodecyl sulfate (SDS). At this stage, solubilized proteins from the membranes can be reduced, if required, by a

reducing agent such as dithiothreitol (DTT). The radioactive solubilized membrane sample is then separated by polyacrylamide gel
electrophoresis (PAGE) in the presence of the detergent SDS. The
technique of SDS-PAGE separates large proteins according to their
size. After this electrophoretic separation, the proteins that have
been photolabeled by the radioactive photoprobe of insulin are revealed by exposing the gel to X-ray film. In order to determine which
of the radioactive bands are specifically labeled by the probe, an excess of native insulin is added to a parallel incubation as a control and
similarly processed. Those labeled bands that are not labeled when
an excess of native insulin is present are considered to be labeled
specifically and to represent receptor proteins.

Both photoreactive probes of insulin specifically labeled three
high molecular weight protein bands of approximately 380, 300, and
230 K in the plasma membranes, as illustrated in lane 1 of Figure 4A.

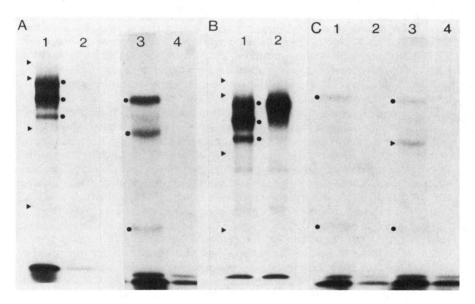

Figure 4 Autoradiographs demonstrating the photoaffinity labeling of
insulin receptor and its subunits. (A) The three unreduced receptor
species labeled by B29-MABI are marked by dots in lane 1. In lane 3
the three receptor subunits labeled by this probe are indicated by the
three solid dots. The four arrows indicate the positions of four
molecular weight protein standards. (B) The three receptor species
(lane 1) were converted to the 380 K form by 0.3 mM PCMPS (lane 2).
(C) The B1-MABI derivative labeled an additional 85 K band (indicated
by the arrow in lane 3 when the fat cells were pretreated with 5 mM DTT.
The dots mark the 130 and 40 K subunits.

The labeling of these protein bands was blocked by an excess of native insulin (lane 2 in Fig. 4A). Lane 3 in Figure 4A shows that when the photolabeled membranes were reduced, the B29-MABI derivative specifically labeled three protein bands of 130, 90, and 40 K; an excess of native insulin blocked the labeling of these three bands (lane 4 in Fig. 4A). In contrast, the B1-MABI probe labeled specifically only a 130 and a 40 K band under similar conditions. It has been possible to establish that the 40 K bands labeled by both photoprobes are different from each other because of their different sensitivity to trypsin digestion. The two distinct 40 K components are not degradation products of the larger subunits (Yip et al., 1982). When we reduce the individual labeled bands of 380, 300, and 230 K, we also obtain the 130, 90 (depending on whether B29-MABI is used), and 40 K bands. These observations demonstrate that these are disulfide-linked subunits of the insulin receptor on the fat cells. These subunits are glycoproteins, as established by their sensitivity to the enzyme neuaminidase (Yip et al., 1982). The relationship between the three high molecular weight forms of the receptor is established by the following experiments. When the photolabeled membrane fraction is reduced by a gradual increase of the reductant, dithiothreitol (DTT), a transition from the higher to the lower molecular weight form is obtained among the 380, 300, and 230 K receptor species leading to the eventual appearance of the fully reduced subunits. A similar transition is observed when the fat cells are first reduced. It is apparent, therefore, that the 380, 300, and the 230 K receptor species represent partially reduced or oxidized forms of the insulin receptor. The reduction or oxidation of these receptor species evidently involves sulfhydryl groups. This is further substantiated by experiments using sulfhydryl reagents, such as N-ethylmaleimide (NEM) and p-chloromercuriphenyl sulfonate (PCMPS). Lane 2, when compared with lane 1 in Figure 4B, shows that the 230 and the 300 K receptor species are converted quantitatively to the 380 K form by 0.3 mM PCMPS. The effect of PCMPS is concentration dependent; NEM has a similar effect.

It is evident from the data discussed thus far that the placement of the photoreactive azidobenzoyl broup on the insulin molecule clearly determines the pattern of subunit labeling: B29-MABI labels a 90 K subunit, whereas B1-MABI does not. Each probe labels a different 40 K subunit, and both probes label a 130 K subunit. The advantage of using two different photoreactive insulin probes with the photoreactive group placed at different functional regions of insulin becomes more evident when the fat cells, before photolabeling, are first exposed to low concentrations of DTT that do not inhibit insulin binding. Under these conditions, the B1-MABI probe now labels specifically an 85 K subunit in addition to the 130 K and the 40 K subunit (Fig. 4C). The labeling of a 85 K subunit by B1-MABI under these conditions may be the result of the partial reduction of the insulin receptor allowing a greater degree of flexibility of this subunit to interact with insulin. The possible allosteric movement of the amino-terminal region of insulin B chain, carrying the photoreactive aryl azide group in this case, as discussed in Section II.B, may also contribute to the labeling of this 85 K subunit.

The probing of the insulin receptor by photoaffinity labeling using the two specifically designed insulin probes has allowed us to conclude (Yip and Moule, 1983) that the 380 K species of the insulin receptor of the rat fat cell is composed of the following five disulfide-linked glycoprotein subunits: one 130 K, one 90 K, one 85 K and two 40 K subunits. This is diagrammatically shown in Figure 5. This proposed subunit structure is minimal since there could be other subunits that may not have been labeled by the probes used. On the other hand, the sum of the molecular weights of the five proposed subunits is in good agreement with the value of 380 K estimated for the largest unreduced receptor species. This model of the insulin receptor differs from a model proposed by other investigators using chemical bifunctional linker; others have concluded that the insulin receptor is composed of two 130 K and two 90 K disulfide-linked subunits (Massague et al., 1980; see also Chapter 4).

Studies on the biosynthesis of the insulin receptor demonstrate that the 130 K and the 90 K subunit are derived from a glycoprotein precursor

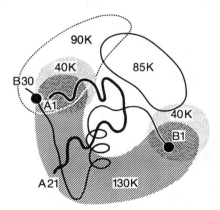

Figure 5 Schematic representation of the subunit structure of the 380 K insulin receptor. The 130 K subunit is shown to interact with the putative receptor binding domain of the insulin molecule and is photolabeled by either B1-MABI or B29-MABI. Normally, the 85 K subunit is not cross-linked by B1-MABI.

of 190 K (see Chapter 12 and Ronnett et al., 1984). Specific proteolytic cleavage of the precursor gives rise to the disulfide-linked subunits.
These observations have been confirmed by the cloning and sequencing
of the complementary DNA of the receptor precursor protein (Ullrich
et al., 1985). The other subunits (the 40 K and 85 K subunits) of the
cell surface insulin receptor detected by the photoreactive insulin
probes therefore do not originate from this receptor precursor protein.
Instead, they may be cell membrane components of different origins
that have become associated with the 130 K and 90 K subunits to form
the insulin receptor complex on the cell surface. Indeed, the 40 K subunit may be identifiable as the Class I antigen of the major histocom-
patibility complex (Chvatchko et al., 1983). While the biological significance of such association is not known, it may have an important
implication in the immunology of insulin-dependent diabetes.

   The most important and significant observation made using the
photoreactive insulin probes is that the insulin receptor of rat fat
cells is present in three forms, of different molecular sizes, and that
the three forms appear to be interconvertible via a redox mechanism
involving sulfhydryl groups. Our current hypothesis (Yip and Moule,
1983) is that the intact insulin receptors of rat fat cells exist as one
physical species of 380 K and that disulfide bonds linking one or two

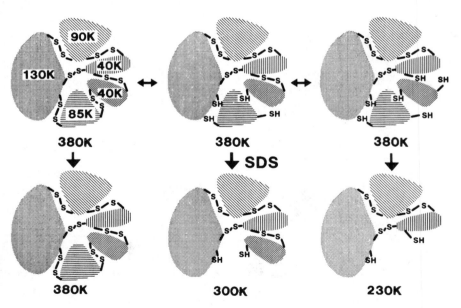

Figure 6 Diagrammatic representation of the interconversion of the
three redox insulin receptor species. From Yip and Moule (1983).
(Reproduced with permission of the American Diabetes Association, Inc.)

specific subunits to other receptor subunits in this physical form can be fully reduced endogeneously. These fully reduced subunits remain associated with the other subunits of the receptor through noncovalent interactions. Upon solubilization by detergents such as SDS, such subunit interactions are disrupted, resulting in the dissociation of these fully reduced subunits and in the appearance of the two lower molecular weight species (300 K and 230 K). Indeed, when the photo-labeled membranes are solubilized in 0.5% instead of 3% SDS (routinely used), relatively more 380 K and 300 K and less 230 K receptor species are detected. This hypothesis is schematically illustrated in Figure 6. Embodied in this hypothesis are the concepts of different redox states of the insulin receptor and the regulation of the redox state by some mechanisms involving sulfhydryl groups. Such mechanisms may be coupled to the redox and thus the metabolic state of the cell. The different redox states of the receptor species may have different binding affinities for insulin. The cellular sensitivity to insulin may therefore be regulated through the redox modulation of the receptor. Thus, peripheral insulin resistance in some diabetics may possibly be the result of a receptor defect in terms of a defective mechanism modulating the redox state of the insulin receptor.

REFERENCES

Blundell, T. L., Dodson, G. G., Hodgkin, D. C., and Mercola, D. A. (1972). *Advan. Protein Chem. 26*:279.

Carpenter, F. H. (1966). *Am. J. Med. 40*:750.

Chvatchko, Y., Van Oberghen, E., Kiger, N., and Fehlmann, M. (1983). *FEBS Lett. 163*:207.

Dixon, G. H. and Wardlaw, A. C. (1960). *Nature 188*:721.

Dodson, E. J., Dodson, G. G., Reynolds, C. D., and Vallely, D. (1980a). In *Insulin: Chemistry, Structure and Function of Insulin and Related Hormones* (D. Brandenburg and A. Wollmer, eds.), p. 9, de Gruyter, New York.

Dodson, G. G., Cutfield, S., Hoenjet, E., Wollmer, A., and Brandenburg, D. (1980b). In *Insulin: Chemistry, Structure and Function of Insulin and Related Hormones* (D. Brandenburg and A. Wollerm, eds), p. 17, de Gruyter, New York.

Emdin, S. O., Gammeltoft, S., and Gliemann, J. (1977). *J. Biol. Chem. 252*:602.

Gattner, H.-G., Danho, W., Behn, C., and Zahn, H. (1980). *Hoppe-Seyler's. Z. Physiol. Chem. 361*:1135.

Geiger, R., Obermeier, R., Teetz, V., Ukmann, R., Summ, H. D., Neubauer, H., Geisen, K., and Regitz, G. (1980). In *Insulin: Chemistry, Structure and Function of Insulin and Related Hormones* (D. Brandenburg and A. Wollmer, eds.), p. 409, de Gruyter, New York.

Gliemann, J., Sonne, O., Linde, S., and Hansen, B. (1979). *Biochem. Biophys. Res. Commun. 87*:1183.

Grant, P. T. and Reid, K. B. M. (1968). *Biochem. J. 106*:531.

Horuk, R., Goodwin, P., O'Connor, K., Neville, R. W. J., Lazarus, N. R., and Stone, D. (1979). *Nature (London) 279*:439.

Horuk, R., Blundell, T. L., Lararus, N. R., Neville, R. W. J., Stone, D., and Wollmer, A. (1980). *Nature (London) 286*:822.

Humbel, R. E. and Renold, A. E. (1963). *Biochim. Biophys. Acta 74*: 84.

Humbel, R. E. and Crestfield, A. M. (1965). *Biochemistry 4*:1044.

Hunt, L. T. (1969). In *Atlas of Protein Sequence and Structure* (M. O. Dayhoff, ed.), Vol. 4, National Biomedical Research Foundation, Silver Spring, Maryland, p. D164.

Kikuchi, K., Larner, J., Freer, R. J., Day, A. R., Morris, H., and Dell, A. (1980). *J. Biol. Chem. 255*:9281.

Massague, J., Pilch, P. F., and Czech, M. P. (1980). *Proc. Natl. Acad. Sci. USA 77*:7137.

McLaughlin, P. J. and Dayhoff, M. O. (1969). In *Atlas of Protein Sequence and Structure*, (M. O. Dayhoff, ed.), Vol. 4, p. 39, National Biomedical Research Foundation, Silver Spring, Maryland.

Moody, A. J., Stan, M. A., Stan, M., and Gliemann, J. (1974). *J. Horm. Metab. Res. 6*:12.

Olefsky, J. M., Saekow, M., Tager, H., and Rubenstein, A. H. (1980). *J. Biol. Chem. 255*:6098.

Peterson, J. D., Steiner, D. F., Emdin, S. O., and Falkmer, S. (1975). *J. Biol. Chem. 250*:5183.

Pullen, R. A., Lindsay, D. G., Wood, S. P., Tickle, I. J., Blundell, T. L., Wollmer, A., Krail, G., Brandenburg, D., Zahn, H., Gliemann, J., and Gammeltoft, S. (1976). *Nature (London) 259*: 369.

Ronnett, G. V., Knutson, V. P., Kahansky, R. A., Simpson, T. L., and Lane, M. D. (1984). *J. Biol. Chem. 259*:4566.

Simon, J., Freychet, P., and Rosselin, G. (1974). *Endocrinology 95*:1439.

Ullrich, A., Bell, J. R., Chen, E. Y., Herrera, R., Petruzzelli, L. M., Dull, T. J., Gray, A., Coussens, L., Liao, Y.-C., Tsubokawa, M., Mason, A., Seeburg, P. H., Grunfield, C., Rosen, O. M., and Ramachandran, J. (1985). *Nature (London) 313*:756.

Yeung, C. W. T., Moule, M. L., and Yip, C. C. (1979). *J. Biol. Chem. 254*:9453.

Yeung, C. W. T., Moule, M. L., and Yip, C. C. (1980). *Biochemistry 19*:2196.

Yip, C. C. and Moule, M. L. (1976). *Can J. Biochem. 54*:866.

Yip, C. C., Yeung, C. W. T., and Moule, M. L. (1980). *Biochemistry 19*:70.

Yip, C. C., Moule, M. L., and Yeung, C. W. T. (1982). *Biochemistry 21*:2940.

Yip, C. C., and Moule, M. L. (1983). *Diabetes, 32*:760.
Zimmerman, A. E., Moule, M. L., and Yip, C. C. (1974). *J. Biol. Chem. 249*:4026.

BIBLIOGRAPHY

Bedarkar, S., Blundell, T. L., Dockerill, S., Tickle, I. J., and Wood, S. P. (1978). Polypeptide hormone-receptor interactions: The structure and receptor binding of insulin and glucagon. In *Ciba Foundation Symposium,* Vol. 60, *Molecular Interactions and Activity in Proteins,* Excerpta Medica, Amsterdam and New York, p. 105–121.

Chowdhry, V. and Westheimer, F. H. (1979). Photoaffinity labeling of biological systems. *Ann. Rev. Biochem. 48*:293-325.

Lwowski, W. (1980). Nitrenes in photoaffinity labeling: Speculations of an organic chemist. In *Ann. N.Y. Acad. Sci. 346*:491-500.

Muggeo, M., Ginsberg, B. H., Roth, J., Neville, D. M. Jr., De Meyts, P., and Kahn, C. R. (1979). The insulin receptor in vertebrates is functionally more conserved during evolution than insulin itself. *Endocrinology 104*:1393-1402.

Raftery, M. A., Witzemann, V., and Blanchard, S. G. (1980). The use of photochemical probes for studies of structure and function of purified acetylcholine receptor preparations. *Ann. New York Acad. Sci. 346*:458-474.

4

Insulin Receptor: Purification and Structure

STEVEN JACOBS *The Wellcome Research Laboratories, Research Triangle Park, North Carolina*

The initial interaction of insulin with target tissues is with specific receptors located on the surface membrane of target cells. These receptors have a dual function. They recognize the presence of the very low concentrations of insulin that are present in the blood under physiological conditions and, depending upon the concentration, generate some graded intracellular signal that initiates a sequence of biological responses. Recognition is accomplished by the high-affinity binding of insulin to its receptor. The precise mechanism by which insulin binding triggers a biological response is not known; however, some clues have recently emerged.

Although insulin receptors were postulated as early as the 1940s, direct evidence of their existence was lacking until the early 1970s, when the perfection of radiolabeled insulin-binding techniques made it possible, for the first time, to detect their presence convincingly and accurately measure their insulin-binding properties. In the following decade, the application of three techniques, affinity chromatography, affinity labeling, and immunoprecipitation by anti-receptor antibodies, along with radiolabeled insulin binding, has resulted in rapid progress in purifying the receptor, determining its structure, and determining its orientation within the membrane (for recent reviews, see Refs. 1—3). This information should provide the preliminaries for a mechanistic understanding of how the receptor functions.

I. RECEPTOR PURIFICATION

The insulin receptor is an integral membrane protein, which means that it is deeply embedded in the cell membrane. In fact, as will be discussed later, it is a transmembrane protein with both an extra-cellular and a cytoplasmic portion. Before it can be purified, it must be extracted from the membrane. This can be accomplished by a variety of nonionic detergents, such as Triton X-100, which solubilize the receptor in a form in which it retains its insulin-binding properties (4).

One problem in purifying insulin receptors is that they are present in extremely small quantities and in a highly impure state. For example, in liver they comprise about 0.01% of total membrane protein. Furthermore, the gross physiochemical properties of the insulin receptor, such as its size, charge, and solubility, are not very different from other membrane proteins. Therefore, conventional methods of protein purification that separate substances on the basis of these properties have only been of limited usefulness in purifying insulin receptors. On the other hand, affinity chromatography, which depends upon the most unique property of the insulin receptor, its high affinity for insulin, has been extremely useful (5,6).

The basic principle of affinity chromatography is illustrated in Figure 1. Insulin is covalently attached to Sepharose beads. Solubilized membranes containing insulin receptors are percolated through the beads that have been packed into a glass column. Insulin receptors, because of their affinity for the immobilized insulin, are tightly adsorbed to the beads, while other proteins pass through. The beads are then thoroughly washed to remove any contaminating proteins, and adsorbed receptor is eluted (i.e., released from the column) by treating it with partially denaturing buffers that dissociate it from the immobilized insulin.

Sodium dodecyl sulfate (SDS)—polyacrylamide gel electrophoresis (a technique that separates polypeptides on the basis of their molecular weights) indicates that the purified material eluted from insulin-Sepharose columns contains predominately three polypeptides: a major polypeptide with a molecular wieght of 135,000 and smaller amounts of 90,000 and 45,000 M.W. polypeptides (6). These three polypeptides, which have been called α, β and β_1 (7), comprise more than 90% of the protein in eluates from insulin-Sepharose, yet they are such minor components of less pure preparations of insulin receptor that they are obscured when these less pure preparations are analyzed on SDS gels.

Since α, β, and β_1 were so selectively retained on an insulin-Sepharose affinity column, it seemed likely that they were components of the purified receptor. One way of demonstrating this would be to determine the specific activity of the purified material to bind insulin. One would expect that one molecule of receptor should bind at least one molecule of insulin. The molecular weight of the insulin receptors, both in crude soluble preparations and after purification, is approximately 350,000. This was determined by the velocity at which insulin

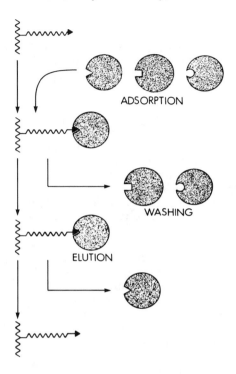

Figure 1 Schematic representation of affinity chromatography. Insulin (▼), immobilized on the Sepharose matrix, binds selectively to the insulin receptor (☻); other receptors can be washed from the column. The selectively adsorbed insulin receptor can then be recovered by dissociation from the immobilized insulin.

receptor sediments through a sucrose density gradient when centrifuged and by its exclusion from the pores of beads whose size have a distribution similar to the dimensions of the receptor. In both types of measurements, insulin receptor was detected by its insulin-binding activity. One nanomole or 350,000 ng of receptor would be expected to bind at least 1 nmol of insulin. Eluates from insulin-Sepharose had a specific activity of only 10−20% of this value. The most likely explanation for this is that a portion of the receptors have been damaged during purification and lost their ability to bind insulin. However, another possibility is that only a small fraction of the protein present in the insulin-Sepharose eluate was receptor and that the major protein bands visible on sodium dodecyl sulfate gels were contaminants.

Although it turns out that this is not the case, and that α, β, and β_1 are receptor subunits, studies using affinity purified material were not sufficient to prove this conclusively. Confirmation from studies using other techniques, in particular affinity labeling and immunopurification, was required.

II. AFFINITY LABELING

The binding of insulin to its receptor is noncovalent and reversible. Many of the procedures used to analyze insulin receptors require denaturing conditions that would dissociate insulin from its receptor. However, insulin binding is the most common means for identifying and detecting insulin receptors. This problem is overcome by affinity labeling techniques in which [^{125}I]insulin is covalently and irreversibly bound to its receptor.

Two types of techniques, photoaffinity labeling (8) and affinity cross-linking (9), have been used to affinity label insulin receptors. In photoaffinity labeling, derivatives of insulin containing ^{125}I and an aryl azide group are synthesized so that they retain the receptor-binding properties of natural insulin. These derivatives are chemically stable in the dark, but when exposed to light of a certain wavelength, they generate highly reactive, free radical nitrenes that can form a covalent bond with a polypeptide chain. These photoaffinity labeling derivatives are then incubated with cells or membranes containing insulin receptors or with solubilized receptor. After they have had sufficient time to bind to the receptor, they are photolysed, and, because they are bound to the receptor, they are likely to associate with it covalently.

In affinity cross-linking, [^{125}I]insulin is allowed to bind to its receptor. Then a bifunctional reagent (i.e., one that has two reactive groups capable of readily forming covalent bonds) is added. If the functional groups have the right geometry, they can react simultaneously with complementary groups on the receptor and on a molecule of insulin bound to the receptor, covalently cross-linking the two.

Each affinity labeling technique has its own peculiar advantages. Affinity cross-linking generally results in a higher efficiency of coupling and avoids the need for synthesis of special photoaffinity labeling derivatives. Photoaffinity labeling is more specific in that cellular proteins other than insulin receptors are not cross-linked; therefore, photoaffinity labeling studies can be carried out in viable cells with minimal disturbance of normal cellular processes.

When cells or membranes are affinity labeled by either technique and the labeled polypeptides are analyzed by SDS-polyacrylamide gel electrophoresis, the results are similar. With both techniques, polypeptides with molecular weights of approximately 135,000, 90,000, and

45,000 are labeled. These are the same polypeptides that are found when insulin receptors are purified by affinity chromatography. However, in affinity labeling studies, there is usually selective labeling of the 135,000 molecular weight polypeptide. The 90,000 and the 45,000 M.W. polypeptides are usually only faintly labeled, and, under certain conditions, they are not labeled at all.

III. IMMUNOCHEMICAL STUDIES

A rare cause of diabetes in humans is due to spontaneously occurring antibodies that, for reasons that are not clear, affected patients produce against their own insulin receptors (10). These antibodies have quite interesting properties. They interfere with the binding of insulin to its receptor, and when tested in vitro in acute experiments, they mimic the biological actions of insulin. Although most patients who have these antibodies are insulin resistant, some go through phases where their sugar becomes dangerously low as a result of the insulin-like activity of these antibodies (11).

Although subsequently, antibodies to insulin receptors have been produced by immunizing animals with purified insulin receptor, antibodies from patients with this syndrome were the first available for studying the insulin receptor. They were particularly useful for confirming studies on the purification and structure of the receptor because they provided, for the first time, a method of directly studying the receptor that was completely independent of its insulin-binding properties. These autoantibodies have been covalently coupled to Sepharose beads (12) and used to purify insulin receptors in a manner analogous to affinity chromatography utilizing insulin-Sepharose described previously. They have also been used in smaller scale immunoprecipitation studies in which membrane proteins are nonspecifically radiolabeled with a variety of techniques, and then labeled insulin receptors are specifically immunoprecipitated with the antibody and analyzed by SDS-polyacrylamide gel electrophoresis (13). The results are in excellent agreement with the previously described affinity chromatography and affinity labeling studies. Peptides corresponding to α, β, and β_1 are identified.

IV. SUBUNIT STRUCTURE

The fact that several different techniques, which depend on two different independent properties of the receptor (its ability to bind insulin and its immunochemical specificity), identify the same polypeptides as components of the insulin receptor indicates that these results are reliable and that α, β, and β_1 are truly components of the receptor.

The next question is, how are these peptides arranged to form the intact receptor?

It appears that β_1 is a fragment of β that is produced when β is clipped by enzymes that digest proteins (14,15). The evidence for this is the following: In different preparations of purified receptor, the relative amounts of β and β_1 vary reciprocally. Precautions to minimize proteolysis result in an increase in β at the expense of β_1. When β and β_1 are extensively digested with proteolytic enzymes, a large number of the small fragments produced from each appears to be the same, suggesting extensive similarities between the two. Furthermore, mild treatment of β with specific proteolytic enzymes, such as elastase or lysozomal proteases, converts it to a polypeptide with a molecular weight similar to β_1.

It is not clear if proteolytic clipping of β is merely an in vitro artifact or if it represents physiologically important processing of the receptor. Following hormone binding, the insulin receptor is internalized and may be exposed to lysozomal proteases, which would provide a possible mechanism for receptor processing.

The molecular size of solubilized insulin receptor can be determined by gel exclusion chromatography. In this technique, solubilized receptor is made to flow through a column packed with porous beads. Large molecules, which are excluded form the pores, will have a shorter probable path to the end of the column, and will therefore flow through the column more rapidly than small molecules, which can enter the pores. The rate at which molecules exit from the column can then be used to calculate their size. By using this technique, the molecular weight of the insulin receptor, after it has been solubilized by nondenaturing detergents, such as Triton X-100, has been found to be approximately 350,000. This, of course, is considerably larger than the individual α and β components and suggests that the intact native receptor is composed of multiple subunits.

In contrast to Triton X-100, sodium dodecyl sulfate is a very denaturing detergent. It tends to unfold proteins and to disassociate subunits unless they are covalently linked by interchain disulfide bonds. When performing SDS-polyacrylamide gel electrophoresis, it is usual to use disulfide-reducing agents to break these bonds so that each subunit migrates independently as a separately staining band. Indeed, these were the conditions under which the α and β polypeptides were identified. If insulin receptor is subjected to SDS-polyacrylamide gel electrophoresis without prior reduction, bands corresponding to the isolated α and β subunits are not present. Instead, the major band has a molecular weight of approximately 380,000, which is quite comparable to the molecular weight of the native receptor as determined by gel exclusion chromatography (16,17). In addition, in some tissues, a less intense band with a molecular weight of approximately 210,000 is also present. This suggests that the subunits that

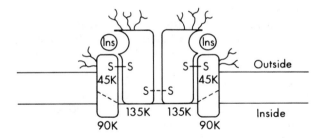

Figure 2 Model of the subunit structure of the insulin receptor. The receptor is shown as a transmembrane disulfide-stabilized heterodimeric glycoprotein with oligosaccharide moieties attached to the extracellular domains of the receptor. The 90 K β-subunit, known to have a transmembrane domain (see Fig. 4), is shown anchoring the receptor in the membrane. The diagonal broken line depicts the proteolytically sensitive site on the β-subunit. The α-subunit, thought to have a large extracellular domain, is shown as the insulin-binding region of the receptor.

compose the intact receptor are linked by interchain disulfide bonds.

The amount of each subunit present in the intact receptor can be determined by two-dimensional sodium dodecyl sulfate-polyacrylamide gel electrophoresis. In this technique, receptor is electrophoresed in the first dimension without disulfide-reducing agents. This separates the 380,000 and the 220,000 molecular weight bands. The gel is then treated with disulfide-reducing agents to disassociate the isolated α and β subunits, and electrophoresis is performed in the second dimension in a direction perpendicular to the first dimension to separate α and β. Both the 380,000 and the 220,000 molecular weight bands generate α and β subunits, and the ratio of α to β derived from each band is the same. It is easy to see that if the 220,000 molecular weight band is composed of both 135,000 molecular weight α subunits and 90,000 molecular weight β subunits, it must contain one copy of each. Since the 380,000 molecular weight band contains α and β in the same ratio as the 220,000 molecular weight band, it is most likely that it is composed of two copies of α and two copies of β. The molecular weights of the proposed subunit components do not add up to exactly 380,000, but that is acceptable since mobility on SDS-polyacrylamide gel electrophoresis does not exactly reflect molecular weight. Other factors, such as the extent of the interaction of the protein with SDS and the shape of the resulting complex, which can be altered by disulfide cross-linking, also effect mobility.

The subunit structure deduced from these studies is summarized in Figure 2. While this model for the structure of the insulin receptor is generally believed to be correct, other models exist (see Chapter 3). According to the model shown in Figure 2, the intact receptor is a tetramer composed of two copies of α and two copies of β. It exists in two states. In one state, all four subunits are linked by disulfide bonds. This is the most prevalent state and corresponds to the 380,000 molecular weight band seen on unreduced SDS-polyacrylamide gels. The other less prevalent state, in which the disulfide bond linking two α−β dimers is reduced, corresponds to the 220,000 molecular weight band on unreduced polyacrylamide gels. The functional significance of these two states is not entirely clear. Some evidence suggests that the partially reduced state may correspond to a low-affinity form of the receptor and that when insulin binds to the receptor, it transforms the receptor to this reduced, low-affinity form (18).

V. MEMBRANE ORIENTATION AND FUNCTIONAL DOMAINS OF THE RECEPTOR

Insulin receptors serve as a relay to transmit information about the concentration of insulin outside the cell to the interior of the cell. The simplest way to envision this occurring would be for the receptor to be a transmembrane protein with an extracellular portion or domain involved in insulin binding and an intracellular portion or domain involved in generating some intracellular signal. Experimental evidence has been gathered to support this model.

It is well known that the insulin receptor is a glycoprotein. Both the α and β subunits contain carbohydrate residues. This is demonstrated by the fact that treatment of the receptor with neuraminidase, an enzyme that digests carbohydrates, alters the mobility of both α and β when they are analyzed on SDS-polyacrylamide gels (19). Furthermore, when cells are incubated in the presence of radioactive carbohydrates, these are incorporated into both α and β subunits of newly synthesized receptors (20). Many membrane proteins are glycoproteins. Their carbohydrate portions are located exclusively on the external surface of the cell membrane. Thus, both α and β have regions that are exposed on the external surface.

Consistent with this, both α and β are affinity labeled by insulin under conditions in which insulin would not be expected to have access to the cytoplasmic surface of the membrane. Although both subunits are affinity labeled, α comprises the insulin-binding site. However, since β is also labeled, it may contribute to the insulin-binding site or at least be in proximity to it.

The β subunit also appears to span the membrane and to be exposed on its internal or cytoplasmic surface. After insulin binds to its receptor on the surface of the cell, the receptor with insulin bound is internalized by an endocytic process and is found in the membrane of intracellular vesicles. Because these vesicles form by invagination and pinching off, the orientation of the vesicle membrane is opposite that of the cell membrane; what was the inside surface becomes the outside surface. When these vesicles are iodinated with lactoperoxidase, a technique in which only proteins that are exposed to the outside and capable of coming in contact with lactoperoxidase are labeled, the β subunit is iodinated. Under these conditions, the α subunit is not labeled. However, if these vesicles are disrupted, both subunits are labeled (21).

In view of these findings, it might be anticipated that the intracellular portion of the β subunit would contain the function portion or domain of the receptor that is involved in generating an intracellular signal. This is supported by the recent finding that the β subunit of the insulin receptor has enzymatic activity that is regulated by insulin binding.

VI. TYROSINE KINASE ACTIVITY OF THE RECEPTOR

In very simple RNA tumor viruses, the information required for tumor production is carried on a single viral gene, called the oncogene. The oncogenes of several viruses in this class code for enzymes that both are phosphorylated on tyrosine residues and can transfer the terminal phosphate of ATP to tyrosine residues of other specific proteins. The activity of these enzymes, called tyrosine-specific protein kinases, is closely correlated with and is presumably responsible for malignant transformation. This is quite interesting because tyrosine is a relatively uncommon site of phosphorylation; serine and threonine are more usual. This became even more interesting when it was discovered that receptors for several growth factors are also phosphorylated on tyrosine residues and are tyrosine-specific protein kinases. As a result of these findings, the hypothesis has developed that tyrosine phosphorylation somehow triggers the processes responsible for both normal cellular growth and the uncontrolled growth associated with some tumors.

The insulin receptor is one such receptor that is phosphorylated (22-25). Phosphorylation occurs on the β subunit of the receptor. The extent of phosphorylation is stimulated by insulin. In solubilized receptor, phosphorylation occurs exclusively on tyrosine residues. In intact cells, the pattern of phosphorylation is more complex; phosphoserine, phosphothreonine, as well as phosphotyrosine are present. The receptor, itself, appears to be a protein kinase. The β subunit binds ATP (26,27) (if the receptor is a kinase, it would have to bind ATP, one of its substrates), and purified receptor will catalyze the tyrosine phosphorylation of exogenous proteins when they are added in vitro (25,28,29).

While the functional significance of the tyrosine kinase activity is not entirely clear, it seems likely that it is somehow involved in the mechanism by which insulin triggers a metabolic response. There are several possible ways this could come about. The receptor could directly phosphorylate some of the terminal enzymes or transport proteins that mediate the effects of insulin (e.g., the glucose transport protein or pyruvate dehydrogenase). This does not seem likely, since several of these ultimate targets for insulin are spatially distant from the receptor and are known not to contain phosphotyrosine, even when stimulated by insulin. An indirect mechanism seems more likely: The kinase activity of insulin receptor may stimulate a cascade of enzymes that ultimately regulate the state of phosphorylation of some of the targets for insulin or, alternatively, the receptor may phosphorylate an enzyme that in turn produces a soluble mediator that will interact with and regulate the various target enzymes of insulin. Such a soluble mediator has recently been reported (see Chapter 9). While it is attractive to implicate the protein kinase activity of the receptor as being involved in its triggering function, it should be pointed out that aside from the receptor, itself, no physiological substrate for the insulin receptor kinase has been identified, and tyrosine phosphorylation has never been clearly shown to alter the function of any protein.

VII. RECEPTOR BIOSYNTHESIS

A considerable amount is known about the biosynthesis of membrane glycoproteins in general (for a review, see Ref. 30). Although much less is specifically known about insulin receptor biosynthesis, it does appear to fit the general pattern, which will be briefly discussed as background.

The initial phase in the synthesis of membrane glycoproteins, like all proteins, is translation of messenger RNA on ribosomes. Translation progresses from the amino end of the protein to the carboxyl end. For membrane proteins, near the amino-terminal end, there is a sequence of amino acids called the signal peptide that recognizes a receptor on the endoplasmic reticulum and causes the ribosome on which translation is occurring to associate with the endoplasmic reticulum. In addition, the signal peptide passes through a pore in the membrane of the endoplasmic reticulum. It is followed by a portion of the remainder of the protein, giving it its transmembrane orientation that is preserved throughout its life span. All this occurs while the newly synthesized protein is still attached to the ribosome and is actively being transalted.

Other processes are also occurring inside the endoplasmic reticulum before translation is complete. For most proteins, the signal peptide

is cleaved by a proteolytic enzyme shortly after it enters the endoplasmic reticulum. Also, a carbohydrate chain, rich in mannose, is
attached as a single unit to specific arginine residues on the protein.
This process, called core glycosylation, is the first stage in the synthesis of the carbohydrate portion of glycoproteins. For most proteins, further modifications of this chain occur, but not until the protein leaves the endoplasmic reticulum.

Core glycosylation is inhibited by the antibiotic, tunicamycin.
Treatment of cells with tunicamycin blocks the expression of newly
synthesized insulin receptors at the cell surface (31,32). Insulin
receptors that are synthesized under these conditions are unable to
bind insulin and do not get transported to the cell membrane. This
indicates that insulin receptors undergo core glycosylation and that
core glycosylation is necessary for both of these processes.

After this preliminary processing, newly synthesized membrane
glycoproteins are transported to the Golgi apparatus where the next
stages of maturation occur. Three types of processes occur in the
Golgi apparatus. Mannose residues are removed from the core carbohydrate chains, and terminal sugar residues are added to form a
complex branched chain. For some proteins, further proteolytic
processing occurs that cleaves high molecular weight precursors to
smaller mature forms. Finally, the mature protein is packaged into
vesicles and is somehow targeted for transport to the cell membrane.

There are two ways in which a multisubunit protein can be formed.
The more common way is for each subunit to be synthesized independently from its own messenger RNA. The subunits then spontaneously
associate shortly after synthesis to form the multisubunit complex.
This, for example, is how the four chains of immunoglobulin G are
synthesized. A less common way is for the various subunits to be
synthesized as a single linear sequence from a single messenger RNA
molecule that is then internally cleaved by a proteolytic enzyme to form
the multiple subunits. Proteolysis occurs in the Golgi apparatus or in
Golgi-derived vesicles en route to the cell membrane. The conversion
of proinsulin to insulin is an example of this type of mechanism.

The biosynthesis of insulin receptors utilizes both types of processes. When cells are incubated with ^{35}S-radiolabeled methionine for
short periods of time (so that newly synthesized proteins do not have
time to fully mature), the earliest identifiable form of the insulin receptor has a molecular weight of approximately 180,000 (33,34). With
slightly longer incubations, a 200,000 molecular weight form appears,
and still later the mature α and β subunits appear. Monensin, which
interferes with Golgi function, blocks the maturation of the receptor
and leads to the accumulation of the 180,000 molecular weight form,
along with small amounts of 115,000 and 85,000 molecular weight peptides (35). The 180,000 molecular weight form appears to be a precursor of both the α and β subunits, since it can bind insulin (a function

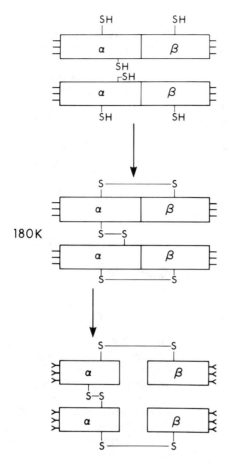

180K

Figure 3 Sequence of steps in insulin receptor biosynthesis. As discussed in this chapter and in further detail in Chapter 12, the receptor is synthesized first as a single polypeptide chain (see Fig. 4). The receptor then undergoes a maturation process, including the addition of oligosaccharide, proteolytic processing, and the formation of disulfide bonds to yield the heterodimeric ($\alpha_2\beta_2$) structure that is incorporated into the cell membrane.

of the α subunit) and is autophosphorylated (a function of the β subunit). In addition, digestion of the 180,000 molecular weight form with proteolytic enzymes generates small peptide fragments that are also generated when both α and β are digested by the same enzymes, which also suggests that the 180,000 molecular weight form is also a precursor for both α and β. The 115,000 and 85,000 molecular weight polypeptides, which are formed in the presence of monensin, are abnormally processed α and β subunits in which terminal glycosylation has not occurred. Presumably, the conversion of the 180,000 molecular polypeptide form to the 200,000 molecular weight polypeptide results from the addition of sugar residues during terminal glycosylation.

The 180,000 molecular weight precursor that accumulates in the presence of monensin exists as a disulfide-linked dimer, since when it is subjected to SDS-polyacrylamide gel electrophoresis without reduction it migrates as a 360,000 molecular weight complex. Only after reduction is it converted to a polypeptide with a molecular weight of 180,000.

From the results discussed above, the normal sequence involved in the biosynthesis of insulin receptors can be deduced (Fig. 3). Insulin receptors are synthesized on the rough endoplasmic reticulum and are core glycosylated to form a 180,000 molecular weight precursor. Shortly after synthesis, two of these precursors form a disulfide-linked dimer. Presumably, intrachain disulfide bonds also form. The receptor is then transported to the Golgi apparatus. There, terminal sugars are added, and the resulting 200,000 molecular weight chain is proteolytically cleaved to generate the mature disulfide-linked tetramer that is then packaged and transported to the cell membrane. The biosynthetic process is dealt with in greater detail in Chapter 12.

VIII. CLONED INSULIN RECEPTOR cDNA

Recently insulin receptor cDNA (DNA complimentary to insulin receptor mRNA) has been cloned and sequenced (36). From this it has been possible to deduce the amino acid sequence of the insulin receptor precursor and the organization of its functional domains (Fig. 4). The results confirm and extend the inferences based upon the biochemical evidence discussed above. At the N-terminus of the polypeptide coded for by insulin receptor mRNA is a sequence of 27 hydrophobic amino acid residues which are not present in the mature receptor and which are characteristic of a signal peptide. This is followed by the alpha subunit (residues 1 to 719). Residues 720 to 723 are four basic amino acids, an excellent target for a proteolytic enzyme with the specificity of trypsin. They are the site at which the insulin receptor precursor is clipped to generate the alpha and beta subunits. Residues 723 to 1343 comprise the beta subunit.

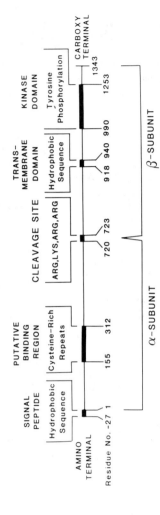

Figure 4 Schematic organization of functional domains of the insulin receptor deduced from the cDNA sequence of its receptor. The numbers indicate the position of amino acid residues, with 1 depicting the N terminus of the mature α-subunit (36). The solid bars indicate the receptor domains for which specific functions can be assigned. The sequence is not drawn to scale.

The beta subunit contains a stretch of amino acids (990 to 1253) that closely resembles corresponding regions in several viral oncogene products having tyrosine kinase activity. There is a homologous region in the epidermal growth factor receptor, which also has tyrosine kinase activity. This region (residues 990 to 1253) is the presumed tyrosine kinase domain of the insulin receptor. The beta subunit also has a run of 23 hydrophobic or nonpolar amino acids (918 to 940) that is characteristic of a membrane-spanning domain. This is the only well defined membrane-spanning domain in the entire receptor. If it is assumed that the tyrosine kinase domain is on the cytoplasmic surface of the membrane, this would imply that the N-terminal portion of the beta subunit (residues 724 to 917) and the entire alpha subunit are on the external surface of the membrane. This is consistent with the lactoperoxidase labeling studies (21) and with other biochemical evidence cited previously. Whether the alpha subunit is anchored to the cell membrane exclusively through its interaction with the beta subunit, or whether there are also direct hydrophobic interactions with the membrane, is not entirely clear.

The alpha subunit, which affinity labeling studies indicate is the major binding subunit, contains a stretch (155 to 312) of not-exactly-repeating sequences that are rich in cysteine residues. Homologous regions are found in the epidermal growth factor receptor and the low density lipoprotein receptor. This region is thought to be a likely candidate for the hormone binding domain.

REFERENCES

1. Czech, M. P. (1981). *Am. J. Med.* 70:14—150.
2. Kahn, C. R., Baird, K. L., Filer, J. S., Grunfeld, C., Harmon, J. T., Harrison, L. C., Karlsson, F. A., Kasuga, M., King, G. L., Lang, U. C., Podskainy, J. M., and Van Obberghen, E. (1981). *Recent Progr. Horm. Res.* 37:477—538.
3. Jacobs, S., and Cuatrecasas, P. (1983). *Ann. Rev. Pharmacol. Toxicol.* 23:461—479.
4. Cuatrecasas, P. (1972). *Proc. Natl. Acad. Sci. USA* 69:318—322.
5. Cuatrecasas, P. (1972). *Proc. Natl. Acad. Sci. USA* 69: 1277—1281.
6. Jacobs, S., Schechter, Y., Bissell, K., and Cuatrecasas, P. (1977). *Biochem. Biophys. Res. Commun.* 77:981—988.
7. Massague, J. and Czech, M. P. (1980). *Diabetes* 29:945—947.
8. Yip, C. C., Yeung, C. W. T., and Moule, M. L. (1978). *J. Biol. Chem.* 253:1743—1745.
9. Pilch, P. F. and Czech, M. P. (1979). *J. Biol. Chem.* 254: 3375—3381.
10. Flier, J. S., Kahn, C. R., Roth, J., and Bar, R. S. (1976). *Science* 190:63—65.

11. Flier, J. S., Kahn, C. R., and Roth, J. (1979). *N. Engl. J. Med.* 300:413—419.

12. Harrison, L. C. and Itin, A. (1980). *J. Biol. Chem.* 255: 2066—2072.

13. Van Obberghen, E., Kasuga, M., Le Cam, A., Hedo, J. A., Itin, A., and Harrison, L. C. (1981). *Proc. Natl. Acad. Sci. USA* 78:1052—1056.

14. Massague, J., Pilch, P. F., and Czech, M. P. (1981). *J. Biol. Chem.* 256:3182—3190.

15. Jacobs, S., and Cuatrecasas, P. (1981). In *Current Views on Insulin Receptor*, (D. Andreane, R. De Piro, R. Lauro, J. Olifsky, and J. Roth, eds.), Academic Press, New York, Vol. 41, pp. 23—28.

16. Jacobs, S., Hazum, E., Schecter, Y., and Cuatrecasas, P. (1979). *Proc. Natl. Acad. Sci. USA* 76:4918—4921.

17. Pilch, P. F. and Czech, M. P. (1980). *J. Biol. Chem.* 255: 1722—1731.

18. Maturo, J. M., III, Hollenberg, M. D., and Aglio, L. S. (1983). *Biochemistry* 22:2579—2586.

19. Jacobs, S., Hazum, E., and Cuatrecasas, P. (1980). *J. Biol. Chem.* 255:6973—6940.

20. Hedo, J. A., Kasuga, M., Van Obberghen, E., Roth, J., and Kahn, C. R. (1981). *Proc. Natl. Acad. Sci. USA* 78:4791—4795.

21. Hedo, J. A., Cushman, S. W., and Simpson, I. A. (1982). *Diabetes* 31(Suppl. 2):2A.

22. Kasuga, M., Karlsson, F. A., and Kahn, C. R. (1982). *Science* 215:185—187.

23. Kasuga, M., Zick, Y., Blithe, D. L., Karlsson, F. A., Haring, H. U., and Kahn, C. R. (1982). *J. Biol. Chem.* 257:9891—9894.

24. Kasuga, M., Zick, Y., Blithe, D. L., Crettaz, M., and Kahn, C. R. (1982). *Nature (London)* 298:667—669.

25. Petruzelli, L. M., Ganguly, S., Smith, C. J., Cobb, M., Rubin, C. S., and Rosen, O. M. (1982). *Proc. Natl. Acad. Sci. USA* 76:6792—6796.

26. Van Obberghen, E., Rossi, B., Kowalski, A., Gazzano, H., and Panzio, G. (1983). *Proc. Natl. Acad. Sci. USA* 80:945—949.

27. Shia, M. A., and Pilch, P. F. (1983). *Biochemistry* 22:717—721.

28. Roth, R. A., and Cassell, D. J. (1983). *Science* 219:299—301.

29. Kasuga, M., Yamaguchi, Y. F., Blithe, D. L., and Kahn, C. R. (1983). *Proc. Natl. Acad. Sci. USA* 80:2137—2141.

30. Sabitini, D. D., Kreibich, G., Morimoto, T., and Adesnik, M. (1982). *J. Cell Biol.* 92:1—22.

31. Rosen, O. M., Chia, G. H., Fung, C., and Rubin, C. S. (1979). *J. Cell Physiol.* 99:37—42.

32. Reed. B. C., Ronnett, G. V., and Lane, M. D. (1981). *Proc. Natl. Acad. Sci. USA* 78:2908—2912.

33. Kasuga, M., Hedo, J. A., Yamada, K. M., and Kahn, C. R. (1982). *J. Biol. Chem. 257*:10392−10399.
34. Deutch, P. J., Wan, C., Rosen, O. M., and Rubin, C. S. (1983). *Proc. Natl. Acad. Sci. USA 80*:133−136.
35. Jacobs, S., Kull, F. C., Jr., and Cuatrecasas, P. (1983). *Proc. Natl. Acad. Sci. USA 80*:1228−1231.
36. Ullrich, A., Bell, J. R., Chen, E. Y., Herrara, R., Petruzzelli, L. M., Dull, T. J., Gray, A., Coussens, L., Liao, Y.-C., Tsubokawa, M., Mason, A., Seeburg, P. H., Grunfield, C. Rosen, O. M., and Ramachandran, J. (1985). *Nature 313*:756−761.

BIBLIOGRAPHY

As indicated in the introductory portion of this chapter, the following references summarize much of the background material dealing with the insulin receptor:

Czech, M. P. (1981). Insulin action. *Am. J. Med. 70*:142−150.
Jacobs, S. and Cuatrecasas, P. (1983). Insulin receptors. *Ann. Rev. Pharmacol. Toxicol. 23*:461−479.
Kahn, C. R., Biard, K. L., Flier, J. S., Grunfeld, C., Harmon, J. T., Harrison, L. C., Karlsson, F. A., Kasuga, M., King, G. L., Lang, U. C., Podskalny, J. M. and Van Obberghen, E. (1981). Insulin receptors, receptor antibodies, and the mechanism of insulin action. *Rec. Progr. Horm. Res. 37*:477−538.

5

Insulin Receptor: Relationship to Receptors for Other Insulinlike Polypeptides

MORLEY D. HOLLENBERG *University of Calgary Faculty of Medicine, Calgary, Alberta, Canada*

I. INSULIN, NONSUPPRESSIBLE INSULINLIKE ACTIVITIES, THE SOMATOMEDINS, AND THE INSULINLIKE GROWTH FACTORS

A. Discovery and Isolation of the Nonsuppressible Insulinlike Activities and the Somatomedins

One remarkable outcome of the development of the immunoassay for insulin relates to the observation that only about 7−10% of the insulin-like activity present in plasma, as measured by bioassay (e.g., on isolated rat fat tissue), can be neutralized by antisera to insulin it-self. The nonneutralizable (by insulin antiserum) insulinlike activity has, in the past, been called nonsuppressible insulinlike activity (NSILA). Shortly after such observations with insulin antiserum, it became apparent, on the one hand, that patients who were clearly insulin deficient, both by clinical and by insulin radioimmunoassay criteria, had an abundance of insulinlike activity that could be meas-ured by a bioassay of their sera, and, on the other hand, it became evident that a large proportion of patients who were diabetic by clini-cal criteria, had insulin present in their sera, measured both by bio-assay and by immunoassay methods, in amounts that were equivalent to or even greater than levels that were present in nondiabetic sub-jects. This second situation, whereby apparently adequate endogen-ous serum levels of insulin are insufficient to control the symptoms of diabetes (so-called "insulin resistance"), is the focus of much of the work described elsewhere in this treatise. The first situation alluded to above, in which substantial insulinlike bioactivity was discovered in the serum of insulin-dependent diabetics, was a stimulus for the discovery of a fascinating family of insulinlike polypeptides, which

have their own distinct receptor systems. This newly emerging family of insulinlike substances will be the subject of this chapter. The
detailed chemistry and biology of the various insulinlike peptides to
be discussed has been dealt with by a number of comparatively recent reviews (1—4).

Over the past two decades, much work in many laboratories has
been directed at the isolation of the factor(s) other than insulin that
are responsible for the insulinlike activities of serum. Although initially a number of peptides were isolated solely on the basis of their
insulinlike bioactivity, it soon became evident that the long sought
after growth hormone-dependent serum "sulfation factors" (or somatomedins) were, in fact, representative of a family of peptides with
insulinlike properties (1,3). Although all of the growth hormone-
dependent polypeptides (or somatomedins) so far examined appear
to have insulinlike properties, in terms of their ability to produce
insulinlike pleiotropic responses in a variety of cell types and to act
as mitogens for multiple tissues (3), it is now evident that at least
some of the insulinlike peptides may not be strictly growth hormone
dependent and may therefore not qualify as "somatomedins." The
isolation and sequence determination of two of the serum-borne peptides with nonsuppressible insulinlike activity (recently named insulinlike growth factors-I and -II or IGF-I and IGF-II) has substantially clarified the situation (2). The strikingly close structural relationship between insulin, proinsulin, and the IGFs provides, at a
glance (Fig. 1), a rationale for the similar biological properties of

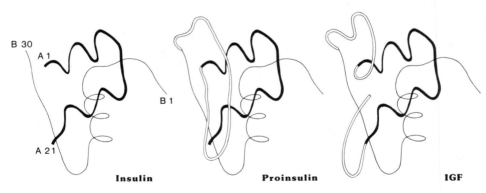

Figure 1 Schematic representations of the conformations of insulin,
proinsulin, and the IGF's. The structure of insulin was based on
X-ray crystallographic analysis; the proposed structures for proinsulin and the IGFs were based on model building (adapted from Blundell et al. quoted in Refs. 2 and 3). The positions of the N- and C-
terminal residues of the A-chain (A-1, 21) and B-chain (B1, 30) are
indicated for reference to Figure 2.

these polypeptides. It is convenient to refer to these polypeptides collectively as IGFs, reserving the term somatomedin to denote those polypeptides for which serum levels are clearly dependent on growth hormone.

B. Acronyms and Synonyms

Given the many laboratories that have been involved in the isolation of the IGFs and given the two initially independent perspectives (growth hormone dependence, on the one hand, and NSILA properties, on the other) that have influenced the isolation efforts, it is perhaps not surprising that the literature is replete with a variety of confusing acronyms that have been used to identify peptides with insulinlike growth-promoting inactivities (Table 1). In brief, it would appear that all of the IGFs so far characterized may fall into two main groups, based on their isoelectric points. The basic group (pIs greater than 7.4; Group 1, Table 1) includes the basic soluble (i.e.,

Table 1 Acronyms and Synonyms for Insulinlike Polypeptides[a]

Group	Polypeptide	Abbreviation
1	Nonsuppressible insulinlike activity-s I	NSILA-s I
	Insulinlike growth factor-I	IGF-I
	Basic somatomedin	basic-SM or B-SM
	Somatomedin C	
2	Nonsuppressible insulinlike activity-s II	NSILA-s II
	Insulinlike growth factor-II	IGF-II
	Somatomedin A	SM-A
	Insulinlike activity-s	ILA-s
	Multiplication stimulating activity	MSA
3	Nonsuppressible insulinlike activity-p	NSILA-p
4	Immunoreactive basic somatomedinlike activity	IRSM

[a]The origins of the terms and their abbreviations are discussed in the text.

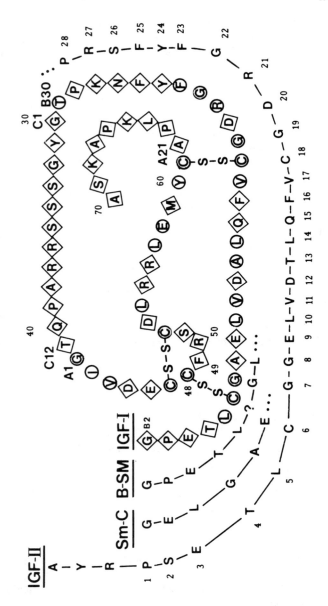

not precipitated by acid-ethanol) nonsuppressible insulinlike activity I (NSILA-s I), that has now been renamed insulinlike growth factor-I (IGF-I), somatomedin-C (SM-C), and basic somatomedin (basic-SM). The acidic-neutral group of peptides (pIs less than 7.4; Group 2, Table 1) includes the acidic soluble nonsuppressible insulinlike activity-II (NSILA-s II), that has now been renamed insulinlike growth factor-II (IGF-II), soluble (i.e., not precipitated by acid-ethanol), acidic insulinlike activity (ILA-s), somatomedin A (SM-A), and the multiplication-stimulating (in cultured cell systems) activities (MSAs) that have been isolated from cultures of buffalo rat liver cells and from calf serum. Except for the MSAs, all of the insulinlike polypeptides characterized to date have come from human serum. The above two groups of insulinlike peptides include those polypeptides with molecular weights close to that of insulin (i.e., in the range 6000 to 9000), but do not include very interesting, but less well-characterized insulinlike substances of higher molecular weight that are either produced by cultured cells (immunoreactive basic somatomedinlike activity, or basic IRSM; Group 4, Table 1) or are precipitated by the acid-ethanol procedure used for the preparation of nonsuppressible insulinlike activity (so-called, NSILA-p; Group 3, Table 1). It may be of considerable significance that only those peptides that are in the basic group appear to be closely associated with the effects of growth hormone and with the development of normal height in humans.

From the sequence data available to date, it is clear that IGF-I and basic-SM have very similar, if not identical, N-terminal sequences, which differ from the N-terminal sequence of IGF-II (Fig. 2). The

---

Figure 2 Comparison of the sequences of proinsulin, IGF-I, basic-SM, SM-C, and IGF-II. The amino acid sequence determined for IGF-I is compared with the sequence for IGF-II and for the published sequences for basic-SM and somatomedin C. The numbering in arabic numerals refers to the sequence of IGF-I, beginning at the N-terminus of the molecule. The analogy of the IGF-I structure with that of human proinsulin is indicated by circles, which indicate those residues that are identical in IGF-I and human proinsulin. The diamond symbols indicate those residues that differ. The portions of the IGF-I molecule corresponding to the A-chain (A1-A21), and to the B-chain (B2-B30) of insulin are shown, as is the IGF-I region corresponding to the connecting peptide (C1-C12) or proinsulin. The sequence can be compared with the conformations illustrated in Figure 1. The abbreviations used for the amino acid residues are as follows: A, alanine; C, half-cysine; D, aspartic acid; E, glutamic acid; F, phenylalanine; G, glycine; H, histidine; I, isoleucine; K, lysine; L, leucine; M, methionine; N, asparagine; P, proline; Q, glutamine; R, arginine; S, serine; T, threonine; V, valine; Y, tyrosine.

preliminary sequence data published for somatomedin C suggest that
the N-terminal sequence may differ from that of IGF-I and basic-SM,
although it is evident that other regions of the SM-C molecule must
be highly homologous with the sequence for IGF-I (3). It is thus as
yet uncertain whether the several peptides within the two main groups
represent different, but closely related peptides, or whether each
"group" will "boil down" to two structures represented by IGF-I and
IGF-II, when the complete sequences are known for all of the various
peptides. Insulinlike growth factors I and II may prove to be representative of two major polypeptides present in a variety of species.
The isolation of a number of insulinlike polypeptides (including insulin
itself) can now be placed in the context of other cell regulatory systems
(e.g., the neurohypophyseal hormones and the interferon system),
wherein closely related polypeptides with overlapping biological activities can be seen to regulate a variety of cell types with distinct
receptor systems.

II. MULTIPLE LIGANDS FOR MULTIPLE RECEPTORS: AN EVALUATION OF RECEPTOR CROSS-SPECIFICITY

A. Receptor Crossover in Biological Systems

Fundamental to an understanding of the multiple actions of the various insulinlike polypeptides in a variety of cell systems is a grasp of
the receptor concept that has developed since the turn of the century.
For insulin, as well as for other peptide hormones, the receptor, as
dealt with in depth elsewhere (5-7), represents the key cell membrane
constituent that has the dual job of (a) recognizing a ligand with high
affinity and specificity and (b) activating a process that ultimately
leads to a cell response. From what has been learned about membrane
receptors over the past decade, it is not unlikely that the recognition
function and activation function of the receptor complex may reside in
distinct receptor domains. Furthermore, it is clear that it is the receptor and not the ligand per se that embodies the information for the
specific cell activation process that ensues upon ligand binding. Thus,
a given receptor, once activated, will stimulate a specific and characteristic cell response that does not depend at all on the nature of the
activating substance. Receptor activation may or may not involve that
receptor's specific ligand (e.g., the insulin receptor can be activated
by plant lectins, anti receptor antibodies, or polymeric insulin derivatives, as well as by insulin itself). This situation can lead to diffi-
culties in data interpretation in situations in which an insulinlike polypeptide causes an insulinlike response (e.g., stimulation of glucose
oxidation) in a particular test system (e.g., the adipocyte). The question that immediately arises is, does the response result form the activation of the insulin receptor or is the response due to the activation

of a distinct receptor system intended for the insulinlike polypeptide itself and not for insulin?

It is the rule, rather than the exception, that biological systems employ multiple receptor systems, responding to multiple, often closely related, if not identical, ligands to regulate cell responsiveness. A classic example of this situation can be seen in the action of acetylcholine, which regulates the contractility of muscle via two totally different receptor systems: the nicotinic receptor for striated muscle and the muscarinic receptor for smooth muscle. For catecholamines, the situation is even more complex; two receptor systems (α and β) responding to catecholamines (either epinephrine or norepinephrine) may coexist within the same cell type (e.g., adipocyte). Even among the two major calsses of receptors for catecholamines (α and β), it is now well recognized that there are a number of receptor subtypes (α-1, α-2, etc. and β-1, β-2, etc.). Similar receptor heterogeneity has been documented for cell regulators, such as histamine, dopamine, adenosine, and serotonin. There is no reason to suspect that a similar situation may not be found for polypeptide receptors. These cases illustrate examples whereby a single ligand can be recognized by multiple distinct receptors. To date, there is not yet evidence for or against the existence of distinct classes of receptors for insulin (e.g., insulin-1, insulin-2) in different tissues.

A useful illustrative example that may more closely parallel the response system for the insulinlike peptides can be seen in the family of neurohypophyseal hormones, represented by oxytocin and vasopressin (also called antidiuretic hormone or ADH). Each of these polypeptides acts via its "own" receptor to cause a specific bioresponse (e.g., smooth muscle contraction in uterine tissue via the oxtocin receptor or increased water permeability in the kidney via the vasopressin receptor). Nonetheless, since the amino acid sequences of oxytocin and vasopressin are so similar (variations are found only at positions 3 and 8 of the sequences), each peptide, at sufficiently high concentrations, can occupy the other's receptor. Thus, oxytocin, at comparatively high concentrations, can cause an antidiuretic response; and vasopressin, in turn, can cause contraction of smooth muscle preparations (e.g., uterus) acting via the oxytocin receptor. What distinguishes the receptor systems in the bioassay systems is the concentration-effect relationship (or dose-response curve) whereby in a vasopressin receptor response system (e.g., antidiuresis), the concentration of vasopressin required for a half-maximal effect (so-called effective dose 50 or ED_{50}) is about tenfold lower than the ED_{50} for oxytocin in the same test system. Exactly the reverse order of potency for oxytocin and vasopressin is observed in oxytocin receptor systems (e.g., uterine contractility). The oxytocin-vasopressin systems are illustrative of the situation where a single receptor can be activated by multiple ligands. By analogy with the oxytocin-vasopressin systems, with the insulinlike polypeptides, one could envision the situation whereby insulin, at sufficiently high concentrations, might activate the IGF-I receptor and vice versa (see below, and Fig. 3). A major area of uncertainty in terms of insulin and the insulinlike polypeptides relates to the lack of a clear-cut distinction of a characteristic bioresponse that can be assigned to each of the several polypeptides that have been described. In this context, it can be pointed out that oxytocin itself, acting via its own receptor in adipocytes, causes an insulinlike response that in many ways mimics exactly the action of insulin (see below, and Ref. 8). Fortunately, the receptor system for oxytocin is sufficiently distinct from those for insulin and the insulinlike polypeptides, so that oxytocin need not be added to the list of insulinlike polypeptides considered in depth in this chapter.

B. Insulinlike Peptides and Receptor Crossover

In terms of the above discussion, insulin and the insulinlike polypeptides can be viewed as homologous polypeptides that can interact with distinct, but related receptor systems. These receptors have been

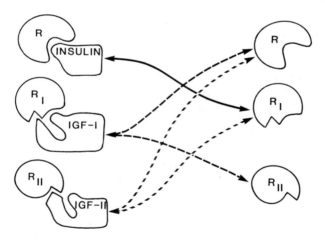

Figure 3 Schematic representation of the crossover in receptor specificity for insulin and the IGFs. The shapes of the ligand-binding regions of the receptors for insulin (R), IGF-I (R_I), and IGF-II (R_{II}) are shown to be complementary to the binding regions of their respective ligands. Neither the ligands nor the receptors are drawn to scale. The ability of each of the three ligands to interact at the receptors for the other two ligands is indicated by the arrows. Insulin is depicted as being unable to bind to the IGF-II receptor.

called isoreceptors, by analogy with the term isoenzymes. The potential crossover of one insulinlike polypeptide with the other receptor systems is illustrated in Figure 3. The different bioresponse profiles of the insulinlike polypeptides in a number of cell systems and the various ligand-binding studies using radioligand probes can now be rationalized partly in terms of the structural relationships illustrated in Figure 1. The broad outline of the receptor specificities for the various insulinlike peptides in a variety of tissues is beginning to emerge.

1. Heterogeneity of Receptors in Different Cell Types

In a tissue such as the human placenta, it appears that there are distinct receptors for insulin, IGF-I (including basic-SM and SM-C), and IGF-II (including SM-A and MSA). The exact cellular localization of these receptors within this tissue has yet to be determined, since the ligand-binding studies employed to document the presence of these receptors have been done primarily with crude membrane preparations. In other human tissues that have been examined, the three receptor types have been found in varying amounts. In some cells, such as skin fibroblasts, receptors for IGF-II appear to predominate, whereas in other cells (e.g., lymphocytes) receptors for insulin and IGF-I appear to be present in amounts greater than those for IGF-II. In rat adipocytes, receptors for insulin and for IGF-II are present, whereas the receptor for IGF-I (basic-SM or SM-C) appears to be absent. The multiplicity of receptors in any particular cell preparation and the multiple radioligand probes that have been used in various studies add complexity to the interpretation of both bioassay and ligand-binding data. To simplify matters, it now appears that one may talk at least in terms of three receptors: one for insulin, one for IGF-I, and one for IGF-II. In any cell type, any combination of these three receptors may be present. For the remainder of this chapter, the discussion will focus on these three receptors.

2. Differential Ligand Affinities of the Three Receptors

The insulin receptor, in addition to binding insulin with a high affinity, also appears to be capable of binding both IGF-I and IGF-II (and presumably, all of the other IGFs). The affinities of the IGFs for the insulin receptor are all one to two orders of magnitude lower than the affinity of insulin for its own receptor. The IGF-I receptor binds IGF-I with the highest affinity, but also exhibits a lower affinity interaction with both IGF-II and insulin. Of the three receptors, the IGF-II receptor seems to display the most selectivity in that it does not appear to bind insulin at all, but does, nonetheless, bind IGF-I, although with a lower affinity than for IGF-II. Since insulin itself lacks the sequence equivalent to the analogous C-peptide loop present

Table 2 Affinity Profiles for Receptors[a]

Receptor	Relative affinity of ligands for receptor
Insulin	insulin >> IGF-II > IGF-I
IGF-I	IGF-I ≥ IGF-II >> insulin
IGF-II	IGF-II > IGF-I >>>> insulin

[a]The affinities of the ligands, based on a composite of binding and bioresponse data reported in the literature (20,21) are listed in order of decreasing receptor affinities.

in proinsulin and in the IGFs (Fig. 1), one may suspect that the absence of this loop in the insulin molecule may explain the inability of insulin to bind to the IGF-II receptor. Thus, one may speculate that the equivalent of the C-peptide loop present in the IGFs may play an important role in the binding of the IGFs to their receptors; the remaining sequence homologies between the IGFs and insulin would enable the IGFs to bind to the insulin receptor. The lower affinity of the IGFs for the insulin receptor may be rationalized further by the potential hindrance of the important receptor-binding region of the insulin molecule (see Chapter 3) that would be caused by the equivalent of the C-peptide loop present in the IGFs (see Fig. 1). In summary, the relative potency series of the three receptors appears to be as follows: For the insulin receptor (e.g., in rat adipocytes), insulin >> IGF-II > IGF-I; for the IGF-I receptor (e.g., in chick embryo fibroblasts), IGF-I ≥ IGF-II >> insulin, and for the IGF-II receptor (e.g., in rat adipocytes) IGF-II > IGF-I >>> insulin. It should be pointed out that, in many of the test systems, the binding affinity of MSA only broadly parallels that of IGF-II; this result may be due to the species difference between these two peptides. The affinity profiles of the three receptors are summarized in Table 2.

III. RECEPTOR STRUCTURES

A. Methodologies

As indicated by the information in Chapter 4, dealing with the isolation of the insulin receptor, a wide variety of methodologies are now available to evaluate many apsects of receptor structure and function (primarily methods summarized in Ref. 9 for ligand-binding properties). Two principal approaches have yielded the most information about the hydrodynamic properties of the soluble receptor and about receptor subunit composition: (a) Gel filtration on columns of Sepharose 6B, in which the receptor is detected either by a polyethylene glycol pre-cipitation procedure (9) or by labeling the receptor either covalently or noncovalently with radiolabeled insulin and (b) gel electrophoresis followed by autoradiography, in which the receptor is first radio-labeled either directly after purification (see Chapter 4) or via affinity labeling methods (both photolabeling and chemical cross-link-labeling methods have been used) in which ^{125}I-labeled peptide (insulin, or IGFs) is coupled specifically to the receptor protein in crude particu-late (cell or membrane) or soluble receptor preparations. In general, there has been remarkably good agreement between the results ob-tained by the photoaffinity and chemical cross-linking approached.

B. Hydrodynamic Properties and General Characteristics of the Receptors

The gel filtration and electrophoretic methods yield data that are com-plementary and provide slightly different perspectives with respect to receptor structure. To date, the most extensive work has been done with the receptors for insulin and for IGF-I (basic-SM, SM-C). Since these two receptors turn out to be very similar, the following discussion will deal with them first, before turning to the IGF-II re-ceptor. In work by us and by others, two hydrodynamic forms (de-noted R_I and R_{II}) of the insulin receptor have been observed both in placenta tissue (Fig. 4 and Ref. 10) and in other tissues (see Hollen-berg et al. in Ref. 11). The two receptor forms observed by gel fil-tration have also been detected by ultracentrifugation methods (Baron et al. in Ref. 11). Surprisingly, the R_{II} form of the receptor is ob-tained when the receptor is isolated using insulin-Sepharose affinity columns, whereas the R_I form of the receptor is yielded by isolation procedures that do not expose the receptor to insulin. Insulin ex-posure appears to convert the receptor from the R_I to the R_{II} form (Ref. 10 and Hollenberg et al. in Ref. 11). The following reaction is thus suggested:

$$INS + R_I \rightleftharpoons INS \cdot R_I \rightleftharpoons INS + R_{II}$$

where INS is insulin and the two receptor forms are designated as R_I and R_{II}.

The two hydrodynamic forms of the insulin receptor have been detected in detergent extracts of a variety of tissue samples, includ-ing liver, fat cells, and cultured fibroblasts. In contrast, the re-ceptor for basic-SM (or IGF-I) obtained from human placenta mem-branes exhibits only one hydrodynamic form on the columns of Se-pharose 6B (Fig. 5) that is equivalent to the R_I form of the insulin

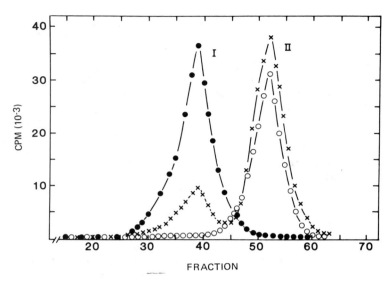

FRACTION

Figure 4 Chromatography of insulin receptor on Sepharose 6B. Comparative analysis of receptor isolated by methods I and II and effect of insulin on R_I form of the receptor. Soluble insulin receptor isolated either without (Method I, ●–●) or with exposure of the receptor to insulin (insulin-Sepharose: Method II, –○–○–) was chromatographed on a column of Sepharose 6B. Receptor material isolated by method 1 that eluted in fraction 39 ($K_{AV} = 0.31$) was subsequently equilibrated with 25 ng/ml of ^{125}I-labeled insulin either in the presence or absence of 50 µg/ml unlabeled insulin. Both samples were rechromatographed, and the radioactivity in effluent fractions was measured. A different plot (–×–×–) is recorded, representing the difference in radioactivity [counts per minute (CPM)] in aliquots from identical fractions from samples preequilibrated either without or with unlabeled insulin prior to chromatography. ●–●, insulin binding (CPM) by receptor prepared without exposure to insulin (method I); –○–○–, binding ($10^{-3} \times$ CPM) by receptor prepared by method II, in which the receptor was exposed to insulin-Sepharose; –×–×–, radioactivity difference plot (CPM) for receptor prepared by method I (fraction 39) that was incubated with 25 ng/ml of [^{125}I] insulin prior to rechromatography. (Data from Ref. 10.)

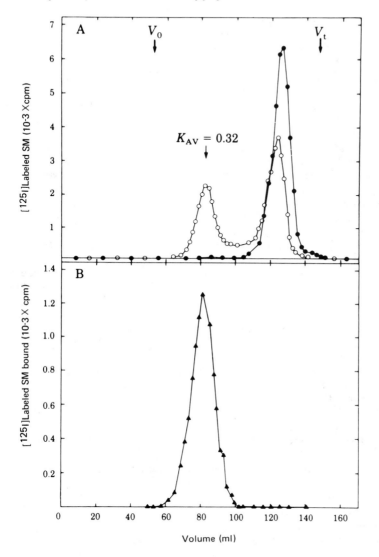

Figure 5 Chromatography on Sepharose 6B of solubilized basic-SM receptor. Aliquots (0.2 ml) of the Triton X-100-soluble extract from placental plasma membranes were subjected to chromatography on a column of Sepharose 6B. (A) Two identical samples were analyzed subsequent to equilibration with ^{125}I-labeled basic-SM either in the absence (●) or presence (○) of unlabeled basic-SM. (B) A second aliquot was chromatographed first, and the specific binding of ^{125}I-labeled basic-SM in the effluent fractions was subsequently measured. (Data from Hollenberg et al. in Ref. 11.)

receptor. To date, we have yet to observe a conversion of the basic-SM receptor from an R_I to an R_{II} hydrodynamic form. On the other hand, the receptor for IGF-II (MSA) appears to exist in two hydrodynamic forms (see below and Ref. 12).

For the insulin receptor, there is now appreciable evidence that the R_I form, present in crude, soluble membrane preparations, may be associated with other non-insulin-binding glycoprotein species that may regulate the receptor-insulin binding affinity. The receptor model proposed by Yip and colleagues (see Chapter 3) takes into account the presence of at least two interesting glycoprotein species that are accessible to insulin receptor photoprobes, but which may not be covalently linked to the receptor-binding subunits. Work by us (summarized by Hollenberg et al. in Ref. 11) and by Harmon and colleagues who used radiation inactivation methodology (Harmon et al. in Ref. 11) has provided indirect evidence for the presence of an insulin receptor affinity regulator that like the receptor may be a glycoprotein. So far, no such affinity regulator has yet been documented for the IFG-I receptor.

Based on the hydrodynamic data, and on work with lectin-agarose affinity columns, both the insulin and the basic-SM (or IGF-I) receptors in detergent solutions behave as slightly assymetric glycoproteins with an apparent Stokes' radius of about 7-8 nm and molecular weights of about 400,000. When the amount of bound detergent is taken into account (see, for example, Pollet et al. in Ref. 11), a molecular weight of about 300,000 can be calculated for the insulin receptor. This value is in reasonable accord with the molecular weights estimated by gel electrophoretic analysis of cross-link-labeled insulin receptor (see below and Chapter 4). There is no reason to believe that the basic-SM (or IGF-I) receptor should differ appreciably from the insulin receptor in terms of detergent binding, and, therefore, the detergent-free basic-SM/IGF-I receptor probably also exhibits a molecular weight of about 300,000 in solution.

The hydrodynamic properties of the IGF-II/MSA receptor, alluded to above, have been best studied in preparations of rat placenta membranes (12). Strikingly, this receptor, like the receptor for insulin, appears to exhibit two hydrodynamic forms, one of which ("Peak 1" receptor) corresponds exactly to the size (apparent Stokes' radius of 7.2 nm) of the major insulin receptor component and of the basic-SM receptor (see Figs. 4 and 5). Also, like the R_{II} form of the insulin receptor, the second form of the IGF-II receptor (apparent Stokes' radius of this "peak 2" receptor is about 4.3 nm) exhibits a somewhat lower affinity for its ligand (K_D = 2.6 nM) than does the "peak 1" receptor species (K_D = 0.5 nM). The molecular weight of the major IGF-II receptor species ("peak 1" receptor) was estimated to be about 290,000 (12). Thus, in many respects, the hydrodynamic properties of the IGF-II receptor (Table 3) appear to parallel closely the properties of the receptors for insulin and basic-SM (or IGF-I).

Table 3 Receptor Properties

Receptor	Molecular weight[a]	Stokes' radius[b] (nm)	Subunit composition	Molecular weight[d]
Insulin	300	R_I form: 7.2 R_{II} form: 3.8	Heterodimer $(\alpha\beta)_2$	α: 125,000-140,000 β: 90,000
Basic-SM, IGF-I, SM-C	300	7.2	Heterodimer $(\alpha\beta)_2$	α': 125,000-140,000 β': 90,000
IGF-II	220-270	N.R.[c]	Single chain	α'': 220,000-270,000
MSA	290	Form 1: 7.2 Form 2: 4.3	?Heterodimer	α'': 220,000-250,000 $?\beta''$: 70,000

[a]Estimate (in kilodaltons) for solubilized, detergent-free receptor based on hydrodynamic measurements for insulin basic-SM (IGF-I), and MSA receptors and on gel electrophoretic measurements (cross-link-labeled receptor) for the IGF-II receptor.

[b]Based on gel filtration estimates in detergent-containing solutions.

[c]N.R., not reported.

[d]Based on gel electrophoretic measurements of cross-link-labeled receptor subunits.

C. Subunit Compositions

Given the cross-specificities of the ligand recognition properties of the receptors for insulin and for the insulinlike polypeptides and given the similarities in the hydrodynamic properties of these receptors, attention has now begun to focus on the detailed compositions of the proteins that make up these receptors. As outlined in Chapters 3 and 4, there appears to be good general agreement that the receptor contains disulfide-linked subunits having molecular weights of about 130,000 (α subunit). In the receptor model proposed by Yip and colleagues (Chap. 3), the α and β subunits are associated with several other membrane proteins (the 40,000 and 85,000 M.W. components) to form the intact receptor oligomer. A more widely accepted model of the receptor (Ref. 15 and Chap. 4) proposes that the α and β subunits are not linked covalently to other membrane proteins, but are linked to each other in a heterodimeric α-β-β-α structure. In either of the two models, the disulfide-linked (α–β) structure would appear to represent the insulin-binding species. It is of considerable interest that the phosphorylation of both the insulin and IGF-I receptor β subunits can be augmented in the presence of their respective ligands and that the receptor may possibly participate in kinase reactions analogous to those described for a variety of receptors, including the epidermal growth factor-urogastrone receptor (for a brief introduction of this topic, see Refs. 13 and 14).

Remarkably, the IGF-I (basic-SM, SM-C) receptor, like the insulin receptor, contains two disulfide-linked subunits having molecular weights of about 130,000 and 90,000. As for the insulin receptor, these species are referred to as the α (130,000) and β (90,000) subunits of the receptor. To date, the data obtained for the IGF-I receptor are most consistent with the heterodimeric (α-β-β-α) insulin receptor model, as illustrated in Figure 6 and summarized in Reference 15. The β subunits of both the insulin receptor and the IGF-I receptor appear to be particularly susceptible to endogenous proteolysis (arrow, Fig. 6). Furthermore, in parallel with observations with the insulin receptor, it is now known that the β subunit of the IGF-I receptor is also a site for ligand-regulated phosphorylation (14).

Despite the overall similarities between the receptors for insulin and IGF-I, it is clear that interesting differences will probably be found in the primary sequences of the α and β subunits of the two receptors. Work with both basic-SM and SM-C radiolabeled probes has revealed that the cross-link-labeled IGF-I receptor differs in its proteolytic mapping profile from the profile obtained for the insulin receptor (Fig. 7 and Ref. 16). A challenge for the future is to determine both the common and distinct receptor domains that are present in the IGF-I and insulin receptors and to look for similar proteolytic domains in the receptor for IGF-II.

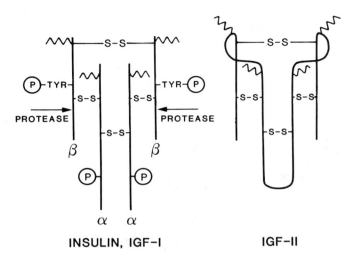

INSULIN, IGF-I   **IGF-II**

Figure 6 Schematic representation of the structures of receptors for insulin, IGF-I (basic-SM, SM-C), and IGF-II. The models represent the known features of the receptors, as discussed in the text. All of the receptors are thought to be glycoproteins, with the oligosaccharide moieties (zigzag lines) exposed at the outer aspect of the plasma membrane. The kinase site on the insulin receptor (and possibly the IGF-I receptor) is thought to reside in the β subunit, where tyrosine can accept a phosphate residue from ATP. The α subunit of the insulin receptor also appears capable of being phosphorylated (amino acid residues unknown) in the presence of ATP and insulin. All receptor structures are stabilized by disulfide bonds. Cleavage of the insulin receptor disulfides, which have differential reactivity toward reducing agents, yields the subunit species observed upon analytical gel electrophoresis.

In contrast with the receptors for insulin and IGF-I, the IGF-II receptor appears to be a single-chain macromolecule (220,000 to 270,000 M.W.) that, upon treatment with reducing agents, behaves as a slightly larger species in polyacrylamide gels. Since the hydrodynamic properties of this receptor (peak 1 form) so closely approximate those of the R_I forms of the insulin and IGF-I receptors, it is not unlikely that the single-chain IGF-II receptor may be stabilized by disulfide bonds in a conformation similar to that of the IGF-I receptor; this possible homology, in keeping with the insulinlike activity by the IGF-II receptor in adipocytes, is illustrated in Figure 6. The molecular properties of the receptors for insulin, IGF-I (basic-SM, SM-C), and IGF-II/MSA are summarized in Table 3. Unlike the

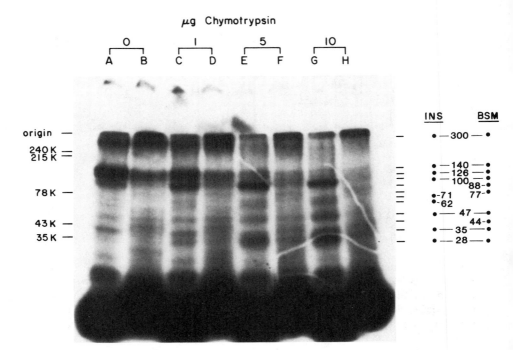

Figure 7 Electrophoretic analysis of disuccinimidyl suberate (DDS) affinity-labeled insulin and basic-SM receptors after proteolytic digestion with chymotrypsin. In lanes A, C, E, and G: insulin receptor specifically cross-link labeled with DSS in the presence of excess unlabeled basic somatomedin. In lanes B, D, F, and H: basic somatomedin receptor specifically cross-link labeled in the presence of excess unlabeled insulin. The proteolytic receptor fragments (chymotrypsin) were analyzed by gradient slab gel electrophoresis to yield the "receptor maps" referred to in the text. The mobilities of molecular weight markers are shown on the left. Mobilities of the chymotryptic fragments from [125I] insulin-labeled receptor and from basic SM-labeled receptor are indicated on the right. In order of decreasing apparent molecular weight, the constituents labeled with 125I-labeled basic-SM had apparent molecular weights of 300,000, 140,000, 126,000, 100,000, 88,000, 77,000, 47,000, 38,000, and 28,000. (Data from Ref. 16.)

insulin and IGF-I receptors, the IGF-II receptor does not exhibit intrinsic tyrosine kinase activity.

D. Receptor Sequence

As pointed out in Chap. 4, the complete sequences of the α- and β-
chains of the human insulin receptor are now known (14a). The clear
homology between the cytoplasmic portion of the β-subunit and the
oncogene family of tyrosine kinases virtually identifies this domain of
the insulin receptor as the site responsible for the tyrosine kinase
activity of the receptor. Undoubtedly, a high degree of homology in
this receptor region will be found between the insulin and IGF-I receptors. Even though the IGF-II receptor appears to be quite distinct from the other two receptors, the close homology between IGF-II
and the other IGFs and the crossover in receptor specificities points
to at least some sequence homology which should become apparent
when the IGF-II receptor sequence is solved.

IV. RECEPTORS AND MEDIATORS: ARE THERE COMMON PATHWAYS OF CELL ACTIVATION FOR INSULIN AND THE INSULINLIKE PEPTIDES?

A. Do Common Receptor Domains Imply Common Cell Activation Pathways?

In view of the homologies of receptor structure described above, a
reasonable question to ask is: Do the three receptors activate similar
processes within the plasma membrane subsequent to ligand binding?
Minimally, one would expect that subsequent to receptor occupation
all three receptors might follow a sequence of events (e.g., microclustering, patching, internalization, and lysosomal degradation)
that is very similar to the one that has been observed for a variety
of membrane receptors and acceptors (see Chap. 6; for brief reviews,
see Refs. 7 and 17).

The similarities between the insulin and IGF-I receptors in terms
of subunit composition, proteolytic domains, and tyrosine kinase activity suggest that the reactions in which the two receptors participate probably go beyond the "general" receptor/acceptor processes
in which many other receptors (including the one for IGF-II) participate. Thus, it would not be surprising if the same multiple mediators
released by insulin, upon binding to the insulin receptor (depicted
in Fig. 8 and discussed in Chap. 9) were also released by IGF-I upon
binding to the IGF-I receptor. The insulinlike actions of the IGFs are
documented (Refs. 2,3, and 18) and summarized (Table 4). As a
corollary, one might also suspect that any hormone that causes an
insulinlike response (e.g., stimulation of glucose oxidation in

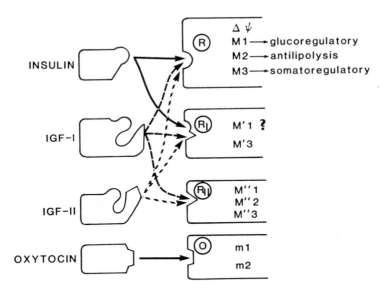

Figure 8 Receptors and mediators. The scheme illustrates the production of a variety of mediators (M, m) via the activation of receptors for insulin (R), IGF-I (basic-SM or SM-C; R_I), IGF-II (R_{II}) and oxytocin (O). The possibility of generation of mediators from activation via ligand cross-specificity is also depicted (arrows). $\Delta \psi$ denotes a change in membrane potential.

adipocytes) might do so by liberating one or more of the same or homologous mediators (as shown for oxytocin, in Fig. 8). The essence of this discussion is that both at the level of the receptor and at the level of postreceptor events regulating metabolic pathways via chemical mediators, there may be biochemical reactions in common for insulin, the IGFs, and possibly for other agents causing "insulinlike" responses in target cells. In terms of the receptors for insulin and IGF-I, it is quite likely that the intrinsic tyrosine kinase (transferring a phosphate from ATP to the receptor β subunits and possibly to other substrates) activity of the receptors will be shown to play a role in receptor function. In contrast, the IGF-II receptor does not display tyrosine kinase activity. Thus, functionally, the IGF-I and insulin receptors may prove to be mechanistically distinct from the IGF-II receptor. Nevertheless, common reactions at points beyond the initial receptor triggering process may yet be found for the actions of all three receptor systems. Potential defects in these common reactions may relate not only to the pathogenesis of diabetes, but also to other disorders involving the IGFs.

B. Insulinlike Activity of Oxytocin: Comparisons with the Actions of Insulin and the IGFs

In view of the above discussion, drawing the parallels between the receptor processes for insulin and the IGFs, it is instructive to examine similar parallels for the action of oxytocin, which via a totally independent receptor system, exhibits an insulinlike action in adipocytes (stimulation of glucose oxidation and lipogenesis as well as inhibition of lipolysis). The insulinlike actions of oxytocin, in the context of the insulinlike actions of the IGFs are summarized in Table 4. In brief, as summarized elsewhere (8), the oxytocin receptor present in rat adipocytes displays the same peptide specificity characteristics as the oxytocin receptor present in "traditional" target tissues like the uterus and mammary gland (i.e., the fat cell receptor is a "bonafide" oxytocin receptor). Since the activation of the oxytocin receptor system causes such a wide spectrum of insulinlike responses in the fat cell (except for stimulation of glucose transport, Table 4), one might, as with the IGFs, suspect the participation of cell regulators similar to the ones involved in insulin action. Several observations with oxytocin relate directly to this area of interest: (1) Oxytocin, like insulin activates the enzyme, pyruvate dehydrogenase (PDH). Thus, the same kind of phosphorylation-dephosphorylation reactions controlling PDH activity, thought to be regulated by the mediators of insulin action, are also very likely involved in the action of oxytocin. (2) In the Brattleboro strain of rat, adipocytes possess an oxytocin receptor fully capable of binding

Table 4 Insulinlike Actions of Oxytocin and Insulinlike Polypeptides

| Action of insulin | Action of | | |
	Oxytocin	IGF-I	IGF-II
Stimulates glucose transport	No	Yes	Yes
Stimulates glucose oxidation	Yes	Yes	Yes
Inhibits Lipolysis	Yes	Yes	Yes
Stimulates pyruvate de-hydrogenase	Yes	Probably	Probably
Stimulates lipogenesis	Yes	Yes	Yes
Stimulates cell growth	Not known	Yes	Yes
Alters membrane potential	Yes	Probably	Probably

oxytocin. Surprisingly, these adipocytes are totally refractory to
the glucoregulatory actions of oxytocin, whereas insulin responsiveness is unimpaired (i.e., insulin-stimulated glucose oxidation, PDH
activation, etc., are normal). Nonetheless, in these adipocytes,
oxytocin does exhibit its full insulinlike antilipolytic activity. (3) In
normal rat adipocytes, where the glucoregulatory actions of oxytocin
are intact, the binding of oxytocin to its receptor renders the adipocyte resistant to the action of insulin (i.e., the insulin dose-response
curve is shifted to the right, as in Fig. 9).

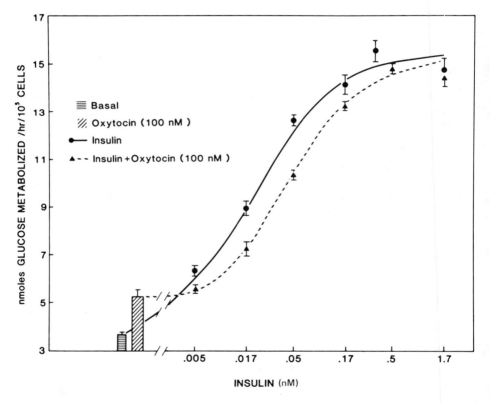

Figure 9 Effect of oxytocin (100 nM) on insulin-stimulated glucose oxidation in adipocytes. The cells were incubated with various concentrations of insulin and various concentrations of insulin plus 100 nM
oxytocin, and the conversion of [U-^{14}C]glucose to $^{14}CO_2$ was measured.
The vertical bars through the data points represent the standard error
of the mean (n = 3). (Data discussed in Ref. 8.)

From the above observations, it would appear that at some point(s) in their action (e.g., antilipolysis or in the initial states of activation of glucoregulatory enzymes) insulin and oxytocin may share common pathways. However, the resistance to the glucoregulatory action of oxytocin in the Brattleboro fat cells, which are fully responsive to insulin, indicates that certain of the oxytocin activation pathways (different glucoregulatory mediators?) must be distinct from those for insulin. Unfortunately, the specifics of the metabolic activation pathways whereby the IGFs cause their insulinlike actions has yet to be examined in any significant detail. Nonetheless, when the data become available for the action of the IGFs, it will be particularly instructive to compare the observations with the information obtained for oxytocin. By such comparisons, the similar and distinct pathways for the action of all polypeptides with insulinlike activities may become apparent. Because of the potential interrelationships between the cell activation pathways for insulin and the pathways for activation by other peptide hormones, it is evident that the disease entity diabetes, which may exhibit defects in the insulin action pathway, may also lead to defects in the activation pathways for peptides as distinct from insulin as is oxytocin. The illustration with oxytocin was elaborated upon to indicate how far-ranging, in terms of other peptide receptor systems, the defect(s) associated with diabetes might prove to be.

C. Implications of Receptor Crossover and Common Cell Activation Pathways for Diabetes

As indicated early on in this chapter, one of the major puzzles of diabetes relates to the apparent resistance of diabetic subjects to the glucoregulatory actions of insulin (so-called "insulin resistance"), whereas certain other responses to insulin (e.g., antilipolysis) are intact in tissues from diabetics. Furthermore, there is as yet little insight into the pathogenesis of the wide variety of complications associated with diabetes, such as the neuropathies, retinopathies, and nephropathies. As alluded to above, information that will be forthcoming related to the structures of the IGF receptors and to their postreceptor processes may relate directly, on the one hand, to biochemical branch points involved in insulin action and in the phenomenon of "insulin resistance" and, on the other hand, to pathological events in diabetic subjects that may involve not only insulin but also the IGFs themselves. It is of interest to speculate a little on the possible pathological interrelationships in the light of information presented in this chapter. The relevance of this speculation is heightened somewhat by the observations that in patients with leprechaunism, who are insulin resistant, there appear to be defects in the receptors for the IGF's as well as for insulin (Knight et al. in Ref. 11).

For instance, it is not unlikely that the "insulin resistance" of diabetic subjects may have its parallel of "resistance" in those tissues that are the major targets for the IGFs. Since the IGF receptor system appears to be quite widespread (receptors are present in tissues as diverse as the kidney, fat cells, skin fibroblasts, and the placenta), one might be able to rationalize some of the untoward complications of diabetes not in terms of insulin per se, but with reference to resistance to the action of the IGFs. In this context, since it is now known that elevated levels of insulin can activate the IGF-I receptor, one may also contemplate the consequence to the IGF receptor systems of elevated insulin levels that may occur in diabetic subjects (either endogenous increases or as a result of the administration of insulin). One could predict that such elevated insulin levels might either activate the IGF receptor system (for instance, this effect might lead to the inappropriate proliferation of retinal vessel cells or of renal glomerular cells) or conversely that the elevated insulin levels might desensitize the IGF receptor system either via a receptor (i.e., down regulation) or postreceptor (i.e., mediator-related) mechanism. In this regard, it may be of more than passing interest that the levels of IGF-I itself appear to be, in part, insulin dependent.

While the previous speculation considered the effect of insulin on the IGF receptor system, it is now clear that the converse is also possible. Thus, the refractory hypoglycemia sometimes associated with certain tumors can now be rationalized in terms of the production of IGF-II-like material that can activate the insulin receptor system. Alternatively, the markedly elevated IGF-I levels associated with excessive growth hormone production (pituitary gigantism) might not only activate insulin receptors acutely, but might, over the long term, desensitize the insulin receptor system in a manner similar to the desensitization caused by the exposure of cells to high insulin levels. In summary, the new information gained about the receptor systems for insulin and the IGFs provides a new context in which the pathogenic mechanisms related to diabetes and allied diseases can be reevaluated. A general scheme summarizing possible sites of interactions between insulin and the IGF's is presented in Figure 8.

V. LOOKING TO THE FUTURE

It was the initial goal of this chapter to illustrate the relationships between the receptor for insulin and the receptors for the insulinlike polypeptides. From the marked similarities that are emerging, it would appear that, in the future, the work on the IGF receptor systems will be of paramount importance to those wishing to unravel the complex problem represented by "insulin resistance" and by the disease entity, diabetes. One looks forward with excitement to the elucidation of the detailed receptor structures, and to the possible discovery of sequence homologies and dissimilarities between the various receptors. Furthermore, one awaits with great interest, the identification of the receptor mechanisms and mediator substance(s) involved in the action of the IGFs, so that these may be compared with the mechanisms and mediator(s) involved in insulin action. In addition, one may hope that as more information becomes available concerning the mechanisms of insulin-mediated enzymatic regulation, greater insight may be possible concerning the regulatory pathways involved in the growth-promoting actions of the insulin-like growth factors; the spinoffs in terms of research in cancer-related areas need not be elaborated upon. Thus, one can anticipate a reciprocal cross-fertilization of the work done in what at first appeared to be two entirely unrelated areas of interest— the one related to diabetes and the other related to disorders of growth. In brief, the future looks both promising and exciting in terms of a combined focus on the IGFs along with insulin; not only in terms of new insights into the pathogenesis of diabetes, but also in terms of molecular mechanisms that may be involved in a much wider number of pathogenic processes.

ACKNOWLEDGMENTS

Work in the author's laboratory has been supported mainly by grants from the Canadian Medical Research Council (MT6859) and from the March of Dimes Birth Defects Foundation (Basic Grant No. 1-677).

ABOUT THE REFERENCES

To minimize the number of references, this chapter, in large part, refers to review articles rather than the individual source references where the original discoveries were described. Thus, the reader is encouraged to consult the bibliographies in the review articles in order to expand on the information presented in this chapter. In particular, Refs. 1—4 review work on the chemical nature of the various insulin-like popypeptides, and the insulin-like properties of oxytocin are summarized in Ref. 8. References 6, 7, 9, and 13 deal in general terms with many aspects of peptide hormone action. Reference 11 serves as a particularly useful collection of many recent research articles dealing with the insulin receptor. Hopefully these review articles will provide a useful up-to-date key to the literature dealing with the insulin-like polypeptides.

REFERENCES

1. Philips, L. S. and Vassilopoulou-Sellin, R. (1980). Somatomedins. *New Engl. J. Med. 302*, 371—380, 438—446.

2. Froesch, E. R., Zapf, J., Rinderknecht, E., Morell, B., Schoenle, E. and Humbel, R. E. (1979). Insulinlike growth factor (IGF-NSILA): structure, function and physiology. In *Hormones and Cell Culture* (G. H. Sato and R. Ross, eds.) Cold Spring Harbor Conferences on Cell Proliferation, Cold Spring Harbor, New York., Vol. 6, pp. 61—77.

3. Clemmons, D. R. and Van Wyk, J. J. (1981). Somatomedin: Physiological control and effects on cell proliferation. In *Tissue Growth Factors: Handbook of Experimental Pharmacology* (R. Baserga, ed.), Springer Verlag, Berlin, Vol. 57, pp. 161—208.

4. Posner, B. I. and Guyda, H. J. (1981). Insulin-like growth factors: Structure and function. In *Plasma and Cellular Modulatory Proteins* (D. H. Bing and R. E. Rosenbaum, eds.) Centre for Blood Research, Boston, pp. 15—34.

5. Goodman, A. G., Gilman, L. S., Gilman, A., Mayer, S. E., and Melmon, K. L. (1980). *The Pharmacological Basis of Therapeutics*, MacMillan, New York, Chap. 2, pp. 28—39.

6. Roth, J. and Grunfeld, C. (1981). Endocrine systems: Mechanisms of disease, target cells and receptors. In *Textbook of Endocrinology*, 6th Ed. (R. H. Williams, ed.), W.B. Saunders Co., Philadelphia, Chap. 2, pp. 15—22.

7. Hollenberg, M. D. (1982). Membrane receptors and hormone action: I. New trends related to receptor structure and receptor regulation and II. New perspectives for receptor-modulated cell function. In *More about Receptors: Current Reviews in Biomedicine* (J. W. Lamble, ed.), Elsevier, Amsterdam, Vol. 2, pp. 1—13.

8. Hollenberg, M. D., Goren, H. J., Hanif, K. and Lederis, K. (1983). Oxytocin, Its receptor and its insulin-like activity: A new look at an old hormone. *Trends Pharmacol. Sci. 4*: 310—312.

9. Cuatrecasas, P. and Hollenberg, M. D. (1976). Membrane receptors and hormone action. *Advan. Protein Chem. 30*:251—451.

10. Maturo, J. M. III, Hollenberg, M. D., and Aglio, L. S. (1983). Insulin receptor: insulin-modulated interconversion between distinct molecular forms involving disulfide: sulfhydryl exchange. *Biochemistry 22*:2579—2586.

11. Andreani, D., DePirro, R., Lauro, R., Olefsky, J. M., and Roth, J. (1981). *Current Views on Insulin Receptors: Proceedings of the Serono Symposia*, Academic Press, New York, Vol. 41.

12. Perdue, J. F., Chan, J. K., Thibault, C., Radaj, P., Mills, B., and Daughaday, W. H. (1983). The biochemical characterization of the detergent solubilized neutral-acidic SM/IGF receptors from rat placenta. *J. Biol. Chem. 258*:7800—7811.

13. Hollenberg, M. D. (1982). Receptor-mediated phosphorylation reactions. *Trends Pharmacol. Sci.* 3:271–273.

14. Jacobs, S., Kull, F. C., Jr., Earp, H. S., Svoboda, M. E., van Wyk, J. J., and Cuatrecasas, P. (1983). Somatomedin C stimulates the phosphorylation of the β-subunit of its own receptor. *J. Biol. Chem.* 258:9581–9584.

14a. Ullrich, A., Bell, J. R., Chen, E. Y., Herrera, R., Petruzzelli, L. M., Dull, T. J., Gray, A., Coussens, L., Liao, Y.-C., Tsubokawa, M., Mason, A., Seeburg, P. H., Grunfeld, C., Rosen, O. M., and Ramachandran, J. (1985). *Nature* 313:756–761.

15. Czech, M. P. and Massague, J. (1982). Subunit structure and dynamics of the insulin receptor. *Fed. Proc.* 41:2719–2723.

16. Armstrong, G. D., Hollenberg, M. D., Bhaumick, B., and Bala, R. M. (1982). Comparative studies on human placental insulin and basic-somatomedin receptors. *J. Cell. Biochem.* 20:283–292.

17. O'Connor-McCourt, M. and Hollenberg, M. D. (1983). Receptors, acceptors and the action of polypeptide hormones: Illustrative studies with epidermal growth factor-urogastrone. *Can. J. Biochem. Cell Biol.* 61:670–682.

18. Zapf, J., Schoenle, E., and Froesch, E. R. (1978). Insulinlike growth factors I and II: Some biological actions and receptor binding characteristics of two purified constitutents of nonsuppressible insulin-like activity of human serum. *Eur. J. Biochem.* 87:285–296.

19. Bhaumick, B., Goren, H. J., and Bala, R. M. (1981). Further characterization of human basic somatomedin: Comparison with insulin-like growth factors I and II. *Horm. Metab. Res.* 13:515–518.

20. Rechler, M. W., Zapf, J., Nissley, S. P., Froesch, R. E., Moses, A. C., Podskalny, J. M., Schilling, E. E., and Humbel, R. E. (1980). Interactions of insulin-like growth factors I and II and multiplication stimulating activity with receptors and serum carrier proteins. *Endocrinology* 107:1451–1459.

21. King, G. L., Kahn, C. R., Rechler, M. M., and Nissley, S. P. (1980). Direct demonstration of separate receptors for growth and metabolic activities of insulin and multiplication-stimulating activity (an insulinlike growth factor) using antibodies to the insulin receptor. *J. Clin. Invest.* 66:130–140.

6

Receptor Dynamics and Insulin Action

MORLEY D. HOLLENBERG *University of Calgary Faculty of Medicine, Calgary, Alberta, Canada*

I. RECEPTOR MOBILITY

One of the more striking outcomes of the study of receptors by ligand binding and by fluorescence probe methods (techniques and approaches sumarized in Refs. 1—3) relates to the development of an understanding of the dynamic processes in which a pharmacological receptor may participate. In the not too distant past, largely due to the influence of classic pharmacological studies dealing with nerve-muscle preparations, receptors were thought of as specifically localized entities (e.g., at the neuromuscular junction) that were tacitly assumed to be in a more or less static state as a consequence of cell differentiation. Now, however, it is realized that, in perhaps the majority of cases, receptors for agents such as insulin are dynamic cell surface entities that can migrate in the plane of the cell membrane. In studies with cultured cells (e.g., mouse fibroblasts), it has been observed that subsequent to the binding of a ligand such as insulin, the receptor may undergo a complex series of protein-protein interactions that can lead to the cellular internalization and degradation of the receptor and the bound ligand (2,3 and see below). The conceptualization of a hormone receptor as a "floating" or "mobile" membrane constituent evolved along with the development of understanding of the general properties of cell surface proteins. In terms of hormone action, receptor mobility is viewed as a most important property that can enable the receptor to interact with a variety of membrane constitutents in the course of cell activation. It is a fundamental assumption of the "mobile" or "floating" receptor paradigm of hormone action (summarized in Refs. 1 and 4), that the ability of the receptor to migrate in the plane of the membrane and

to interact with other membrane constituents is dramatically altered
when the receptor is occupied by its specific ligand (e.g., insulin).
This situation is illustrated schematically in Figure 1 where the formation of the insulin-receptor complex (IR') is depicted as causing a
conformational change in the receptor, permitting the interaction of
the receptor with hypothetical "effector" molecules in the plane of
the membrane in order to form ternary complexes such as IR'E or
IR'E$_1$. In principle, it is possible that the insulin-receptor complex
may interact with multiple effectors located in the membrane. This
chapter deals with several aspects of the dynamic pathways that
have been observed for receptors such as the one for insulin. The
chapter will present a composite picture of information obtained with
a number of peptide hormone probes in order to give a general overview of the dynamic receptor events that can occur in the course of
the activation of cells by insulin. It is important to note that the
generalized picture that will be presented is derived in large part
from studies done with cultured cells (e.g., normal fibroblasts or
tumor-derived cells). As will be pointed out in the following chapter (Chap. 7), there may be cell to cell variation in terms of the
dynamic processes in which various receptors may participate (e.g.,
microclustering, localization in coated pit regions, endocytosis, recycling to the cell surface, and degradation).

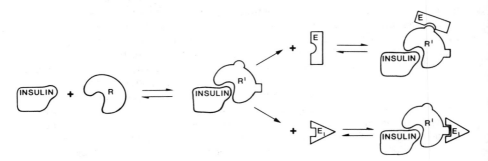

Figure 1 Interaction of mobile insulin receptors with multiple membrane effectors. In terms of the "mobile" or "floating" receptor
paradigm of hormone action (1,4), the insulin receptor, upon binding insulin, is depicted as changing its molecular conformation. The
conformation of the insulin-receptor complex is shown to be capable
of interacting in the plane of the membrane with two separate membrane effector molecules (E and E$_1$). Neither insulin nor the receptor and effector molecules are drawn to scale.

II. RECEPTOR MICROCLUSTERING AND PATCHING

Largely stimulated by the "floating" or "mobile" receptor model, recent work has turned from simple ligand-binding studies to measurements of the surface mobility of receptor-bound fluorescently labeled
hormone probes. Much of the information to be discussed below has
been obtained with derivatives [either fluorescent (5) or radio-
labeled] of insulin and of epidermal growth factor-urogastrone (EGF-
URO) in fibroblast culture systems. Epidermal growth factor-urogastrone is a polypeptide that, in humans and in other species, is
a potent inhibitor of gastric acid secretion and a stimulator of cell
division (for reviews describing EGF-URO and its receptor see
Refs. 5–8). Using very sensitive image-intensification cameras (or
fluorescence monitors) attached to a fluorescence microscope, it has
become possible to visualize receptors on the cell surface and to
estimate receptor mobility quantitatively (summarized in Refs. 2 and
3). With the fluorescence photobleaching recovery (FPR) method,
a laser beam is focused briefly on receptor-bound fluorescently
labeled ligand in order to bleach a very small cell surface area.
Subsequent to the bleaching episode, the rate of migration of neighboring fluorescent receptor-bound ligand into the previously bleached area can be measured. From the rate of recovery of fluorescence into the bleached area, a diffusion coefficient for the ligand-
receptor complex can be calculated. When the FPR method was used
in fibroblast cultures to measure the mobility of a number of receptors, including the one for insulin, lateral diffusion coefficients in
the range of $5 \times 10^{-10}/cm^2/sec$ were observed. This value, typical
of a number of membrane proteins, indicates that the insulin receptor can migrate rapidly in the lipid bilayer and that it could, in a
very short time period (e.g., tens of milliseconds), collide with many
other membrane constituents.

From observations in a number of studies with several ligands,
including insulin, it has become evident that in many cells, in the
absence of their specific ligands, receptors can be diffusely distributed over the cell surface. However, as depicted in Figure 2,
at physiological temperatures, the binding of ligand can lead to a
rapid (within about 10 min) reduction in receptor mobility, accompanied by the progressive aggregation of ligand-receptor complexes
into immobile patches that can be visualized on the cell surface using the videofluorescence monitoring technique (VIM) (Refs. 2, 3,
and 5 and Fig. 2). In cultured fibroblasts, it is believed that a
microclustering event takes place prior to the aggregation of receptors into the visible patches that can be seen by the VIM techniques
(In terms of the processes that lead to cell activation, to be discussed below, the microclustering event is viewed as a phenomenon
related to but separate from the aggregation process, whereby

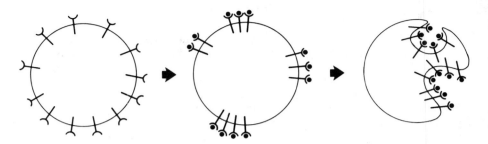

Figure 2 Microclustering and patching of receptors: early events related to cell activation. The scheme illustrates the ligand-mediated microclustering and patch formation processes described in the text. Upon going from the predominantly diffuse distribution (hormone-free state) to the ligand-occupied microclustered state, it is thought that in many cells, such as fibroblasts, ligand-receptor complexes coalesce in coated pit regions prior to cellular internalization. It is important to note that in some cell types receptors may exist in a preclustered state and that in certain cells, receptor internalization can occur predominantly at sites distinct from the coated pit region (see Chap. 7).

comparatively large receptor aggregates form in order to be visualized by the VIM technique.) Subsequent to the formation of comparatively large receptor aggregates, or patches, the complexes can be either shed into the medium or taken into the cell (internalized). Receptor internalization appears to be an ongoing process that is accelerated when a ligand such as insulin binds to its receptor. It is not clear whether or not receptor occupation is a prerequisite for receptor microclustering in all cell types. For instance, in adipocytes (see Chap. 7), there are data to indicate that the insulin receptors exist as clusters prior to the addition of insulin. Furthermore, the receptors for epidermal growth factor-urogastrone in certain cultured cells appear to be present as microclusters in the absence of the ligand. The mechanism(s) that leads to the microclustering, aggregation, and internalization of receptors is poorly understood. In many cells, such as fibroblasts, receptor internalization appears to occur at specific sites on the cells surface—the so-called "bristle-coated pit" (2). Subsequent to cell surface binding in fibroblasts, ligands as diverse as insulin, epidermal growth factor-urogastrone, and α_2-macroglobulin all seem to localize preferrentially at the coated pit region. However, receptor internalization in many cell types need not occur in coated pit regions. For instance, data obtained with adipocytes (see Chap. 7) indicate that the majority of receptors may be localized and internalized at sites other than the "coated pit" regions. As will be discussed below, the initial phases of insulin receptor dynamics, comprising the microclustering and initial patching of receptors, are events that occur concurrently with the process of insulin-mediated cell activation.

III. RECEPTOR INTERNALIZATION AND PROCESSING

The events that have been observed in fibroblasts, which very likely reflect processes that occur in many (but not all, see Chap. 7) cell types, can be summarized as follows: Subsequent to receptor micro-clustering and aggregation, the receptor can become internalized via an endocytotic process into a cellular compartment that appears to be distinct from the lysosome (Fig. 3). The intracellular receptor-bearing vesicles, which in contrast with lysosomes are not phase dense in the electron microscope and are acid phosphatase negative, have been termed "endosomes," "prelysosomes," or "receptosomes" (see Ref. 2). The latter term emphasizes the role of these specialized endocytotic vesicles in the process of receptor-mediated

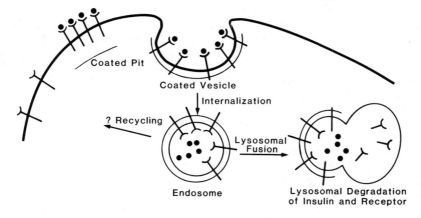

Figure 3 Formation and migration of receptor-bearing vesicles. As discussed in the text, after aggregation, receptors may become trapped in an endocytic vesicle that buds inward forming an intracellular vesicle, the endosome (or receptosome). The internalized receptor-bearing vesicles are thought to change their shape (possibly by fusing with other nonlysosomal intracellular constituents) and to migrate to a variety of cellular locations. Two further possibilities are depicted: (1) fusion with lysosomal structures and (2) recycling of the receptor to the cell surface.

endocytosis. The endosome (or receptosome) that has been observed in cultured fibroblasts and in liver cells appears, at the
electron microscopic level, as a smooth continuous membrane-lined
vesicle with an inner proteinaceous layer, tubular protrusions, and
a central region of lower density. Recent evidence indicates that the
internal environment of the endosome becomes rapidly acidified,
favoring the dissociation of many ligands such as insulin from their
receptor. The morphology and cellular location of the endosomal
structures are thought to change rapidly as the receptor-bearing
vesicles migrate inward from the cell surface. One possible fate of
such receptor-bearing endosomes is the ultimate fusion with lysosomes, followed by the lysomomal degradation of the receptor (so-
called "receptor processing") and of the bound ligand. From several
studies, it appears that a limited amount of receptor processing may
also occur at a prelysosomal site (possibly in the endosome). An
alternative route that the endosome may follow leads back to the
cell surface via a recycling process that reintegrates the receptor
into the plasma membrane. At present, little is known about the
factors that control either the internalization process or the traffick-
ing process that may lead, on the one hand, to lysosomal receptor
degradation or, on the other hand, to a recycling of the receptor
back to the cell surface (Fig. 3). Likewise, little is known about
the possible role(s) for the degradation products (degraded insulin
or insulin receptor fragments) that may be released into the cytoplasm as a result of the endosomal and lysosomal processing (degradation) events.

It would appear that the internalization of receptors for various
ligands may occur at varying rates and to varying degrees. Furthermore, a given receptor in one cell type may be internalized,
whereas in another cell type, internalization may be a minor event
subsequent to ligand binding (see Chap. 7). For instance, in the
presence of ^{125}I-labeled insulin, about 25−40% of the receptor-bound
ligand can be degraded by adipocytes (presumably either at a cell
surface or at a lysosomal site) over a 2- to 3-hr period; for epidermal growth factor-urogastrone, over twice this proportion of
bound ligand can be degraded by fibroblast cultures over a 2- to
3-hr period. The internalization of occupied receptors for insulin
and epidermal growth factor-urogastrone can occur rapidly (over a
period of tens of minutes, up to 1 hr); in contrast, the internalization of receptors for human chorionic gonadotropin appears to pro-
ceed at a much slower rate (hours to tens of hours). In fibroblast
cultures, in the absence of insulin, the unoccupied receptors can
be internalized with a half-life of about 7-13 hr (see Chaps. 7 and
12). This rate of internalization is about one-third to one-fifth the
disappearance rate of the insulin-occupied receptors. The rate of
receptor internalization does not appear to affect the rate of receptor

resynthesis and insertion into the plasma membrane (this topic is dealt with in detail in Chap. 12). Thus, the continued exposure of cells to a ligand such as insulin, causing accelerated receptor internalization, can lead to a marked diminution of the steady-state level of receptors present at the cell surface (a phenomenon that has been termed "receptor down-regulation"). The replenishment of the deficit of receptors at the cell surface may in certain cases require de novo protein synthesis, and possibly (as appears to be the case for EGF-URO receptors) the participation of factors other than insulin that are present in the bloodstream. In other instances, the internalized receptor may be recycled back to the cell surface.

The process of insulin receptor internalization (or down-regulation) that occurs in the presence of insulin may represent a homeostatic mechanism, whereby the cell can partially adjust to different ambient levels of insulin. As will be discussed below, receptor number per se can be an important factor in determining the sensitivity of cells to insulin. Although receptor down-regulation is by no means a complete explanation of the reduction in insulin sensitivity observed in the diabetic state, it has been suggested that this process may contribute significantly to the cellular desensitization process mediated by high blood levels of insulin.

IV. RECEPTOR MICROCLUSTERING AND CELL ACTIVATION

It is perhaps ironic that studies of patients highly resistant to the action of insulin have led in large part not to a complete understanding of the mechanism(s) of insulin resistance, but rather to a more in-depth picture of the cellular activation process itself. In a rare subset of insulin-resistant patients, exhibiting marked hyperinsulinemia, severe insulin resistance with hyperglycemia, and benign acanthosis nigricans (a characteristic thickening and hyperpigmentation of the skin), autoantibodies directed against the insulin receptor have been discovered (9). Such antibodies were initially detected because of their ability to block the binding of insulin to its receptor. However, when the effects of the patient-derived antibodies were evaluated in intact adipocytes, it was observed that, rather than blocking the action of insulin, the intact anti-receptor antibodies themselves exhibited intrinsic insulinlike activity (Fig. 4). Since their initial discovery, the anti-insulin receptor antibodies, obtained from insulin-resistant patients, have been observed to mimic most, if not all of the actions of insulin in target cells except for the stimulation of DNA synthesis in fibroblast cell cultures (9). It is important to note that antibodies directed against crude fat cell membranes can also cause insulinlike responses, and thus it was most important that the work with patient derived anti-receptor

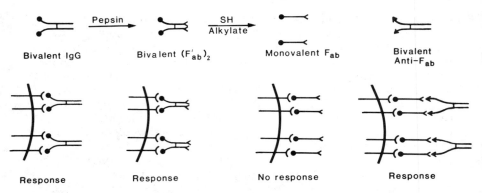

Figure 4 Effects of bivalent and monovalent anti-receptor antibodies. The scheme illustrates results obtained with bivalent and monovalent polyclonal anti-insulin receptor antibodies as outlined in the text (summarized in Ref. 9). A role for receptor microclustering in generating a cell response has been postulated on the basis of these experiments. (Adapted from Ref. 9.)

antibodies was supported by concurrent work with bivalent poly-clonal antibodies, prepared in rabbits using highly purified rat liver insulin receptor preparations (work summarized in Ref. 3). Interestingly, the polyclonal antibodies prepared using pure rat liver insulin receptor did not interfere with insulin binding. The rabbit antibodies thus appear to be directed at a receptor site dif-ferent from the site(s) at which a number of the patient-derived antibodies bind.

In brief, the results with the polyclonal anti-receptor antibodies are illustrated in Figure 4. Intact antibody (IgG) and the bivalent antibody derivative generated by pepsin cleavage (Fab)$_2$ were cap-able of stimulating cells. [Intact antibodies possess two antigen-binding sites (i.e., they are bivalent). Chemically modified anti-bodies can be prepared (Fab) that have only one antigen combining site (i.e., they are monovalent). Both bivalent and monovalent anti-body molecules are depicted in Figure 4.] Most importantly, how-ever, it was observed that the monovalent anti-receptor Fab anti-body fragment, prepared from the intact patient-derived bivalent antibody molecule, was not biologically active even though this Fab fragment could compete for the binding of insulin to the receptor. In fact, the monovalent Fab fragment proved to be an excellent com-petitive antagonist of insulin action in an intact cell system (9). Strikingly, the biological activity of the monovalent Fab fragments can be restored in the presence of a second set of bivalent anti-bodies that are directed against the Fab fragment (Fig. 4). In essence, the cross-linking of the receptor-associated Fab fragments by the second set of bivalent anti-Fab antibodies appears to be required for cell activation. Although it had been appreciated for some time that bivalency or multivalency and cell-surface clustering were critical factors in the activation of cells by antigens or by plant lectins, only recently has it become apparent that receptor cross-linking (or microclustering) may be a key event in the process of cell activation caused by hormones such as insulin (Fig. 4).

Evidence implicating receptor microclustering as a key event for cell activation has now been obtained for two other hormones in independent studies done in several laboratories. In one series of experiments, it was observed that a chemically modified derivative of epidermal growth factor-urogastrone (CNBr-EGF-URO, see below), that of itself bound to the EGF-URO receptor but was not mitogenic, became mitogenic when aggregated by anti-EGF-URO antibody (10). In other work, studying the action of luteinizing hormone releasing hormone (LHRH, also called gonadotropin-releasing hormone or GnRH), two independent laboratories (11-13) have observed that LHRH antagonists (biologically nonstimulatory derivatives that bind to the receptor and that block the LH-releasing activity of intact LHRH) can be caused to stimulate LH release by bivalent antibodies directed against the LHRH antagonists. Dimerization of the occupied LHRH receptors (the monovalent Fab antibody derivatives did not activate the antagonist) would thus appear to be a prerequisite for the stimulation of LH release from pituitary cells. The ability of ferritin derivatives of LHRH to cause the microclustering and internalization of LHRH receptors has also been observed at the electron microscopic level (13). Thus, the microclustering event, associated with cell activation, is probably involved in the activation of a variety of cells by a number of hormones, including insulin.

In the adipocyte, the exact relationship between insulin-mediated receptor microclustering and cell activation is not entirely clear. Recently, monoclonal antibodies directed against the human insulin receptor have been developed (14). (Monoclonal antibodies, prepared by specialized hybridoma cell culture methods, are homogeneous immunoglobulins directed against a unique site on an antigen such as the insulin receptor. Polyclonal antibodies, raised in animals such as the rabbit, comprise a set of heterogeneous immunoglobulins that can be directed against multiple regions of an antigen such as the insulin receptor.) Because of their nature, the monoclonal bivalent IgG antibodies are thought to react with a single receptor locus, whereas the polyclonal IgG antibody preparations previously used (derived both from insulin-resistant patients and from receptor-injected rabbits) would presumably contain IgG molecules capable of interacting at several receptor loci. In contrast

with the polyclonal antibodies, one of the monoclonal anti-insulin receptor antibody preparations that has been described (14) blocks insulin receptor binding, but does not itself possess intrinsic insulinlike activity in human adipocytes. There is no reason to suspect
that the intact bivalent monoclonal antibodies could not simultaneously
cross-link two separate insulin receptors, as is thought to happen
with the bivalent polyclonal antibodies (illustrated in Fig. 4). Further work will be required to resolve the apparent discrepancies
between the observations with the polyclonal and monoclonal antibodies, in terms of the requirement for antibody bivalency to cause
adipocyte activation. Other observations that relate to the question
of receptor microclustering and adipocyte activation will be described
in some detail in the following chapter (Chap. 7). In brief, studies
with insulin-ferritin reveal that a substantial proportion of adipocyte insulin receptors appear to be present in groups of two or
more prior to insulin binding. Furthermore, the presence of insulin-
ferritin does not lead to an increase in the degree of receptor clustering. These results can be contrasted with the effect of ferritin-
LHRH, which clearly caused the microaggregation of previously dispersed LHRH receptors in anterior pituitary cells (13). Thus, although receptor microaggregation may be a general phenomenon associated with cell activation, the exact mechanism whereby the preclustered insulin receptors in adipocytes are triggered upon occupation by either polyclonal anti-receptor antibody or by insulin (or
the insulin-ferritin derivative) remains to be determined. Taken
together, the data suggest that the receptor may not only have to
be clustered but that in addition, the receptor may also require a
special conformational perturbation (e.g., caused only by insulin or
by a subset of antireceptor antibodies) to generate the reaction that
leads to cell activation. In summary, receptor clustering may be necessary but not necessarily sufficient to initiate a response in a target cell for insulin.

Despite the reservations outlined above, concerning the precise role of insulin receptor microclustering in the process of cell
activation, work with the anti-insulin receptor antibodies has led
to the following conclusions: (a) Evidently it is the receptor and
not insulin per se that embodies the information that directs cellular responsiveness; (b) insulin receptor microclustering appears to
be an important factor in initiating a cellular response; and (c) perturbation of receptor sites other than the insulin binding region can
cause an insulinlike response. This last observation raises the possibility that it may be feasible to develop agents other than insulin
to act via the insulin receptor for therapeutic purposes.

The discovery of the insulinlike activity of the anti-insulin receptor antibodies has led to new insights concerning possible mechanisms for the pathogenesis of insulin resistance in the patients who

have receptor antibodies in their bloodstream. Why, one may ask, would these patients need insulin at all, since the cell-activating antibodies might be able to substitute for insulin in triggering the receptor? The answer to this paradox very likely lies in the stimulatory properties of the antibodies themselves. For instance, if the antibodies simply blocked the access of insulin to its receptor in a competitive manner, then raising the insulin concentration high enough should be able to overcome the antibody blockade. Nonetheless, in the patients with the anti-receptor antibodies, clinical experience has demonstrated that even extremely high levels of insulin are unable to control the blood glucose concentration. Thus, one is forced to conclude that the antibodies must act in a "noncompetitive" manner to block insulin action. This noncompetitive mechanism can very likely be attributed to the intrinsic biological activity of the antibodies, which can mimic most of the actions of insulin (9). The persistent triggering of the receptors by the anti-receptor antibodies would lead to the same kind of cellular densensitization that has been documented for the persistent triggering of the receptor by elevated (well above physiological) insulin concentrations. Thus, at the receptor level, the antibodies could induce receptor activation and down-regulation, resulting in a reduced steady-state concentration of receptors at the surface of target cells, and the persistent triggering of cells by antibody could also call into play the postreceptor mechanisms that can lead to cellular desensitization, with respect to insulin action. Since the antibodies present in the patients' serum can also cross-react with receptors for the insulinlike growth factors (IGFs) (see Chap. 5), one might also suspect that some of the pathophysiology in these patients may also stem from activation or densitization of the IGF receptor systems.

The other side of the coin, with respect to the symptomatology of anti-receptor antibody-bearing patients, relates to the inexplicable episodes of refractory hypoglycemia that have been documented in a few of these individuals. Given the new understanding of the bioactivity of the anti-receptor antibodies, one can rationalize the hypoglycemia in terms of a persistent unopposed antibody-mediated triggering of the receptor, during a period where the normal mechanisms leading to insulin resistance may have disappeared. In sum, the studies with antibodies directed against the insulin receptors have led both to new insights relating to the general process of hormone-mediated cell activation and to new perspectives in understanding the pathophysiology of the subset of diabetic patients who exhibit extreme insulin resistance and benign acanthosis nigricans.

V. INTERNALIZED RECEPTOR AND CELL ACTIVATION

It is recognized that insulin causes a wide spectrum of cellular responses, ranging in time course from the immediate (seconds to

minutes) stimulation of glucose transport to the much delayed (hours
to tens of hours) effects on DNA synthesis and cell division (for a
summary, see Table V in Ref. 9). How, one may ask, might the
receptor dynamics discussed in this chapter bear on the varied time
courses of the multiple actions of insulin? In part, the answer to
this question comes not from studies with insulin, but from work in
fibroblast cell culture systems with the mitogenic/acid-inhibitory polypeptide, epidermal growth factor-urogastrone (EGF-URO) (see Refs.
3, 5—8, 15 for more details). Under normal circumstances, EGF-URO
can, like insulin, activate a large number of cell responses that occur over periods of seconds to minutes (e.g., stimulation of membrane transport and inhibition of acid secretion), up to tens of hours
(e.g., stimulation of RNA and DNA synthesis and cell division). A
chemical derivative of mouse EGF-URO has been prepared in which
the molecule has been cleaved at methionine residue 21 using cyano-
gen bromide (CNBr). This cleavage results in an opening of one of
the disulfide-maintained loops of the EGF-URO molecule. The derivative, denoted CNBr-EGF, still binds to the receptor, but is unable
to stimulate DNA synthesis and cell division. It has also been observed that although microclustering presumably still occurs, the
CNBr-EGF derivative is unable to cause gross aggregation of the
EGF-URO receptor. Nonetheless, the nonmitogenic CNBr-EGF derivative is still able to stimulate a number of the rapid cellular responses caused by intact EGF-URO (e.g., stimulation of ion flux
and induction of morphological changes). The data obtained with
CNBr-EGF have been considerably amplified by work with monoclonal antibodies directed against the EGF-URO receptor (5,15). In
brief, those antibodies capable of causing receptor aggregation (and,
consequently, internalization) were able to mimic both the short-
term as well as the long-term (mitogenesis) effects of EGF-URO.
However, monovalent Fab antibody derivatives that were not capable
of inducing receptor aggregation and that were unable to stimulate
DNA synthesis, were nonetheless capable of stimulating an early
event (membrane phosphorylation) associated with EGF-URO action.
A number of hypotheses have thus been put forward concerning
the possible role(s) of aggregated receptor and of internalized receptor or internalized receptor fragments in the long-term processes
of cell growth or cell differentiation (see Ref. 3 for a synopsis).
The short-term membrane-localized reactions may be related to the
receptor microclustering process. As discussed above, it is now
realized that in many cell types appreciable amounts of both insulin
and the insulin receptor can be taken up and degraded by insulin-
responsive cells. Furthermore, there is evidence that binding sites
for insulin can be found on Golgi elements, on smooth and rough
endoplasmic reticulum, as well as on the nuclear membranes of selected cells. Thus, it has been suggested that an internalized

degradation product either of insulin or of the insulin receptor may act at an intracellular site to cause at least some of the biological responses triggered by insulin. A role for internalized insulin or insulin fragments appears to be ruled out, in view of the remarkable effects of the anti-receptor antibodies and in view of the stimulatory actions of macromolecular insulin derivatives (e.g., insulin-Sepharose) that cannot enter the cell. Nonetheless, it is quite possible that there is a role for internalized receptor in directing some of the delayed actions of insulin (e.g., gene regulation and stimulation of cell division).

In keeping with the data that have been described in connection with EGF-URO action, it is possible to speculate on a series of events that may occur during the course of insulin-mediated cell activation. Although very hypothetical, the scheme proposed (Fig. 5), derived largely from experiments done with fibroblast cells, places in a feasible context both the receptor dynamics described in this chapter and the intrinsic kinase activity of the insulin receptor (16) that has recently been described in work from a number of laboratories. (The receptor can become phosphorylated and may also phosphorylate other cellular substrates.) It must also be kept in mind that the scheme presented is a generalized picture that synthesizes information obtained from a number of cultured cell systems using several peptide hormone probes. For a specific ligand such as insulin acting on a particular cell type (e.g., the adipocyte), some but not all of the processes outlined in the generalized scheme may in fact occur.

It is quite likely that the rapid actions of insulin (change in membrane potential, stimulation of glucose transport and release from the membrane of chemical mediators that rapidly regulate enzyme activity) are caused by biochemical reactions in which the receptor participates within the plane of the plasma membrane. The initial receptor microclustering event probably represents a key process that is directly related to these membrane-localized reactions. One exciting possibility is that the intrinsic tyrosine kinase activity of the receptor (16) may initiate some of these key reactions. As indicated above, the rapid modulation of cellular activity may require a special receptor conformation that would permit effective interactions between the receptors that associate in microclusters. In this context, insulin can be viewed as an essential allosteric regulator that can modulate membrane-localized reactions (and thereby cell response) on a minute-to-minute basis. Cells would thus be very responsive to extracellular changes in insulin concentrations.

Once internalized, however, the receptor would no longer be exposed to the variations in insulin concentrations that might occur in the extracellular milieu. Thus, the time course of reactions in which the internalized receptor might participate could differ

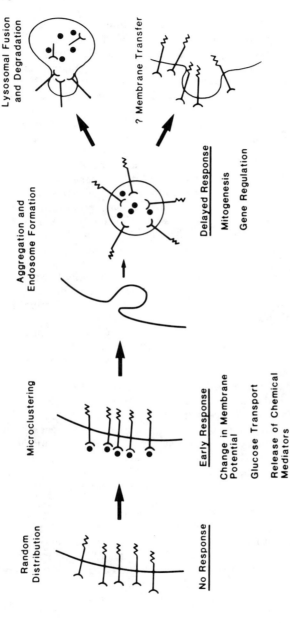

Figure 5 Receptor dynamics and cell activation. As discussed in the text, cell responses that are rapidly regulated by insulin probably involve the initial microclustering event. Delayed effects of insulin may be caused by receptor that is internalized in the endosomal organelle. The topography of the endosome would permit the intracellular portion of the receptor (zigzag line) to interact with a variety of intracellular constituents located at considerable distances from the plasma membrane. In the course of its intracellular migration, the receptor-bearing endosome could ultimately fuse either with lysosomes or with other membrane structures (e.g., Golgi elements or nuclear membranes), resulting in a further relocation of the receptor.

considerably from the time frame of those reactions occurring in the plasma membrane. One role for the internalized receptor may be to regulate some of the delayed effects (hours to tens of hours) that insulin has on its target cells.

As hypothesized in Figure 5, the internalized receptor-bearing endosome [or "receptosome" (2)] may do more than simply function as a way station for the receptor, en route either to the lysosome or, via recycling, back to the cell surface. Rather, the endosome may function as a site-directed receptor-kinase-bearing vesicle that may regulate enzyme activity by phosphorylation reactions that could occur in regions quite distant form the cell surface. In addition, by membrane fusion, the endosome may even transfer the receptor to a new membrane environment, such as the nuclear membrane. Since the endosome-associated receptors are subject to inactivation by lysosomal degradation, a constant influx of fresh receptor-bearing endosomes sustained over a prolonged time period may be required to bring about some of the delayed cellular effects of insulin. The essence of the above discussion is that the temporally distinct actions of insulin may relate directly to the topographically distinct receptor dynamic events that, subsequent to ligand binding, occur over quite different time frames. In this context, the continued internalization of receptor may play a key role in the activation of the delayed effects of insulin.

VI. RECEPTOR REGULATION AND THE CONTROL OF CELL SENSITIVITY

In addition to the potential role for the internalization process in terms of providing intracellular receptor for possible cell activation events, the internalization process may also be a factor in regulating cell sensitivity. For instance, because of the mass action law governing the interaction between insulin and the receptor,

$$R + INS \rightleftharpoons INS-R$$

$$K = \frac{[INS-R]}{[R][INS]}$$

a reduction in receptor concentration would, at the same ambient insulin concentration, lead to a reduction in the concentration of insulin-receptor complexes. Furthermore, since the cell response is in some way proportional to the number of occupied receptor, i.e., respons $\alpha[INS-R]$, the occupation of fewer receptors by insulin would lead to a reduced signal for cellular response. Put another way, it can be said that in an abnormal situation, where the numbers of cellular receptors are reduced, it will require a higher

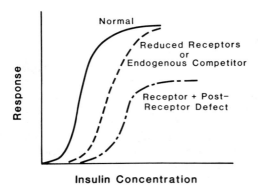

Insulin Concentration

Figure 6 Effects of receptor regulation and postreceptor defects on dose-response curves. A hypothetical situation is depicted for a cell that normally has insulin receptors in excess of the number required for a maximal cell response. The consequences of reducing receptor number down to or below the number required for a maximum response are illustrated, as well as the situation wherein a post receptor defect is present. A combination of reduced receptors and a postreceptor defect would lead to a rightward shift of the dose-response curve as well as a reduction in the maximum response (right-hand response curve).

insulin concentration to occupy the same number of receptors that in the normal cell cause a "normal" response; that is, the cells will appear to exhibit "insulin resistance." Nonetheless, because there appears to be a "receptor reserve" situation, insofar as insulin receptors are concerned (i.e., many cells have more receptors than are required for generating a maximal cell response), in the abnormal situation where receptor numbers are somewhat reduced, it should still be possible, by raising the insulin concentration high enough, to occupy enough receptors to generate a maximal cell response. This situation is illustrated in Figure 6 (middle response curve). The same response curve might be observed if an endogenous reversible competitor of insulin binding were present.

In the event that the cellular receptor number falls below the level required for a maximal cell response, then the dose-response curve would be effected not only by a shift to the right, but also by a reduction in the maximum response (right-hand curve, Fig. 6). The reduction in the maximum response could also be caused by postreceptor mechanisms that affect cell activation. Clearly, a combination of postreceptor and receptor-related events can both play an important role in the phenomenon of "insulin resistance," and in regulating the sensitivity of the cell to insulin.

VII. FUTURE PROSPECTS FOR RECEPTOR DYNAMICS AND INSULIN ACTION

The dynamic aspects of receptor properties have only recently been appreciated. This aspect of receptor pharmacology adds tremendous flexibility to the possible processes in which receptors such as the one for insulin may participate, not only in terms of multiple membrane reactions, envisioned by the mobile receptor paradigm of hormone action (outlined in Ref. 1), but also in terms of processes at multiple geographic sites, at which surface receptors may act subsequent to cellular internalization. The challenge for the future is to identify the critical cellular locales involved in the cellular activation process. The cell surface is perhaps the easiest location at which receptor activation processes may be understood. However, the focus on the potential intracellular sites of receptor function may reveal processes related not only to the problem of diabetes, but also to the complex processes of cellular division and differentiation, where insulin very likely plays an important role. Thus, the studies bearing on the dynamics of the receptor for insulin will shed light not only on the factors related to diabetes, but may, in a wider context, also illuminate biological mechanisms fundamental to a variety of normal and pathological processes.

ABOUT THE REFERENCES

As with Chapter 5, to minimize the number of references, I have in many cases referred the reader to review articles rather than the individual source references where the original observations were described. It is hoped that by consulting the review articles, the reader will be able to expand upon the reference material provided in this chapter. References 1 and 4 provide a large amount of background material related to mechanisms of hormone action. References 2 and 3 summarize some of the recently described observations related to receptor mobility and internalization. Much information about the mechanism of insulin action as it relates to the effects of antireceptor antibodies is summarized in Reference 9. Since so much knowledge about the way peptide hormones work is coming from studies of the action of epidermal growth factor-urogastrone (EGF-URO), a number of useful reviews summarizing work with this very interesting polypeptide are cited (Refs. 5—8). Overall, the bibliographies in the cited reviews will provide the reader with ample additional information related to the topics dealt with in this chapter.

REFERENCES

1. Cuatrecasas, P. and Hollenberg, M. D. (1976). Membrane receptors and hormone action. *Advan. Prot. Chem. 30*:251–451.
2. Pastan, I. H. and Willingham, M. D. (1981). Journey to the center of the cell: Role of the receptosome. *Science 214*: 504–509.
3. King, A. C. and Cuatrecasas, P. (1981). Peptide hormone-induced receptor mobility, aggregation and internalization. *N. Engl. J. Med. 305*:77–88.
4. Hollenberg, M. D. (1979). Hormone receptor interactions at the cell membrane. *Parmacol. Rev. 30*:393–409.
5. Schlessinger, J., Schreiber, A. B., Levi, A., Lax, I., Libermann, T. A., and Yarden, Y. (1983). Regulation of cell proliferation by epidermal growth factor. *CRC Crit. Rev. Biochem. 14*:93–112.
6. Carpenter, G. and Cohen, S. (1979). Epidermal Growth factor. *Ann. Rev. Biochem. 48*:193–216.
7. Hollenberg, M. D. (1979). Epidermal growth factor-urogastrone, a polypeptide acquiring hormonal status. *Vit. Horm. 37*:69–110.
8. Carpenter, G. (1981). Epidermal growth factor. In *Handbook of Experimental Pharmacology*, Vol. 57, *Tissue Growth Factors* (R. Baserga, ed.). Springer Verlag, Berlin, pp. 98–132.
9. Khan, C. R., Baird, K. L., Flier, J. S., Grunfeld, C., Harmon, J. T., Harrison, L. C., Karlsson, F. A., Kasuga, M., King, G. L., Lang, U. C., Podskalny, J. M., and van Obberghen, E. (1981). Insulin receptor, receptor antibodies and the mechanism of insulin action. *Rec. Progr. Horm. Res. 37*: 477–538.
10. Shechter, Y., Hernaez, L., Schlessinger, J., and Cuatrecasas, P. (1979). Local aggregation of hormone-receptor complexes is required for activation by epidermal growth factor. *Nature (London) 278*:835–838.
11. Conn, P. M., Rogers, D. C., Stewart, J. M., Niedel, J., and Sheffield, T. (1982). Conversion of a gonadotropin-releasing hormone antagonist to an agonist. *Nature (London) 296*:653–655.
12. Gregory, H., Taylor, C. L., and Hopkins, C. R. (1982). Leuteinizing hormone release from dissociated pituitary cells by dimerization of occupied LHRH receptors. *Nature (London) 300*: 269–271.
13. Hopkins, C. R., Semoff, S., and Gregory, H. (1981). Regulation of gonadotropin secretion to the anterior pituitary. *Phil. Trans. Roy. Soc. London B 296*:73–81.
14. Roth, R. A., Cassell, P. J., Wong, K. Y., Maddux, B. A., and Goldfine, I. D. (1982). Monoclonal antibodies to the human insulin receptor block insulin binding and inhibit insulin action. *Proc. Natl. Acad. Sci. USA 79*:7312–7316.

15. Schreiber, A. B., Libermann, T. A., Lax, I., Yarden, Y., and Schlessinger, J. (1983). Biological role of epidermal growth factor-receptor clustering. Investigation with monoclonal antireceptor antibodies. *J. Biol. Chem. 258*:849–853.
16. Kasuga, M., Zick, Y., Blithe, D. L., Grettaz, M., and Kahn, C. R. (1982). Insulin stimulates tyrosine phosphorylation of the insulin receptor in a cell-free system. *Nature (London) 298*:667–669.

7

Tissue-Specific Variations in Insulin Receptor Dynamics

ROBERT M. SMITH and LEONARD JARETT *University of Pennsylvania School of Medicine, Philadelphia, Pennsylvania*

I. INTRODUCTION

The importance of understanding the biological processes involved in the events following the binding of insulin to its receptor is evident by the number of recent symposia on this subject (see Suggested Reading List) and the publication of this treatise. It is clear from the previous chapters, as well as the literature, that specific areas of both agreement and disagreement exist among various investigators concerning fundamental conceptual aspects of insulin's interaction with target tissues. Many of these disparities reflect the interpretation of data obtained from the investigation of different cell systems, suggesting that diversity of cell structure and function may result in such variations. There is growing evidence that differences between cell types must be taken into account. Other apparent conflicts, which involve similar cell types, may be caused by seemingly trivial differences in experimental conditions and techniques used in the studies.

This chapter presents morphological and correlative biochemical data accumulated on various cell types in an attempt to clarify some of the complicated events following insulin binding. Figure 1 depicts some of the events that may occur subsequent to the interaction of insulin with its receptor and that are the subject of this and previous chapters.

Figure 1 is not typical of any single cell type, but presents some of the variations observed during the course of the studies described in this chapter. Panel (1): Insulin (▲) binds to receptors (■) in the glycocalyx of the plasma membrane. The receptors may be naturally grouped as depicted in (a) or dispersed as in (b). In some cells, dispersed receptors microaggregate after occupancy of insulin,

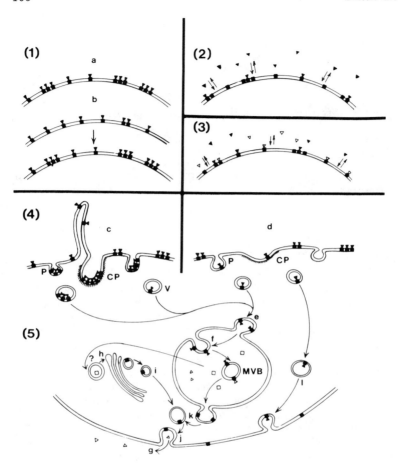

Figure 1 Schematic representation of the events following binding of insulin to its receptor. For explanation of figure, see text.

resulting in a grouped distribution of receptors as shown in the lower
portion of (b). Panel (2): Insulin in the media binds to and dissociates from receptors on the plasma membrane and this process attains
an equilibrium. Panel (3): Complicating the determination of the
equilibrium noted above is the fact that insulin bound to the receptor
can be degraded (△) and dissociate into the media. Membrane-associated
degradation may be a substantial, or even major, source of hormone
degradative activity in some cells. Panel (4): Endocytosis of the
insulin-receptor complex may be preceeded by concentration of the
occupied receptors, as shown in (c), into specialized membrane structures such as pinocytotic invaginations (P) or coated pits (CP). On
other cells, endocytosis appears randomly to remove occupied receptors from the cell surface (d) without concentrating the hormone-
receptor complex. Specialized endocytotic structures vary from cell
to cell in their relative contribution to the total uptake process. This
variation is affected by the density of receptors in the structure and
the number of those structures on a given cell type. Endocytosis proceeds via small cytoplamic vesicles that may or may not be coated.
Panel (5): Once the hormone-receptor complex is endocytosed in the
cytoplasmic vesicles, there are various routes that it may take. As
shown (e), vesicles may fuse with multivesicular bodies (MVB) or lysosomes. The vesicles usually evert as shown (f), exposing the
hormone-receptor complex to the proteases in the lysosomes. The
hormone apparently is degraded (△) at this point in many cells. It
is possible that the receptors, or some proportion of the receptors,
may be degraded as well (□). Degraded insulin is released into the
extracellular media (g). Fragments of insulin receptors may be re-
utilized (h) to form new receptors. Newly synthesized receptors are
probably transported to the cell surface (i) in vesicles morphologically
indistinguishable from the endocytotic cytoplasmic vesicles. The vesicles fuse with the membrane by forming invaginations (j) similar to
endocytotic invaginations. Receptors which are not degraded in the
lysosome may be recycled to the plasma membrane (k). It is apparent
that in some cell types a substantial amount of the internalized insulin
does not go to the lysosomes. Other organelles that have been reported to accumulate insulin include the Golgi apparatus, nuclei, and endoplasmic reticulum. In adipocytes, we have observed the apparent recycling of intact insulin-receptor complexes in vesicles and exocytotic
invaginations (1).

  High-resolution electron microscopic studies on several structurally
and functionally different cell types have shown that insulin receptor
distribution, mobility, and internalization differ on these various cell
types. Along with the differences are some similarities that are shared
by some, but not all cells in these studies. The biochemical analysis
of insulin binding and processing has also demonstrated tissue-specific
variations; these variations will be described. The morphological

studies utilized a unique monomeric ferritin-insulin conjugate (Fm-I).
The preparation and characterization of this conjugate have been described in detail (Smith and Jarett, 1982a). The Fm-I conjugate is indistinguishable from native insulin in its ability to bind to insulin receptors and to elicit insulin-sensitive responses. The Fm-I conjugate
can provide complimentary and distinct information not available from
that obtained using either [^{125}I]insulin radioautography or fluorescently labeled insulin techniques. These latter methods have provided
substantial information about insulin receptor dynamics as reviewed in
Chapter 6. One of the primary advantages of Fm-I is that the extremely small distance between the ferritin particle and the occupied
insulin receptor provides a substantial improvement in the localization
of the occupied receptor both on the cell membrane and in intracellular
structures as examined with high-resolution electron microscopy.
With Fm-I, both individual as well as grouped receptors can be seen
and, more importantly, distinguished and quantitated. In addition,
the Fm-I conjugate retains full biological potency, whereas some other
ligands have potencies of 1-5% of the native hormone. The Fm-I ultrastructural marker has permitted quantitative high-resolution studies
to be performed on the occupied insulin receptor, including determination of the native distribution, mobility, and internalization of the
insulin-receptor complex. The most striking observation from these
studies of various insulin-responsive cells is the extent of the variations in insulin receptor dynamics.

II. INSULIN RECEPTOR DISTRIBUTION AND ORGANIZATION IN CELL MEMBRANES

As described in the previous chapter, mobility of receptor molecules
within the plane of the membrane appears to be a widespread characteristic of various hormone receptors on different cell types. In some
cells, the ability of hormones, such as insulin, to alter receptor mobility or to change the distribution patterns of their receptors may be
important in the cellular response to hormonal stimulation. Microaggregation of ligand-receptor complexes may be caused by at least two
mechanisms: (a) microaggregation of randomly mobile receptors due
to occupancy and cross-linking by multivalent ligands or (b) an or-
chestrated migration and microaggregation of the receptor molecules as
an induced response of the cell or cell membrane to receptor occupancy
by either multivalent or monovalent ligands. In the first case, the
multivalent ligand actively participates by cross-linking its mobile receptors, and the cell may be a passive participant in this process until
large membrane deformations have occurred. Molecules of multivalent
ligands have two or more active binding regions that permit the ligand
simultaneously to occupy multiple receptor molecules. The occupancy

of multiple receptors by multivalent ligands leads to the microaggregation, and, under appropriate conditions, clustering and capping of receptors. Examples of multivalent ligands include lectins (such as concanavalin A and wheat germ agglutinin), holoantibodies, and their Fab_2 fragments. The aggregation or capping caused by multivalent ligands usually results in the endocytosis and/or sloughing of the receptors in the affected area of the cell membrane. In the second case, microaggregation of receptors probably is due to an induced response of the membrane to receptor occupancy. The ligand binding to the receptor may trigger a biochemical reaction or other stimuli that results in movement of the receptors to specific domains on the cell surface. This microaggregation may also result in clustering and substantial membrane deformation with results similar to multivalent ligand-induced aggregation, i.e., endocytosis or sloughing of occupied receptors. Illustrative of this second type of aggregation would be that caused by insulin. There is no direct evidence suggesting that insulin can bind to more than one receptor simultaneously, and, therefore, it would probably not cross-link receptors and cause redistribution of receptor sites as do multivalent ligands. The preparation of Fm-I has not altered the monovalent characteristics of the hormone. Consequently, postbinding redistribution of insulin receptors as visualized with Fm-I would suggest that a specific cellular or membrane response was generated as a result of receptor occupancy.

Studies were designed to determine the original or native distribution of occupied insulin receptors on various tissues and to determine the subsequent postoccupancy distribution of receptor molecules. These experiments were performed by incubating glutaraldehyde-fixed or unfixed cells or membrane fractions with Fm-I and comparing the distribution patterns of insulin receptors that were found. Fixation of the tissue must be performed so that insulin binding is not impaired, and receptor migration is prevented. Under these conditions the binding of Fm-I will demonstrate the native distribution of the insulin receptors. Biochemical studies showed that appropriate fixation and subsequent inactivation of aldehyde groups with Tris-HCl or lysine eliminated microaggregation of multivalent concanavalin A, indicating that membrane proteins were immobilized. The same fixation conditions did not affect specific or nonspecific [^{125}I]insulin binding (Jarett and Smith, 1977). Subsequent ultrastructural studies with Fm-I have shown that both the native distribution of insulin receptors and the ability or extent of receptors to redistribute on unfixed tissue subsequent to hormone binding differed on the various cell types investigated. The results of such studies are presented below.

A. Rat Adipocytes

Adipocytes are exquisitely insulin sensitive and are obtained as a homogenous cell preparation, making them ideal for studies of insulin action.

Our laboratory has used this cell type and its subcellular fractions for biochemical studies for a number of years. Therefore, it was the natural choice for our first, and most detailed, ultrastructural studies using Fm-I as a marker for the occupied insulin receptor.

Initial studies (Jarett and Smith, 1975) on the adipocyte showed that the receptor sites occurred either as single receptors or in small groups of two to six occuppied receptors.

Isolated adipocytes were incubated with 40 ng/ml Fm-I for 30 min at 37°C in Krebs-Ringer phosphate buffer, pH 7.4. The cells were prepared for electron microscopy as described (Jarett and Smith, 1975). The ferritin molecules were found in the glycocalyx portion of the plasma membrane, indicating that the receptor was glycoprotein and projected from the surface of the membrane bilayer. Figure 2 is an electron micrograph that demonstrates the binding of Fm-I in the glycocalyx of the intact adipocyte plasma membrane and shows representative groups of insulin receptor sites. The receptors were found to be randomly distributed over the entire cell surface. Quantitative studies (Jarett and Smith, 1977) showed that about two-thirds of the receptors occurred in small groups of two to six receptors per group while one-third occurred as single receptors. These data were similar whether insulin receptors on intact cells or isolated plasma membranes were analyzed. These observations raised the question as to whether occupancy of the insulin receptor by Fm-I caused the groups to form or whether they existed prior to insulin binding. This question was

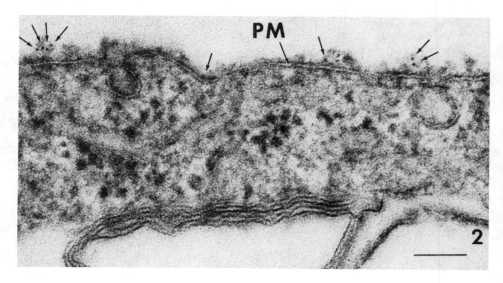

Figure 2 Electron micrograph of Fm-I receptor sites on rat adipocytes. PM = plasma membrane. Bar = 0.1 μm.

addressed by comparing the receptor organization on fixed and unfixed tissue. The organization of Fm-I occupied receptors was the
same on fresh cells or membranes as on fixed tissue, indicating that
the groups occurred naturally, existed prior to the binding of insulin,
and were not due to receptor microaggregation secondary to occupancy. The percentage of the total occupied receptors found in
groups of various sizes, or the absolute size of the groups, was not
related to the total number or density of occupied receptors on the
plasma membrane. When rat adipocytes were incubated for 60 min at
37°C with increasing concentrations of Fm-I, from 10 to 200 ng/ml,
and prepared for electron microscopy as described (Jarett and Smith,
1975), the organization of receptors into groups, as a percentage of
the total number of occupied receptors, stayed relatively constant as
shown in Table 1. The total number of occupied receptor sites per
square micrometer of cell surface increased with increasing concentrations of Fm-I until the receptors sites were saturated. The number of receptor sites per square micrometer of surface area was approximately the same whether calculated from the ultrastructural data
or [125I]insulin binding assay results, adding further validity to the
ultrastructural studies. These data have been confirmed by computer-
assisted analysis (Gershon, et al., 1981) of the receptor organization
which in addition showed that there was a maximum distance of 400 Å
between occupied receptors in a group and a mean distance of about
150 Å. Computer modeling also confirmed that the maximum number
of receptors sites per group was about four to six receptors per group.

During prolonged incubations of intact adipocytes at 37°C, which
resulted in a significant amount of hormone-receptor complex internalization (see below), there was no evidence that the individual or
grouped receptors redistributed into larger clusters or caps or migrated to specific areas of the cell prior to internalization. The random distribution of the Fm-I over the entire cell was the same on both
fixed and fresh cells, which provided additional evidence that the receptor groups were not aggregating. Studies were done where aggregation of the groups of occupied receptors was attempted by using
multivalent anti-insulin or anti-ferritin antibodies. These antibodies
should bind to the insulin or ferritin molecule of the Fm-I bound to
the insulin receptor and cause multivalent ligand-induced aggregation
and cross-linking if the receptors or groups of receptors were mobile.
No effect of anti-insulin antibody was seen on adipocyte membranes
(Lyen et al., 1983a), although anti-insulin antibody caused significant
aggregation of insulin receptors on liver plasma membranes (see below).
Anti-ferritin antibodies also failed to alter the number of Fm-I receptors in groups of the distribution of groups. The lack of aggregation
of the receptor sites suggested that the mobility of the insulin receptor on the adipocyte was at least partially restricted.

Investigations have been performed to help determine the mechanism responsible for holding the groups of adipocyte insulin receptors

Table 1 Organization and Concentration of Occupied Fm-I Receptors on Rat Adipocytes Determined with Various Concentrations of Fm-I

Concentration		Receptor sites per group (% of total occupied receptor sites)					
Fm-I (ng/ml)	Receptors[a] (receptors/μm^2)	1	2	3	4	5	6
10	8.3	37.3	22.7	17.9	13.5	6.6	2.0
20	17.4	36.8	25.7	22.9	10.1	3.0	1.5
40	21.6	35.3	23.6	18.9	11.0	7.0	4.2
200	25.7	35.1	27.2	22.6	11.2	2.4	1.5

[a]Receptor concentration was calculated from the total number of Fm-I particles observed along the total measured length of plasma membrane, and surface area was calculated by including the section thickness in the computations. The analysis of grouping was performed by measuring the distance between nearest-neighbor particles, with the maximum distance between grouped molecules defined as 400 Å as previously reported by Gershon et al. (1981).

together. A logical mechanism for regulating the structural arrangement of intramembraneous proteins is the cytoskeleton network of actin and microfilaments found immediately beneath the plasma membrane. Disrupting the cytoskeleton often results in gross structural alterations in the membrane and affects the mobility of protein molecules within the membrane. For this reason, we incubated intact adipocytes for 15 min at 37°C with either control buffer, 1 μm cytochalasin B or 1 μm cytochalasin D, prior to the addition of 20 ng/ml Fm-I. After an additional 30 min at 37°C, the cells were washed and prepared for electron microscopy as described (Jarett and Smith, 1975). Analysis of receptor grouping was performed as described in Table 1.

The groups of insulin receptors were partially disrupted by cytochalasin B but were unaffected by cytochalasin D (Jarett and Smith, 1979) as shown in Fig. 3. Disruption of the groups of receptor sites by cytochalasin B had virtually no effect on insulin binding or stimulation of glucose oxidation. The differences in the effects of these two agents on the disruption of receptors indicated that neither microfilaments nor actin were directly responsible for holding the groups of receptors together. The major difference between these two agents is that only cytochalasin B binds to thiol groups. This unique property suggested to us that disulfide bonds might play a role in the maintenance of the groups of receptor sites in the adipocyte plasma membrane.

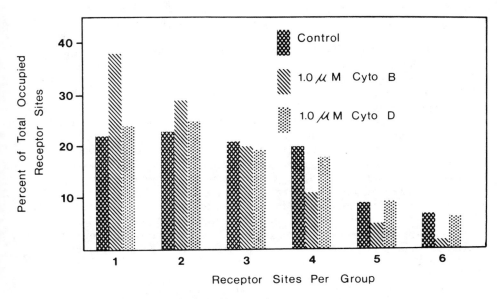

Figure 3 Comparison of the effects of cytochalasin B and D on the organization of insulin receptors on rat adipocyte plasma membranes.

A series of biochemical and ultrastructural studies utilizing reducing, alkylating, and oxidizing agents were undertaken to determine the role of disulfide bonds in holding groups of insulin receptors together on adipocyte membranes (Schweitzer et al., 1980; Jarett and Smith, 1983). Treatment of adipocyte plasma membranes with dithiothreitol (DTT), a potent reducing agent, affected subsequent [^{125}I]-insulin binding to the membrane in a biphasic manner. Dithiothreitol concentrations of 0.1 to 1.0 mM caused an increase in insulin binding at low hormone concentrations to a maximum of threefold over control, while 5 mM DTT caused a marked decrease in binding. The Scatchard analysis of [^{125}I]insulin binding data obtained after treatment of 1 mM DTT revealed a marked change in the affinity profile with a straight line, rather than the normal curvilinear plot and with a resulting K_a of 1.0×10^8 M^{-1}. These effects could be reversed by incubating the tissue with oxidized glutathione after the DTT treatment and before measuring [^{125}I]insulin binding. When N-ethylmaleimide (NEM) alkylation was performed between the DTT and oxidized glutathione incubations, the DTT effect was not reversible by oxidized glutathione. Neither NEM nor oxidized glutathione had an effect on insulin binding. The data suggest that the DTT effect on insulin binding to adipocytes may be related to the disulfide bonds proposed to be involved in holding the subunits of the insulin receptor together (see Chapters 3 and 4). The low concentrations of DTT that altered the binding affinity of the receptor are the same concentrations that can dissociate the receptor into two $\alpha, \beta - \alpha, \beta$ subunit pairs. The higher concentration of DTT that inhibited insulin binding can dissociate the α subunit from the β subunit in the solubilized receptor. However, it is quite possible that high concentrations of DTT cause relatively major alterations in the entire plasma membrane and that the effects of 5 mM DTT on [^{125}I]insulin binding reflect these changes rather than a limited and direct effect on the insulin receptor per se. The effect of these same agents on insulin binding to receptors on adipocytes was not the same in other tissues (see below).

Ultrastructural observation of the Fm-I receptors on adipocyte membranes treated in the same manner as the biochemical experiments revealed that DTT caused a partial and dose-dependent disruption of the groups of insulin receptors (Jarett and Smith, 1983). The maximum effect on the disruption of the receptor groups was approximately equal to the maximum effect seen with cytochalasin B (Table 2). Oxidized glutathione reversed the DTT-mediated disruption. However, the reversal was prevented when alkylation with NEM was performed after DTT treatment but prior to oxidized glutathione treatment. Interestingly, NEM itself caused a partial disruption of the receptor groups virtually identical to that found with both cytochalasin B and DTT; the effects of DTT and NEM were slightly additive.

Table 2 Organization of Occupied Fm-I Receptors on Rat Adipocyte Plasma Membranes after Various Treatments[a]

Treatment[b]	Receptor sites per group (% total occupied receptor sites)					
	1	2	3	4	5	6
None	35.3	23.6	18.9	11.0	7.0	4.0
Cyto B (5 µM)	44.6	30.3	14.1	5.1	3.1	2.3
DTT (1 mM)	50.6	30.5	12.8	3.6	2.0	0.4
NEM (1 mM)	59.9	22.6	9.9	5.2	1.3	1.0
GSSG (50 mM)	32.6	22.2	20.8	15.0	7.3	2.0
DTT (1 mM) followed by GSSG (50 mM)	39.7	25.8	15.4	9.3	6.3	3.5
DTT (1 mM) followed by NEM (1 mM)	63.2	27.2	7.0	1.7	0.7	0.0
DTT (1 mM) followed NEM (1 mM) followed by GSSG (50 mM)	58.7	23.6	8.4	4.8	3.1	1.4

[a]Fm-I was added at a final concentration of 20 ng/ml to the plasma membranes and incubated for 20 min at 24°C, washed and prepared for electron microscopy. Analysis of grouping was as described in Table 1.
[b]Cyto B, cytochalasin B: DTT, dithiothreitol; NEM, n-ethylmaleimide; GSSG, oxidized glutathione.

The differences in the effects of dithiothreitol, N-ethylmaleimide, and cytochalasin B on insulin binding and on the disruption of groups of insulin receptors on adipocyte plasma membranes suggested that these agents were affecting two functionally different sets of disulfide bonds. A proposed model is illustrated in Figure 4. One set of disulfide bonds appeared to be relatively unstable, spontaneously undergoing reduction to sulfhydryl groups and reoxidation to the disulfide state, with the disulfide bond and grouped receptors favored at equilibrium. All three reagents tested could decrease the number of disulfide bonds that formed grouped receptors either by direct disruption of disulfide bonds (DTT) or by shifting the equilibrium through alkylation (NEM) of or reversible binding (cytochalasin B) to the sulfhydryl groups. The effect of DTT could be reversed by oxidized glutathione;

A. Unstable Disulfide Bond—Related to Receptor Grouping

1. S-S $\rightleftharpoons$ 2(SH)
   Normal condition; insulin receptors naturally grouped

2. S-S $\xrightleftharpoons{DTT}$ 2(SH)
   DTT reduction shifts equilibrium; insulin receptor groups dispersed

   Followed by

   a. 2(SH) $\xrightleftharpoons{GSSG}$ S-S
      GSSG oxidation reverses DTT effect; insulin receptors grouped

   b. SH $\xrightarrow{NEM}$ S-NEM
      NEM alkylation prevents oxidation of thiols and therefore reversal of DTT effects; insulin receptors dispersed

3. S-S $\rightleftharpoons$ 2(SH)

   a. SH $\xrightleftharpoons{Cyto\ B}$ S-Cyto B
      Cyto B binding to thiols shifts equilibrium; insulin receptor groups dispersed; reversible in absence of Cyto B

   b. SH $\xrightarrow{NEM}$ S-NEM
      NEM alkylation of thiols shifts equilibrium; insulin receptor groups dispersed; irreversible

B. Stable Disulfide Bond—Related to Insulin Binding Properties

1. S-S $\rightleftharpoons$ 2(SH)
   Normal condition; normal curvilinear insulin binding affinity profile

2. S-S $\xrightleftharpoons{DTT}$ 2(SH)
   DTT reduction shifts equilibrium; insulin binding affinity profile altered

   Followed by

   a. 2(SH) $\xrightleftharpoons{GSSG}$ S-S
      GSSG oxidation reverses DTT effect; normal insulin binding affinity profile restored

   b. SH $\xrightarrow{NEM}$ S-NEM
      NEM alkylation prevents oxidation of thiols; DTT effect preserved

3. S-S $\rightleftharpoons$ 2(SH)

   a. SH $\xrightarrow{Cyto\ B}$
   b. SH $\xrightarrow{NEM}$
      Cyto B and NEM have little or no effect without prior DTT treatment; normal insulin binding affinity profile

Figure 4 The role of disulfide bonds in rat adipocyte membranes.

the effect of cytochalasin B could be reversed by removal of cytochalasin B. However, the effect of NEM could not be reversed because of the permanent nature of alkylation. The additive effects of NEM and DTT may have been the result of alkylation of the sulfhydryl groups and consequent prevention of the normal spontaneous reoxidation to the disulfide state that follows the removal of DTT from the incubation medium. Therefore, in adipocytes these unstable disulfide bonds appeared to be involved in maintaining the grouped arrangement of the insulin receptor.

The second type of disulfide bond in our model would be more stable and not susceptible to spontaneous reduction. These disulfide bonds were involved in the effect of DTT on [^{125}I]insulin binding and the reversal caused by oxidized glutathione. N-Ethylmaleimide and cytochalasin B would have little, if any, effect on these bonds because of the lack of spontaneous reduction and availability of sulfhydryl groups.

It is not clear where these two sets of disulfide bonds are located. It is possible that the unstable bonds are between neighboring protein molecules in the plasma membrane itself, surrounding the insulin receptors and helping to hold them together in the aggregated state. Similar disulfides may play a role in the receptor model developed by Yip and colleagues (Chap. 3). The morphological observations imply that these bonds have some tissue specificity because of the variations in insulin receptor aggregation found in different tissues. The stable disulfide bonds that are affected only by DTT may be the type I disulfide bond proposed to hold the two identical halves of the insulin receptor together in the model discussed in Chap. 4. Comparatively low concentrations of dithiothreitol disrupt the insulin receptor into two identical pairs containing both α and β subunits. It is conceivable that separation of the insulin receptor complex into monovalent components through disruption of the type I disulfide bond changes the affinity profile of the receptor for insulin without changing the absolute number of total receptors. This model would be consistent with the data on the effects of DTT on insulin binding to adipocyte plasma membranes. Dithiothreitol would also be expected to alter the binding of insulin to liver and placental membranes in the same manner as the adipocyte, since the subunit structure of the receptor from all three tissues appears to be the same. However, as will be discussed below, DTT had no effect on insulin binding to liver plasma membranes (Schweitzer et al., 1980; Jacobs and Cuatrecasas, 1980). Although DTT changed the affinity profile in the placental membranes without altering the total number of receptor sites, receptor occupancy at low hormone concentrations was markedly reduced compared to the control (Jacobs and

and Cuatrecasas, 1980). This was exactly opposite to the DTT
effect in the adipocyte where receptor occupancy was increased
at low hormone concentrations. These findings suggest several
possible explanations. The most obvious explanation would be
that the local membrane environment affects the ultimate insulin-
binding characteristics once the receptor subunits are disrupted.
The second suggestion would be that DTT affected disulfide bonds
not between the receptor subunits but between the receptor and
other membrane constituents surrounding the insulin receptor (e.g.,
see the receptor model of Yip and colleagues in Chap. 3). These
membrane constituents or their interactions with insulin receptors
may be different in various cell types. Finally, despite similar
electrophoretic behavior of labeled insulin receptor subunits, there
may be subtle differences between receptors from different cell
types, e.g., their molecular structure, including oligosaccharide
composition, may vary from cell to cell causing differing binding
properties for insulin once the subunits are disrupted.

The biochemical and morphological findings concerning the insulin receptor on the adipocyte are in many respects unique to
this cell type when compared to other cells studied and discussed
below. Such findings are not unexpected considering the unique
morphological features and biochemical functions of the adipocyte
in comparison to these other cell types.

B. Human Placental Syncytial Trophoblast

Analysis of the distribution of Fm-I bound to insulin receptors on
human placental syncytial trophoblast (Nelson et al., 1978) revealed
a pattern of receptor distribution with similarities to and differences
from the adipocyte. These studies provided our first evidence that
insulin receptors can have distinct tissue-specific ultrastructural
arrangements. As on the adipocyte, receptors were grouped together in small groups as well as some single receptor molecules.
However, instead of being randomly distributed over the cell surface, the insulin receptors were restricted entirely to the distal
portion of the microvillous projections of the cell. No specific insulin receptors were found on the intervillous cell surface. This
restricted distribution of Fm-I was consistent with the unique distribution pattern of various glycoproteins on the surface of the
microvilli. The receptors were shown to exist in groups prior to
the binding of Fm-I since fixed tissue showed the same pattern of
receptor organization as did unfixed tissue. During incubations
of unfixed tissue at 24° and 37°C there were no indications of migration of the occupied insulin receptors to other areas of the cell.

There was also no indication that the size of the receptor groups increased. These data suggested, but did not prove, that (as with the adipocyte) receptor mobility was restricted.

Because of the ultrastructural similarities of the organization of insulin receptors on the adipocyte and placenta and the widespread similarities in receptor subunit composition, one might expect that DTT treatment of the placenta would have effects on [125I]insulin binding similar to those found on adipocytes. Jacobs and Cuatrecasas (1980) investigated the effects of DTT on insulin binding to the placenta and showed that the Scatchard plot was linearized with a significant change in the affinity profile without affecting the total number of insulin receptors. However, over a wide concentration range of DTT, insulin binding at low hormone concentrations was decreased on the placenta. This decrease in binding at low hormone concentrations was the opposite of the effect seen on adipocytes. It is apparent that disulfide bonds play an essential role both in the ultrastructural organization and kinetic binding properties of insulin receptors. However, the data obtained with adipocytes, placenta, and, as will be seen below, the liver, prevented the design or proposal of a comprehensive model correlating the ultrastructural organization of insulin receptors with their insulin-binding kinetics or affinity profiles.

C. Isolated Liver Plasma Membranes

Attempts to study the distribution of insulin receptors on isolated or cultured hepatocytes were not feasible due to the high concentration of endogeneous ferritin in those cells. The insulin uptake process and possible cell regulated redistribution of insulin receptors prior to internalization could not be addressed. It was nevertheless possible to determine the native organization of insulin receptors on the cell membrane by using an isolated plasma membrane fraction. The Fm-I binding to the isolated liver plasma membranes (Jarett et al., 1980) showed a receptor organization pattern distinct from both the placenta and adipocyte. Over 60% of the receptor sites were single receptors. This organization pattern, as was the case with the adipocyte, appeared to be independent of the concentration of Fm-I used in the incubation, and there appeared to be no preferential localization of Fm-I to any portion of the membrane. After prolonged incubation at 24° or 37°C, there was no indication that the Fm-I receptors were microaggregating. Fixation of the membranes had no effect on the observed receptor organization. As stated above, these observations were made on an isolated membrane fraction; therefore, it

was not possible to determine whether insulin occupancy of receptors
on the intact hepatocyte would cause cell-induced receptor mobility
that might result in receptor aggregation.

In an analysis of [^{125}I]insulin binding to liver plasma membranes,
Shechter et al. (1979) demonstrated that bivalent anti-insulin antibody at selected concentrations increased insulin binding to the high-
affinity site and linearized the Scatchard plot of the binding data.
These effects also were observed on 3T3-C2 fibroblasts. They showed
that anti-insulin antibody was unable to increase insulin binding or
affect insulin receptor affinity on adipocytes. Since monovalent Fab
anti-insulin antibody failed to increase insulin binding on liver membranes and fibroblasts, Shechter postulated that the mechanism involved in the increased binding caused by the holoantibody required
multivalent ligand-induced cross-linking and microaggregation of dispersed mobile receptors. This explanation was compatible with our
ultrastructural observations that adipocyte insulin receptors were
naturally grouped and relatively immobile and, therefore, as we subsequently showed, unlikely to be affected by the anti-insulin antibody.

Our laboratory confirmed Shechter's biochemical finding that anti-
insulin antibody increased [^{125}I]insulin binding to liver plasma membranes but had no effect on insulin binding to its receptors on the
adipocyte. We extended these biochemical studies to an ultrastructural analysis of the effect of anti-insulin antibody on Fm-I-occupied
receptor organization on liver plasma membranes (Lyen et al., 1983b).
Bivalent anti-insulin antibody resulted in a dramatic microaggregation
of the dispersed insulin receptor sites on liver membranes resulting
in an organization pattern similar to the organization pattern seen on the
adipocyte. Monovalent antibody and normal immunoglobulin G (IgG)
had no effect on the receptor organization pattern on either tissue.
It was possible that the apparent reorganization of single receptors
into groups on the liver membranes could simply be due to the increased binding of insulin to the membrane and the subsequent increase in the density of occupied receptors caused by the antibody.
This possibility was eliminated by showing that increasing the receptor
occupancy by increasing Fm-I concentrations did not increase the
percentage of grouped insulin receptors.

The insulin receptors on liver membranes could be further distinguished from the insulin receptors on adipocyte and placenta membranes by the use of reducing and oxidizing agents. Neither DTT
nor oxidized glutathione had a significant effect on [^{125}I]insulin binding to liver membranes. This contrasts to the changes in affinity profiles seen in both adipocyte and placenta receptors caused by DTT.
The organization pattern of Fm-I on liver membranes was unaltered by
either DTT or oxidized glutathione in contrast to the findings reported
above for the adipocyte.

D. 3T3-L1 Adipocytes

After treatment with dexamethasone and isobutylmethylxanthine, murine 3T3-L1 fibroblasts differentiate into cells (3T3-L1 adipocytes) that exhibit many of the morphological and biochemical properties of adipocytes. Various factors have been shown to regulate the number and affinity of the insulin receptors on these cells. The 3T3-L1 adipocytes have been a useful model for studies of insulin binding and internalization using both biochemical and morphological techniques. The initial distribution of Fm-I receptors was determined in a recent series of studies in collaboration with Drs. M. Cobb and O. Rosen. The 3T3-L1 adipocytes were fixed with 0.1% glutaraldehyde for 5 min at 24°C and washed with 50 mM Tris-HCl, pH 7.4, in 0.9% NaCl. The cells were resuspended in Krebs-Ringer phosphate buffer, pH 7.4, with 3% bovine serum albumin. Both fixed and unfixed cells were incubated 30 min at 37°C with 40 ng/ml Fm-I, washed, and prepared for electron microscopy.

Comparison of the Fm-I organization pattern in Figure 5A and B of the fixed and unfixed tissue reveals that substantial microaggregation of occupied insulin receptors occurred. On the fixed cells (Fig. 5A), the majority of Fm-I (indicated with arrows) bound to single dispersed receptor sites and a few small groups of two to three molecules. These receptors were found primarily on the microvillous projections of the cell surface. When unfixed cells (Fig. 5B) were examined, Fm-I was also found in the microvilli, but much larger amounts of Fm-I were found in large groups of six or more receptor sites on the intervillous cell surface and in the numerous pinocytotic invaginations (I) of the plasma membrane, and the coated pits. As will be discussed in the following section, this microaggregation preceeded internalization of the hormone-receptor complex via invaginations and coated pits into cytoplasmic vesicles (V). These observations agree in part with those found using [125I]insulin autoradiography (Fan et al., 1982).

Even though this cell line has many characteristics in common with the adipocyte, it is clear from our studies that the distribution and handling of the insulin receptors have many differences from that found on the adipocyte. The adipocyte has a truly random distribution of insulin receptors; the data on 3T3-L1 adipocyte indicate that the majority of receptors on that cell are initially found on microvilli. The 3T3-L1 adipocyte is capable of aggregating dispersed or small groups of receptors into larger clusters. The groups of insulin receptors on the adipocyte do not aggregate. The receptors on the 3T3-L1 adipocyte apparently migrated from the microvilli and were found on the intervillous membrane and in both pinocytotic invaginations and coated pits. Insulin receptors on the adipocyte did not migrate and were virtually excluded from coated pits. The concentration

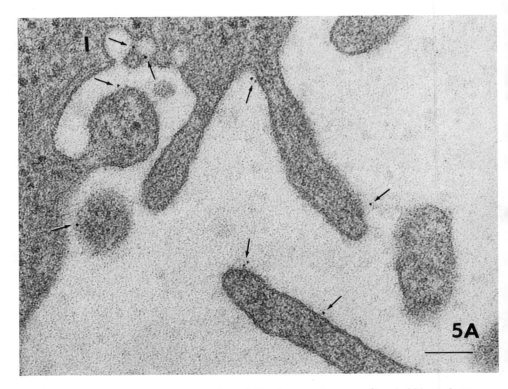

Figure 5 Electron micrographs of Fm-I receptors on fixed (A) and unfixed (B) 3T3-L1 adipocytes. Bar = 0.1 μm. Arrows indicate Fm-I
bound. I, pinocytotic invagination; V, cytoplasmic vesicle.

of Fm-I receptors in the invaginations and coated pits of the 3T3-L1
indicated that a cell-induced concentrative endocytotic process had
occurred, whereas the adipocyte did not concentrate the Fm-I receptors prior to endocytosis. The uptake process in the adipocyte and
3T3-L1 have distinct differences as will be discussed in more detail
below.

E. IM-9 Lymphocytes

Insulin-binding characteristics of the cultured human IM-9 lymphocyte
have been extensively studied in many laboratories. While it is generally agreed that these cells have no insulin-mediated cellular responses, much of our current knowledge about insulin receptor molecular structure, binding kinetics, down-regulation, and negative

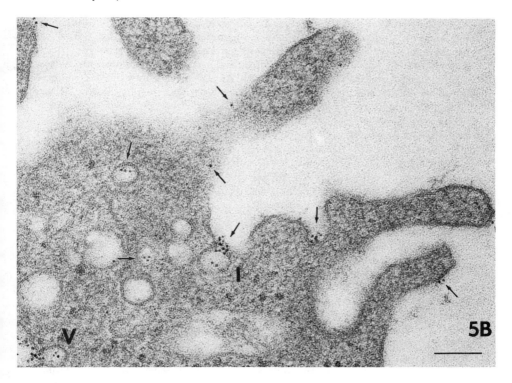

cooperativity was obtained from studies using the IM-9 lymphocyte.
Biochemical and morphological studies in our laboratory were designed
to document the initial and subsequent distribution of insulin receptors on the cell and to determine whether insulin was internalized by
the IM-9 lymphocyte. Conflicting reports have been published concerning the uptake phenomenon. Biochemical studies have suggested
that internalization of insulin was minimal in the IM-9 cell (Sonne and
Gliemann, 1980; Marshall and Olefsky, 1979; Olefsky and Kao, 1982),
that the insulin receptor was shed (Gavin et al., 1972), and that insulin degradation occurred extracellularly (Berhanu and Olefsky, 1982).
In contrast, evidence from morphological studies showed that internalization of [^{125}I]insulin occurred after prolonged incubation at 37°C
with localization of autoradiographic grains in the Golgi area of the
cell (Carpentier et al., 1981). Other studies (Goldfine et al., 1976,
1977, 1978) showed insulin was internalized and concentrated in the
endoplasmic reticulum and nuclei of the IM-9 lymphocyte. Our studies
hoped to resolve these differences.

The initial distribution of Fm-I receptors on the IM-9 lymphocyte,
as shown on fixed cells, was essentially the same as observed on the

3T3-L1 adipocyte. The majority of occupied receptors were found on the microvillous projections of the cell surface and were primarily single receptor sites with a few small groups of two to three receptor molecules. Fewer receptors were found on the intermicrovillous cell surface than on the microvilli. When the IM-9 lymphocytes were incubated at 15°C (the temperature at which most biochemical studies have been performed and where specific binding is most pronounced), little or no change in receptor distribution was found over a 60 min time period. Most of the receptors were located on the microvilli after 60 min, and the size of the groups had not changed. When the cells were incubated for 2 hr at 37°C (a temperature that has been reported to increase nonspecific and total insulin binding but decrease calculated specific binding), the Fm-I was found in large aggregates in electron-dense material that was often entirely removed from the cell surface. These Fm-I particles represented 70 to 90% of the total Fm-I observed and were not displaced by excess unlabeled insulin. The remainder of the Fm-I receptors were found as single molecules and groups of two to six Fm-I particles on all portions of the cell, including the microvilli. The Fm-I on these receptors was displaced by excess insulin. These data suggest that the specific receptors for Fm-I are initially limited to the microvilli and, after occupancy by the hormone, aggregate on the microvilli; some receptors move laterally to the cell surface. A high percentage of the Fm-I "receptor" sites appeared to be sloughed from the cell surface. This fraction was seen as the aggregated, nonspecifically bound, Fm-I in the electron-dense material loosely attached to the cell or separated entirely from it. This material contributed substantially to the total amount of Fm-I molecules, which were internalized by the IM-9 lymphocyte as will be shown in the next section of this chapter. The studies to date have not been able to determine whether the sloughing process is due to receptor occupancy or whether it occurs in the absence of insulin at 37°C. Biochemical studies of [^{125}I]insulin binding would suggest that sloughing occurs at a basal rate of 37°C but that insulin occupancy may accelerate the sloughing, leading to the well-known observations of insulin receptor down-regulation (Gavin et al., 1974). These phenomena will be the subject of further morphological investigations.

F. H4(IIEC3) Cultured Hepatoma Cells

This cell line was chosen because of its reported ability to bind and internalize [^{125}I]insulin (Terris et al., 1979; Hofmann et al., 1980) and because our initial observations revealed that the cell contained little if any endogenous ferritin. The lack of endogenous ferritin would permit studies of insulin uptake to be performed. Using the same types of protocols as with the previous cells, the initial distribution of insulin receptors was found to be similar to the IM-9 lymphocyte and 3T3-L1 adipocyte. Most of the receptor sites were single molecules or small groups of two to four receptor sites primarily localized on the microvilli of the cell surface. On fixed cells, only a small percentage of the Fm-I particles were found on the nonvillous surface, and most of these were found as dispersed receptors. When unfixed cells were incubated at 37°C, within 5−10 min, most of the receptors were found in clusters of up to ten Fm-I particles primarily on the nonvillous portions of the cell, although the microvilli still had single and small groups of receptor sites. Our observation with the cultured hepatoma cell was almost identical to that found in the cultured 3T3-L1 adipocyte, but entirely different than on the isolated liver plasma membranes. The observation that microaggregation and migration of the occupied insulin receptor sites occurred on the cultured hepatocyte raised the possibility that the same phenomena would occur on the intact hepatocyte. Migration and microaggregation may not have been observed on the isolated plasma membrane because the mechanisms for generating the signal or responding to the signal to aggregate the receptor sites were missing in the isolated membrane fraction.

G. Summary

Table 3 summarizes the characteristics of insulin receptor distribution found on six cells or tissues that bind insulin. Four cells were found with a nonrandom distribution of insulin receptor. All four of these cells had microvilli, and the initial binding sites appeared on the microvilli. On three of these four cells (3T3-L1 adipocyte, IM-9 lymphocyte, and H4 hepatoma cell), the receptors appeared to aggregate and migrate from the microvilli. On the placenta, the receptors did not migrate. The IM-9 lymphocyte receptors, unlike the hepatoma and 3T3-L1 adipocyte, did not stay closely associated with the cell surface but appeared to slough from the cell. The receptors on the 3T3-L1 adipocytes and H4 hepatoma cell microaggregated into clusters two to five times larger than the initial groups found on the microvilli. While five of the six tissues showed predominantly single and small numbers of grouped receptors initially, the adipocyte had the largest percentage of naturally grouped receptors and the largest number of receptors per group on the fixed cells. The cultured cell lines all had predominantly single receptors, with a small percentage of receptors in small groups of two to three receptors. These data convincingly demonstrated that the distribution of insulin receptors and the dynamic processes involved in receptor migration subsequent to receptor occupancy depend to a large extent on the specific structural and biological uniqueness of the cell type. It also is apparent that no single cell line can be used to define a universal model of insulin receptor dynamics due to these rather significant variations.

Table 3 Initial and Subsequent Distribution of Occupied Insulin Receptors on Various Tissues[a]

Cell type	Initial receptor distribution		Subsequent receptor distribution	
	Localization	Primary organization	Localization	Organization
Adipocyte	Random	Groups >> singles	No change	No change
Placenta	Nonrandom; microvilli	Groups > singles	No change	No change
Liver plasma membrane	Random	Singles >> groups	No change	No change
3T3-L1 adipocyte	Nonrandom; microvilli	Singles > groups	Nonrandom; relocated to cell surface, invaginations and coated pits	Clusters > groups > singles
IM-9 lymphocyte	Nonrandom; microvilli	Singles > groups	Nonrandom; relocated to extracellular material, cell surface and invaginations	Aggregates > groups > singles
H4(IIEC3) hepatoma cell	Nonrandom; microvilli	Singles > groups	Nonrandom; relocated to cell surface, invaginations and coated pits	Clusters > groups > singles

[a]Based on observations of Fm-I receptors on these tissues under a variety of incubation conditions including the use of fixed tissue, to determine the initial distribution of insulin receptors. The details are discussed in the text. For the purpose of this table we have arbitrarily defined various sizes of receptor groups as follows: singles, 1 receptor; groups, 2–6 receptors per group; clusters, 6–12 receptors per group; aggregates, greater than 12 receptors per group.

III. INSULIN AND INSULIN RECEPTOR UPTAKE, PROCESSING, AND RECYCLING

Until recently, there was little direct evidence that insulin was internalized, and in some cases such a prospect was entirely discounted.
It is now apparent from both biochemical and morphological analysis
that many cells that bind insulin have processes for internalizing the
hormone-receptor complex. In other cells, notably the IM-9 lymphocyte, the question of internalization is still disputed. The biochemical
aspects of hormone-receptor internalization are dealt with in some detail in other chapters. Our laboratory has performed combined morphological and biochemical studies directed at answering several questions: (a) Does a particular cell type internalize the insulin receptor
complex? (b) If so, is the process random or does internalization occur via concentrative endocytosis? (c) What structures on the cell
membrane are associated with the internalization? (d) What intracellular structures receive and presumably process the complex? (e) To
what extent does the insulin-receptor complex recycle to the cell membrane?

The Fm-I particle is used to localize insulin molecules precisely on
the cell surface and in intracellular structures. We presume that under specific conditions the Fm-I molecule will also demonstrate the location of the insulin receptor. The Fm-I particle, when bound to the
insulin receptor is found within the glycocalyx, 75 to 100 Å from the
membrane bilayer. This orientation is preserved when Fm-I is found
in invaginations, coated pits, cytoplasmic smooth or coated vesicles,
and, in some cases, multivesicular bodies. When the distance between
the Fm-I particle and the membrane structure is less than 100 Å, the
hormone-receptor complex is probably intact. When the Fm-I dissociates from the receptor, and the distance between the membrane and
ferritin particle exceeds 100 Å, the fate of the insulin receptor cannot
be followed. The hormone can still be traced unless it becomes degraded. In lysosomes, where insulin dissociates from its receptor and
is probably degraded, the ferritin molecule is also degraded and is no
longer visible as a discrete particle. Our analyses using Fm-I can determine the location of binding, mode, and sites of internalization and
recycling and the point of degradation of the intact hormone and possibly the hormone-receptor complex. Other techniques will be required
to follow the degradation or possible recycling of the unoccupied insulin
receptor.

A. Uptake and Recycling on Intact Adipocytes

Studies were initially performed with Fm-I concentrations that required
about 5 min to reach steady-state binding to the adipocyte plasma membrane. While it was evident from these experiments that insulin was

rapidly taken up by cells, we were unable to do quantitative analysis of the uptake process. Since pulse-chase types of experiments were impractical due to the rapid and virtually complete dissociation of insulin from its receptor on the cell surface, experiments were performed with very high concentrations (200—400 ng/ml) of Fm-I (Smith and Jarett, 1983). This concentration of ligand saturated the plasma membrane receptors within 1 min at 37°C. The experimental conditions for these studies included fixed cells incubated for 30 min and unfixed cells incubated for 2 to 90 min at 37°C. The concentration of Fm-I receptors per square micrometer and the organization of receptors into groups of various sizes was determined on various membrane components and intracellular structures.

Analysis of receptor concentration was performed by determining the total number of Fm-I particles in various cellular organelles, i.e., invaginations, cytoplasmic vesicles, and lysosomes, and on the plasma membrane of the cell at each time point. The details of the method of analysis are described elsewhere (Smith and Jarett, 1982b, 1983). Briefly, since the concentration of receptors remained constant on the plasma membrane during the time course (see below and Table 4), the number of Fm-I particles observed on the plasma membrane in a set of electron micrographs was used to standardize the data and allow

Table 4 Concentration of Occupied Fm-1 Receptors on Rat Adipocyte Plasma Membrane, Pinocytotic Invaginations, and Coated Pits as a Result of Incubation Time[a]

	Receptors/μm^2		
Time (min)	Plasma membrane	Invaginations	Coated pits
Fixed tissue	25.3	13.6	1.1
5	24.5	20.6	1.5
10	26.7	24.8	1.2
30	25.7	26.2	1.6
90	27.8	26.8	1.5

[a]Adipocytes were fixed with 0.1% glutaraldehyde, washed with 50 mM Tris-HCl, pH 7.4, in 0.9% NaCl and incubated with 200 ng/ml Fm-I for 30 min at 37°C. Fresh, or unfixed, rat adipocytes were incubated for 5 to 90 min at 37°C. The cells were washed and prepared for electron microscopy. At least 100 high-magnification micrographs were taken of Fm-I receptor sites at randomly selected portions of the cell surface. Receptor concentration was calculated as in Table 1.

a direct comparison between the amount of Fm-I in one organelle (relative to the plasma membrane) to the amount of another organelle.

The first observation was that the number of receptors per group on the plasma membrane did not increase during the time courses studied. This reconfirmed that microaggregation of the receptors was not occurring. The entire plasma membrane was divided into three structural components, pinocytotic invaginations, coated pits, and the remainder of the membrane. An analysis of the concentration of receptor sites per square micrometer of each of these membrane segments is shown in Table 4. The concentration of receptors remained stable over the 90-min incubation period on the plasma membrane area. The concentration of insulin receptors in the coated pits, whose surface area accounted for less than 0.3% of the total cell surface area, had a Fm-I concentration that was about 5% of that found on the rest of the plasma membrane (1.3 versus 25.7 receptors/μm^2, respectively). It was also noted that the concentration of Fm-I molecules associated with the coated pits did not increase with time. These data are convincing evidence that coated pits, at the very best, had only a minor role in internalizing receptor-bound insulin since very few coated pits existed and they did not concentrate insulin receptors. In fact, coated pits appear to exclude the insulin receptor in comparison to the concentration of receptor sites found on the rest of the plasma membrane. The concentration of receptors in the pinocytotic invaginations increased with time until the concentration reached a level equal to, but not greater than, that found on the plasma membrane. The data that showed this increase were the result of a larger percentage of the invaginations at later time points containing at least one Fm-I particle. This suggested that the Fm-I receptors were not being aggregated and concentrated in the invaginations by a cell-induced, time-dependent migration of the receptors. Instead, the data suggest that recycling of the invaginations and the Fm-I receptor complex from an intracellular pool was occurring. This is more fully explained and supported by additional data below. The relative concentration of receptor sites on all portions of the adipocyte plasma membrane, the absence of an increase in the size of the groups of receptor sites, and the lack of a higher concentration of receptor sites in the pinocytotic invaginations are consistent with a random uptake process rather than a migratory and concentrative cell-induced response to receptor occupancy. The pinocytotic invaginations, which constitute about 17% of the total surface area of the cell, were the primary and virtually sole route of insulin uptake in the adipocyte.

Quantitative determinations showed that by 5 min about 16% of the membrane associated Fm-I was found in invaginations. These structures rapidly pinched off to form cytoplasmic vesicles. In Figure 6, it can be seen that substantial amounts of Fm-I were found in the cytoplasmic vesicles by 2 min and equilibrium had been reached by 10—15 min. About 10—12% of the membrane-associated insulin was found in the

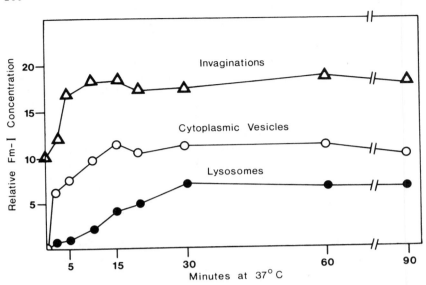

Figure 6 Time course of Fm-I uptake in rat adipocytes.

cytoplasmic vesicles. The invaginations contained substantially more Fm-I than the vesicles. There are several possible explanations for this finding. It is possible that some degradation of the Fm-I might occur in the vesicles, which would make the ferritin molecule undetectable. This seems unlikely but it cannot be ruled out. If the number of endocytotic invaginations were overestimated, then the amount of Fm-I reportedly being endocytosed also would be overestimated. We believe this is a very likely possibility. It is currently impossible to tell the difference between an endocytotic and an exocytotic invagination. If, in fact, a substantial proportion of the invaginations are exocytotic, then the time curve that showed an increase in the Fm-I concentration in the invaginations and the excess amount of Fm-I in the invaginations relative to the vesicles could be accounted for by exocytotic recycling of vesicles, invaginations and Fm-I to the cell surface. As stated earlier the increase with time in the percentage of invaginations that contained Fm-I supports the concept of internalization of Fm-I in endocytotic invaginations and the time-dependent recycling of Fm-I by morphologically similar exocytotic structures to the cell surface. After 10 to 15 min at 37°C, about 7% of the Fm-I appears in multivesicular bodies or lysosomelike structures within the cytoplasm. Again the discrepancy between the amount of Fm-I found in the lysosomes and the cytoplasmic vesicles has at least two explanations. In this case, however, degradation of the Fm-I is a viable and contributing cause, along with recycling of some of the Fm-I in the

vesicles to the cell surface. Recycling or exocytosis of intact insulin
from adipocytes has been shown by biochemical [^{125}I]insulin studies
(Olefsky et al., 1982). The time course and relative amounts of insulin being internalized, recycled, and degraded were virtually identical in both the ultrastructural and biochemical studies.

One of the most commonly used agents to study insulin uptake is
the lysosomatotropic agent chloroquine. This agent has been shown
to increase cell-associated insulin in adipocytes (Hammons and Jarett,
1980; Marshall and Olefsky, 1979), presumably by preventing lysosomal
degradation of the hormone that, in turn, results in an increase in the
intralysosomal concentration of the hormone. Studies were designed to
document the effect of chloroquine on the insulin-receptor uptake process in adipocytes (Smith and Jarett, 1982b). Chloroquine had no effect on the amount or distribution of Fm-I binding to the adipocyte
plasma membrane or its components. Nor did chloroquine affect the
time course of Fm-I association with the membrane or cytoplasmic vesicles. Quantitative analysis of the Fm-I in the lysosomes revealed that
the amount of Fm-I increased in a time-dependent manner (Fig. 7) as
compared to the control, which reached a steady state within 30 min.
However, the effects of chloroquine were not simply explained by an
apparent inhibition of degradation within the lysosomes. Morphological

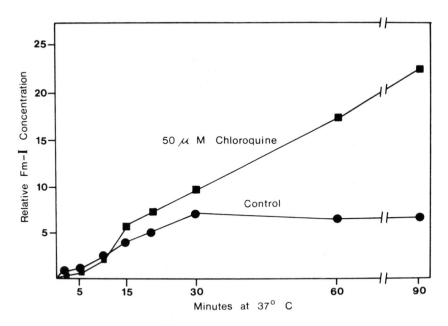

Figure 7 The effect or 50 μm chloroquine on Fm-I uptake into rat
adipocyte lysosomes.

comparison of control and chloroquine-treated adipocytes showed that
chloroquine had pronounced effects on the cell's ultrastructure. These
effects included a significant 50% increase in the number of multivesicular bodies and a 120% increase in the number of lysosomes. When
these two structures were examined separately, and the concentrations
of Fm-I in each type of structure were compared to the control, it was
found that chloroquine had virtually no effect on the number of Fm-I
particles per multivesicular body. At the same time chloroquine caused
significant increases in the percentage of lysosomes with detectable
Fm-I and in the concentration of Fm-I per lysosome. It has, therefore, been determined that chloroquine had two effects that in combination result in a marked increase in the intracellular concentration
of insulin. Chloroquine apparently inhibited membrane fusion or lysosomal cycling, resulting in an increase in the number of multivesicular bodies and lysosomes. In addition there was an inhibition of proteolysis that results in an increase in the amount of insulin trapped in
the lysosomes. These data suggested that little if any chloroquine-
sensitive degradation occurred in cytoplasmic vesicles or multivesicular
bodies, which adds further to the evidence that recycling, rather than
degradation of Fm-I, was responsible for the difference in the amounts
of Fm-I bound in the invaginations, vesicles, and lysosomes.

In summary, adipocytes internalized approximately 10—15% of the
membrane-associated hormone-receptor complex almost exclusively in
smooth pinocytotic invaginations in a random, nonconcentrative manner.
Coated pits were not involved. The uptake process began immediately
and reached equilibrium quickly. Approximately half of the internalized
insulin was transported through smooth vesicles to multivesicular bodies
and subsequently to lysosomes where the hormone was degraded; the
other half of the insulin was recycled in the smooth vesicles to the cell
surface as intact hormone.

B. Uptake in 3T3-L1 Adipocytes, H4(IIEC3) Cultured Hepatoma Cells, and IM-9 Lymphocytes

In an attempt to further our knowledge of the specialization and variation among cell types in their mechanisms for processing occupied insulin receptors, we have extended our ultrastructural studies to several cell lines in addition to the adipocyte. The nature of these studies
is such that the acquisition of quantitative data is extremely time-
consuming, and, at the time this chapter was prepared, only qualitative
data were available. However, these qualitative data allow the determination of the structural elements involved in the endocytotic process.

When 3T3-L1 adipocytes were incubated at 37°C, there appeared
to be a rapid migration of insulin receptors from the microvilli toward
the intervillous cell surface and microaggregation of the single receptors and small groups of 2—3 receptors into clusters of up to 12 Fm-I

molecules. These clusters of receptors were found both on planar portions of the plasma membrane and in smooth pinocytotic invaginations and coated pits. The invaginations appeared to contribute more to the endocytosis of Fm-I than did coated pits, primarily because the latter were less frequently observed. Both the pinocytotic invaginations and the coated pits contained a higher concentration of Fm-I occupied receptors per square micrometer after 5 min of incubation than did the plasma membrane, which suggested that presence of a cell-induced concentrative endocytotic process. This observation differs from that seen with adipocytes. On the 3T3-L1 adipocyte, Fm-I has been found in multivesicular bodies, lysosomelike structures, and cytoplasmic vesicles resembling Golgi, within 5 to 15 min at 37°C. On the basis of currently available data, it is not possible to determine whether these intracellular locations represent a series of organelles along a single processing pathway or if more than one pathway exists. More detailed analysis will hopefully resolve this issue. In the absence of quantitative analyses the possibility of hormone-receptor recycling cannot be addressed.

The 3T3-L1 adipocytes treated with 100 μm chloroquine demonstrated the same morphological alterations as did adipocytes, i.e., chloroquine caused an increase in the number of multivesicular bodies and lysosomes. In addition, some swelling of endoplasmic reticulum and apparent Golgi vesicles was noted. Analysis of the number of Fm-I particles suggested that lysosomal accumulation on Fm-I was enhanced in chloroquine-treated 3T3-L1 adipocytes in much the same manner as in the adipocyte.

The Fm-I uptake into H4(IIEC3) cultured hepatoma cells was investigated both biochemically and ultrastructurally. Reports had suggested that insulin was internalized by a chlorquine-sensitive process (Hofmann et al., 1980). However, a later publication suggested that insulin receptor processing did not occur in this cell line (Hofmann et al., 1981). In our studies, chloroquine failed to increase the amount of cellular associated [125I]insulin or inhibit insulin degradation. However, techniques designed to remove membrane-associated [125I]insulin, including acid washing and trypsin digestion, suggested that the H4 hepatoma cells accumulated intracellular insulin in a time- and temperature-dependent manner.

Ultrastructural studies showed that after the initial binding of Fm-I to single receptors or groups of two to four molecules on the microvilli of the hepatoma cells, the receptors microaggregated and migrated to the intervillous cell surface and formed clusters of up to 12 receptors molecules. These clusters were internalized in both smooth vesicles and coated pits, the former being more predominant in terms of the total insulin uptake. The Fm-I molecules were observed in cytoplasmic vesicles and multivesicular bodies within the first 5 min of incubation. Very few lysosomal structures were observed

in comparison to intact liver or isolated hepatocytes. Few Fm-I particles were seen in the lysosomes that were observed.

Incubation of the H4 hepatoma cells with chloroquine resulted in
swelling of the endoplasmic reticulum and an increase in the size but
not the number of multivesicular bodies. The number of lysosomes
was marginally increased, if at all, but their size increased dramatically. These observations were not the same as were found with chloroquine-treated adipocytes or 3T3-L1 adipocytes, but are essentially the
same as we have found with other liver-derived cells. It was not possible to show an increase in the amount of Fm-I associated with the
multivesicular bodies or the lysosomes. Although this analysis is
preliminary, it does correlate with our biochemical data. It would
appear that the H4(IIEC3) hepatoma cells internalized insulin. However, the majority of the internalized hormone was not taken to the
lysosomes for degradation. Based on published biochemical data, this
would appear to be different from the isolated hepatocytes.

As discussed earlier, there is considerable disagreement about insulin processing by IM-9 lymphocytes. Most biochemical studies have
shown little if any insulin uptake and degradation, but has shown considerable amounts of receptor sloughing and extracellular degradation
of insulin (Sonne and Gliemann, 1980; Marshall and Olefsky, 1979;
Olefsky and Kao, 1982; Gavin et al., 1972). On the other hand,
[125I]insulin autoradiography suggested that insulin was taken up by
cells after prolonged incubation (Carpentier et al., 1978, 1979, 1981;
Goldfine et al., 1976, 1977, 1978). A series of biochemical studies in
our laboratory demonstrated that a majority of the labeled material
taken up into the IM-9 lymphocytes after prolonged incubations at
37°C was the result of covalent binding of 125I-labeled products to a
high molecular weight, extracellular material that was subsequently
endocytosed in a insulin nonspecific and nonsaturable but time- and
temperature-dependent manner.

When IM-9 lymphocytes were incubated with Fm-I at 37°C under
conditions identical to those used in the biochemical studies, we observed a rapid aggregation of Fm-I particles to an electron-dense
material that was often removed from the cell surface. Apparently
internalized Fm-I particles were also attached to the same material inside large membrane-bound structures. Although on all other cell
types we have studied, excess unlabeled insulin prevented Fm-I binding and uptake, the unlabeled hormone did not prevent the aggregated
Fm-I observed on the IM-9 lymphocyte. Biochemical studies had shown
that excess unlabeled insulin did not prevent the internalization of the
125I-labeled high molecular weight material. The combination of the
biochemical and morphological data suggest that insulin binds primarily
to dispersed receptors on the microvilli that subsequently aggregate
and migrate to other areas of cell surface. Some of the insulin-receptor
complexes may be shed from the cell surface. At the same time, large

Table 5 Summary of the Characteristics of the Fm-I Internalization Process in Various Cell Types

Cell type	Concentrative or random endocytosis[a]	Endocytotic structure(s)[a]	Confirmed intracellular localization(s)[a,b]
Rat adipocytes	R	PI	VES, MVB, LYS
3T3-L1 adipocytes	C	PI > CP	VES, MVB, LYS, GOL
IM-9 lymphocytes[c]	C	Phagocytosis >> PI	VES, MVB
H4(IIEC3) cultured hepatoma cells	C	PI > CP	VES, MVB, LYS

[a]R, random endocytosis of dispersed or grouped receptor sites; C, endocytosis of receptors which micro-aggregate and concentrate into endocytotic structures; PI, smooth pinocytotic invaginations; CP, coated pits; VES, smooth or coated cytoplasmic vesicles; MVB, multivesicular bodies within the cytoplasm; LYS, lysosomes; Gol, Golgi.

[b]The presence of Fm-I receptor complexes have been consistently observed in the specified structures. Omission of other structures, e.g., endoplasmic reticulum and nuclei, from the description does not imply that insulin could not be associated with such structures, only that we have not been able to demonstrate such association with a significant degree of reliability.

[c]The IM-9 lymphocytes are a special case where Fm-I appears to be phagocytosed in a nonspecific manner bound to extracellular debris as described in the text. Specific uptake of Fm-I is a small percentage of the total intracellular Fm-I, and its localization is restricted to probable vesicles.

amounts of insulin associate with the high molecular weight material
in the extracellular media, which may or may not be composed of insulin receptors (Saviolakis et al., 1981). This material adsorbs to
the cell membrane or binds to a receptor other than the insulin receptor and is phagocytosed. Only a very small percentage of the Fm-I
seen intracellularly was associated with apparent cytoplasmic vesicles
in a manner similar to that seen on any of the other cells studies, that
is bound in the glycocalyx portion of the membrane. In those limited
instances where this was seen, the vesicles were very close to the
cell surface, raising the possibility that they were not actually vesicles but merely cell surface which, by virtue of its orientation, appeared to be vesicular in nature. These Fm-I particles were entirely displaced with excess unlabeled insulin.

C. Summary

The accumulated evidence clearly demonstrates that a great deal of
diversity exists in the mechanisms involved in the endocytosis and
intracellular processing of insulin. These variations should not, in
retrospect, appear unusual. All types of cells have both common and
specific functions. The former may be described as those functions
that maintain the life of the individual cells (i.e., protein synthesis
and maintenance of required intracellular processes). The unique and
specific functions of cells maintain the metabolism and health of the
entire organism, and, in order to be both efficient and effective, the
individual cells must interact in concert. It would appear reasonable
that all insulin-responsive cells would share some common features,
such as the molecular structure of the insulin receptor and binding
affinity. On the other hand, the specialized functions of individual
cells, such as glucose metabolism, synthesis of proteins for exocytosis, and degradation or utilization of circulating hormones, nutrients,
and other substances could result in specialized structural or biochemical adaptations. Our data have shown that insulin can bind to specific
receptors that have unique organizations within the membrane on different cells. The cell, depending on its structure and function, in-
ternalizes and processes the insulin and the insulin-receptor complex
in a variety of manners. Table 5 presents some of the variations
observed.

IV. Conclusions and Comments

In this chapter, we have presented data describing the binding of insulin to several cell types, and we have tried to focus on one aspect
of the morphological investigation of insulin-receptor dynamics: variability in the binding and processing of insulin by different target

tissues. By comparing the ultrastructural characteristics of insulin binding and processing in different cells using identical morphological and analytical methods, the evidence presented demonstrates that variations in the native distribution of insulin receptors and microaggregation, internalization, and processing of the insulin-receptor complex are apparently the result of structural and functional specificities of individual cell types. A comprehensive review of the morphological studies of insulin binding and internalization is beyond the scope of this chapter. Several recent reviews of this subject have been published (Goldfine et al., 1981; Gorden et al., 1980). Those reviews have revealed a number of apparent inconsistencies. A review of the studies of other ligands, such as epidermal growth factor, thrombin, α-2-macroglobulin, and low-density lipoprotein, to name but a few, would demonstrate similar degrees of variability. In most instances, the studies that came to substantially different conclusions with identical ligands used different types of cells. There are also instances where the binding and internalization of different receptors on a single type of cell has been studied with unique and specific patterns of receptor distribution, microaggregation, internalization, and processing for a particular ligand-receptor complex being shown. The ultrastructural study of receptors is a relatively new field. Yet the well-established area of biochemical analysis of ligand binding and processing has demonstrated that unique characteristics exist when detailed comparisons are made. The observations of these differences, whether they be between similar ligands on different cells or different ligands on the same cell, and whether the differences are determined by morphological or biochemical methods, lead to several possible conclusions. If technical errors, inappropriate experimental design, and overinterprepation of insufficient data are eliminated as reasons for the variabilities, one must conclude that the biological process itself must contain a certain degree of variability depending on the extent of specialization of the cell type. These biological variations, while of great value to the well-being of complex organisms, add to the difficulty in determining the "normal condition" by extrapolating the data from one presumably normal tissue and applying to it another. It is appropriate, therefore, that independent investigations continue in a widely diversified manner in the anticipation that such an approach will eventually lead to the recognition of the ultrastructural and/or biochemical abnormalities that are manifested in the diabetic state. While it was our original hope, and that of other investigators as well, to find a model system that would describe the normal condition that would vary dramatically from the diseased state, it would appear that the unitary "normal" model will not be found.

REFERENCES

Berhanu, P. and Olefsky, J. M. (1982). *Diabetes* 31:410.

Carpentier, J.-L., Gorden, P., Amherdt, M., Van Obberghen, E., Kahn, R. C., and Orci, L. (1978). *J. Clin. Invest.* 61:1057.

Carpentier, J.-L., Gorden, P., Freychet, P., LeCam, A. and Orci, L. (1979). *J. Clin. Invest.* 63:1249.

Carpentier, J.-L., Van Obberghen, E., Gorden, P., and Orci, L. (1981). *Exp. Cell Res.* 134:81.

Fan, J. Y., Carpentier, J.-L., Gorden, P., Van Obberghen, E., Blackett, N. M., Grunfeld, C., and Orci, L. (1982). *Proc. Natl. Acad. Sci. USA* 79:7788.

Gavin, J. R., III, Buell, D. N., and Roth, J. (1972). *Science* 178:168.

Gavin, J. R., III, Roth, J., Neville, D. M., Jr., DeMeyts, P., and Buell, D. N. (1974). *Proc. Natl. Acad. Sci. USA* 71:84.

Gershon, N. D., Smith, R. M., and Jarett, L. (1981). *J. Memb. Biol.* 58:155.

Goldfine, I. D. and Smith, G. J. (1976). *Proc. Natl. Acad. Sci. USA* 73:1427.

Goldfine, I. D., Smith, G. J., Wong, K. Y., and Jones, A. L. (1977). *Proc. Natl. Acad. Sci. USA* 74:1368.

Goldfine, I. D., Jones, A. L., Hradek, G., Wong, K. Y., and Mooney, J. (1978). *Science* 202:760.

Goldfine, I. D., Jones, A. L., Hradek, G., Kriz, B. M., and Wong, K. Y. (1981). In *Hormones in Normal and Abnormal Human Tissue.* (K. Fotherby and S. B. Pal, eds.). Walter de Gruyter, New York, p. 503.

Gorden, P., Carpentier, J.-L., Freychet, P., and Orci, L. (1980). *J. Histochem. Cytochem.* 28:811.

Hammons, G. T., and Jarett, L. (1980). *Diabetes* 29:475.

Hofmann, C., Marsh, J. W., Miller, B. and Steiner, D. F. (1980). *Diabetes* 29:865.

Hofmann, C., Ji, T. H., Miller, B., and Steiner, D. F. (1981). *J. Supramol. Struct. Cell. Biochem.* 15:1.

Jacobs, S. and Cuatrecasas, P. (1980). *J. Clin. Invest.* 66:1424.

Jarett, L. and Smith, R. M. (1975). *Proc. Natl. Acad. Sci. USA* 72:3526.

Jarett, L. and Smith, R. M. (1977). *J. Supramol. Struct.* 6:45.

Jarett, L. and Smith, R. M. (1979). *J. Clin. Invest.* 63:571.

Jarett, L. and Smith, R. M. (1983). *Proc. Natl. Acad. Sci. USA* 80:1023.

Jarett, L., Schweitzer, J. B., and Smith, R. M. (1980). *Science* 210:1127.

Lyen, K. R., Smith, R. M., and Jarett, L. (1983a). *Diabetes* 32:648.

Lyen, K. R., Smith, R. M., and Jarett, L. (1983b). *J. Receptor Res.* 2:523.

Marshall, S. and Olefsky, J. M. (1979). *J. Biol. Chem.* 254:10153.

Nelson, D. M., Smith, R. M. and Jarett, L. (1978). *Diabetes* 27:530.

Olefsky, J. M. and Kao, M. (1982). *J. Biol. Chem.* 257:8667.

Olefsky, J. M., Marshall, S., Berhanu, P., Saekow, M., Heidenreich, K., and Green, A. (1982). *Metabolism* 31:670.

Saviolakis, G. A., Harrison, L. C., and Roth, J. (1981). *J. Biol. Chem.* 256:4924.

Schweitzer, J. B., Smith, R. M., and Jarett, L. (1980). *Proc. Natl. Acad. Sci. USA* 77:4692.

Shechter, Y., Chang, K., Jacobs, S., and Cuatrecasas, P. (1979). *Proc. Natl. Acad. Sci. USA* 76:2720.

Sonne, O. and Gliemann, J. (1980). *J. Biol. Chem.* 255:7449.

Smith, R. M. and Jarett, L. (1982a). *J. Histochem. Cytochem.* 30:650.

Smith, R. M. and Jarett, L. (1982b). *Proc. Natl. Acad. Sci. USA* 79:7302.

Smith, R. M. and Jarett, L. (1983). *J. Cell Physiol.* 115:199.

Terris, S., Hofmann, C., and Steiner, D. F. (1979). *Can. J. Biochem.* 57:459.

SUGGESTED READING LIST

These selected publications are provided as additional literature that may be of value to the readers of this chapter. They include material specifically dealing with biochemical and morphological studies of insulin receptors, as well as other hormone receptors. Also listed are publications dealing in a more general fashion with cell membrane dynamics, including mobility, endocytosis, and membrane recycling.

D. Andreani, R. DePirro, R. Lauro, J. M. Olefsky and J. Roth, eds. (1981). *Current Views on Insulin Receptors, Proceedings of the Serono Symposia*, Vol. 41. Academic Press, New York.

R. F. Beers, Jr., and E. G. Basset, eds. (1976). *Cell Membrane Receptors for Viruses, Antigens and Antibodies, Polypeptide Hormones, and Small Molecules*. Raven Press, New York.

Besterman, J. M. and Low, R. B. (1973). Endocytosis: a review of mechanisms and plasma membrane dynamics. *Biochem. J.* 210:1–13.

R. A. Bradshaw, W. A. Frazier, R. C. Merrel, D. I. Gottlieb, and R. A. Hogue-Angeletti, eds. (1976). *Surface Membrane Receptors*. Plenum Press, New York.

J. L. Middlebrook and L. D. Kohn, eds. (1981). *Receptor-Mediated Binding and Internalization of Toxins and Hormones*. Academic Press, New York.

Schlessinger, J. (1980). The mechanism and role of hormone-induced clustering of membrane receptors. *Trends. Biochem. Sci.* 5:210–214.

8

Membrane Polarization and Insulin Action

KENNETH ZIERLER *The Johns Hopkins University School of Medicine, Baltimore, Maryland*

I. INTRODUCTION

In 1957, I found that insulin increased the electrical potential difference between the Krebs-Ringer solution bathing rat extensor digitorum longus (EDL) muscles and the aqueous phase in the interior of muscle fibers (Zierler, 1957). An increase in electrical potential difference across a cell membrane is called hyperpolarization.

Insulin hyperpolarizes rat skeletal muscle. We have observed it in EDL (Zierler, 1959a,b; Hazlewood and Zierler, 1967) and in caudofemoralis (Zierler and Rogus, 1981a,b), as well as in other rat muscles. Clausen and colleagues have reported insulin-induced hyperpolarization in rat soleus (Flatman and Clausen, 1979), Otsuka and Ohtusuki (1965), Bolte and Lüderitz (1968), and Takamori et al. (1981), in rat diaphragm, and Zemkova et al. (1982) in mouse diaphragm. De Mello (1967) and Moore and Rabovsky (1979) found insulin-induced hyperpolarization in frog sartorius muscle. Insulin-induced hyperpolarization has also been reported in canine heart muscle in situ (LaManna and Ferrier, 1981) and in cultured chick myocardial cells (Lantz et al., 1980). Beigelman and Hollander (1962) first reported insulin-induced hyperpolarization in epididymal fat pads.

All of the above measurements were made with electrodes sensing the difference between an intracellular electrode and an extracellular reference electrode. By other means of estimating membrane potential, two groups reported insulin-induced hyperpolarization of adipocytes isolated from fat pads and suspended in a Krebs-Ringer solution (Petrozzo and Zierler, 1976; Cheng et al., 1981; Davis et al., 1981).

In addition, insulin has been reported to hyperpolarize toad bladder (Crabbé, 1969), rat gastric mucosa (Rehm et al., 1961), toad colon mucosa (Crabbé, 1969), rabbit ciliary epithelium (Miller and Constant, 1960), and pancreatic β cells (Pace et al., 1977).

Insulin does not hyperpolarize hepatocytes. Friedmann et al. (1971) reported that insulin prevented liver cell hyperpolarization that glucagon would have produced in the absence of insulin. Wondergem (1983) has more recently reported that insulin depolarizes liver.

Williams et al. (1982) reported that insulin does not hyperpolarize pancreatic acinar cells, although it increases glucose uptake in those cells.

There have been three apparently contrary reports that insulin does not hyperpolarize tissues in which others have found hyperpolarization. In none of these reports was it demonstrated that the insulin used was biologically active on the tissues studied under the circumstance of its use. These include reports by Malinow (1958) on isolated rat papillary muscle and by Stark and O'Doherty (1980) and Stark et al. (1982) on rat fat pad and rat soleus muscle. In these two reports there were also obvious errors in technique and in experimental design.

II. WHAT IS A MEMBRANE POTENTIAL AND HOW IS IT MEASURED?

A. Definitions

For convenience, I shall, as is the custom, refer to the difference in electrical potential between the two aqueous phases, separated by the complex cell membranes, as the membrane potential (Fig. 1). In excitable cells, nerve, and muscle, it is essential to normal function that the membrane potential be altered by a more or less abrupt decrease in the electrical potential difference between the two phases. The complicated, relatively rapid pattern over which the membrane potential moves from its basal state and returns to that state is designated the action potential. The basal state potential in excitable cells is the resting membrane potential, ψ_m, and it is this with which we are concerned. (In nonexcitable cells, such as adipocytes, there is no action potential, and it is gratuitous to refer to adipocyte potentials as resting, since they do not seem to have the ability to have action potentials.)

When there is a nonzero membrane potential, we say that the membrane is polarized, meaning that it is electrically polarized, tending to accumulate electrical charges of opposite sign at the interfaces between membrane and aqueous phase. For the observed resting membrane potential, the interior aqueous phase is considered, arbitrarily, electrically negative with respect to the exterior phase. When the magnitude of electrical potential difference is increased, the degree of

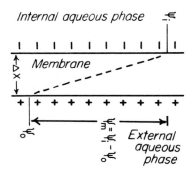

Figure 1 The difference in electrical potential between the aqueous phase inside a cell and the aqueous phase outside it. Neither absolute electrical potential is measured, only the difference between them. Electrical charges are separated across the cell membrane; the interface between membrane and internal aqueous phase is negatively charged and that between membrane and external aqueous phase is positively charged.

polarization is increased. The membrane is said to be hyperpolarized; the interior becomes more negative with respect to the exterior aqueous phase.

B. Methods

Direct electrical measurements are made by impaling a cell (or a cluster of cells in the case of cultured chick myocardium) with a glass pipette called an intracellular electrode. The pipette, drawn to a tip with an inner diameter of a few tenths of a micrometer, is filled with 2 or 3 M KCl or potassium acetate, which serves to conduct from the interior of the cell to a poorly polarizable Ag-AgCl electrode. A reference electrode is in the exterior aqueous phase. The potential difference between the two electrodes is led to an electrometer and displayed or recorded.

Other methods have been used to estimate membrane potentials, particularly in cells that are difficult to impale with microelectrodes, either because they are free floating, such as erythrocytes or suspensions of adipocytes prepared by collagenase digestion of fat pads, or because they are very small or fragile. These methods depend on the use of a substance having some measurable property sensitive to an electrical field or to an electrical potential difference between two aqueous phases. The two most widely used types are (a) ions whose equilibrium distribution between internal and external aqueous phases depends only on the electrical potential difference (i.e., there are no pumps for the substance, operating in addition to the thermodynamic equilibrium potential) and (b) fluorescent dyes whose signal is voltage dependent either because they fall in the same class as ions in group (a) above or because the fluorescence quantum yield is, in ways not well understood, dependent on either electrical fields or membrane surface charges. Substances in this latter category, such as merocyanine dyes, can follow the rapid time course of muscle action potentials, of the order of milliseconds, whereas substances in the former category, such as cyanine dyes, require as much time as is necessary (of the order of minutes or tens of minutes) to equilibrate in the two aqueous phases on either side of the membrane.

The ions used to estimate membrane potential, in addition to the fluorescent ions, are usually protected by relatively large nonpolar portions of the molecule to facilitate solubility in and "diffusion" through the lipid phase of the cell membrane. Both cations and anions have been used, but cations are preferable because the direction of the electrical difference is such that cations that are distributed only in accordance with the electrical potential (i.e., have zero electrochemical potential difference at equilibrium) are concentrated inside the cell, in accordance with the Nernst equation for monovalent ions.

$$E_N = - (RT/F) \ln [(c^+)_i/(c^+)_o] \tag{1}$$

where E_N is the Nernst potential (the electrical potential difference at zero electrochemical potential difference) of the solute molecule. R is the gas constant, T the temperature, F the Faraday's constant, ln the natural logarithm, and (c^+) the activity of the cation. The subscript i or o refers to inside or outside of cell, respectively. It is assumed that, because there is no active transport for these test ions, the Nernst potential for that ion is the membrane potential, ψ_m. It is, of course, not the ratio of activities of the test ion that causes the membrane potential, but the other way around, it is ψ_m that determines the ratio of activities, if all assumptions are met. With E_N set at ψ_m, raising both sides of Equation (1) to powers of the base of natural logarithms, we find

$$(c^+)_o/(c^+)_i = \exp (F\psi_m/RT) \tag{2}$$

Therefore, if one measures the ratio of activities (or of concentrations, assuming that activity coefficients are the same in the two aqueous phases) one can calculate ψ_m. Usually, the test ion is radiolabeled.

There are pitfalls, traps, or violations of underlying assumptions with all methods of estimating ψ_m. Discussion of these problems is beyond the scope of this chapter, but the subject is of major importance. If the measurements were not made properly or if assumptions were violated, the conclusions are best forgotten. It is essential that readers understand the limitations and vulnerabilities of these methods in order to assess reports or carry out experiments. Recommended critiques are by Armstrong and Garcia-Diaz (1981) and Leader (1981).

C. Distribution and Causes of Bioelectrical Potentials

A membrane potential is a property of all cells. In amphibian and mammalian nerve and muscle resting potentials vary from about -70 to -95 mV, inside negative with respect to outside. In inexcitable cells, such as hepatocytes or adipocytes, basal membrane potentials vary from about -40 to -70 mV, the same order of magnitude as those of excitable cells. Electrical field strength is the gradient of electrical potential. If we consider some small element of surface of a cell membrane as a plane and the x direction as that normal to the plane, the electrical field strength at rest or in the basal state is considered to be nonzero only in the x direction, and its sign and magnitude are given by the gradient $d\psi/dx$. The external aqueous phase is isopotential and so is the internal aqueous phase. The electrical potential difference is exerted from the interface between membrane and outer aqueous phase to the interface between membrane and inner aqueous phase. ψ_m of -70 mV through a 70 Å membrane gives a field strength of 100,000 V/cm. This is powerful. When one separates proteins by electrophoresis in the laboratory, one uses field strengths of about 200—600 V/cm, less than 1% of the field strength of biomembrane potentials.

Bioelectricity is static electricity. It is due to spatial separation of charges. This occurs in three general ways:

1. There are surface charges on cell membranes. Although biomembranes have both positive and negative fixed charges, they are predominantly anionic, owing largely to carboxylic groups of surface glycosides. These surface charges have been treated as though they obey the same laws governing a system of a metal electrode in a salt solution. Membrane surface charges command organization of counterions in the aqueous phase. This order dies away exponentially with distance from the interface. The distance at which the counterion charge density is 1/e maximum is about 8 Å for cells in normal buffered salt solutions, such as Krebs-Ringer. These are neither long-range nor strong forces. Roles of cell surface potentials are not well understood. They may be involved in many processes. One of these is likely to deal with interrelation between surface potential and membrane potential. Indeed, it is an old, but still unproven, conjecture that it is a change in surface potential that is responsible for the great increase in Na^+ conductance that initiates action potentials. It is not conceivable that association between insulin and its receptors may alter cell surface charges and so initiate events leading to hyperpolarization.

2. The first of two factors contributing to the membrane potential may be called the diffusion potential, ψ_D. This may be thought of as

the electrical component of the electrochemical potential difference that is caused by separation of ion species in the two aqueous phases. At some time in the development of a cell, an energy-expensive process occurs that pumps Na^+ ions out of the cell and K^+ ions in. For the process under consideration, it makes no difference what the ratio is of number of Na^+ ions out to K^+ ions in. It can be 1:1. What matters is that charges are separated; there is a greater concentration of Na^+ outside than in and a greater concentration of K^+ inside than out. Work had to have been done on the system to achieve these nonunity concentration ratios, and work must continue to maintain them. However, the work on the system not only moved chemical species in such a way as to establish a chemical potential difference for Na between the two aqueous phases and a chemical potential difference for K, but, because Na^+ and K^+ are charged, the work also moved electrical charge setting up an electrical potential difference. When a steady state is reached, there is no net change in concentration of either (or any) ion in either aqueous phase, and there is no net change in distribution of electrical charge, no net ion flow, and no net electrical current across the membrane. The electrochemical potential difference for the system as a whole is zero, although for any given ion species it may not be.

Quantitative expression for the contribution of monovalent ions to the diffusive component of the resting membrane potential is the classic Goldman-Hodgkin-Katz equation (Goldman, 1943; Hodgkin and Katz, 1949).

$$\psi_D = -\frac{RT}{F} \ln \frac{P_K[K^+]_i + P_{Na}[Na^+]_i + P_{Cl}[Cl^-]_o}{P_K[K^+]_o + P_{Na}[Na^+]_o + P_{Cl}[Cl^-]_i} \qquad (3)$$

where P is the permeability coefficient, with dimensions of velocity, for the ion indicated by the subscript. Permeability coefficients are functions of mobility of the given ion through the membrane, "solubility" of the ion in the membrane, and membrane thickness. For amphibian and mammalian skeletal muscle, P_{Cl} is about twice P_K, and P_K is about 30–100 times P_{Na}. An analogue of the contributions of concentration differences and permeabilities (Fig. 2) is a sliding board. Its steepness is concentration gradient. Its width is P_K. Both determine the quantity of matter that can be delivered down it per unit time.

There is no metabolically active Cl^- pump in skeletal muscle, and therefore Cl^- appears to be distributed between the two aqueous phases so that its concentration ratio is the function of membrane potential, ψ_m, given in Equation (2), with the sign reversed to account for the fact that the effect of the electrical field on Cl^- anion is opposite that on the cation of Equation (2). If the membrane potential is due

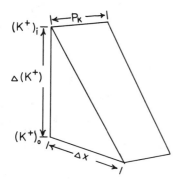

Figure 2 A sliding board, an analogue of a diffusive component of a membrane electrical potential. The quantity of charge, per unit time, in the form of net flow of specified ion, for example, K^+, which a given membrane can permit to have moved across it from one side to the other, depends not only on the concentration gradient of the ion across the membrane, represented by the vector which is the slope and length of sliding board, but also on the permeability of the membrane to that ion, represented by the width of the sliding board.

entirely to the diffusive component, ψ_D, then the equality between E_N for Cl^- and ψ_m means that the Cl^- has no influence on the magnitude of ψ_D, even though P_{Cl} is the largest permeability coefficient. [This is proved by recasting Equation (3) in exponential form and noting that $[Cl^-]_i/[Cl^-]_o = \exp(F\psi_D/RT)$.] This permits simplification of Equation (3) (Hodgkin and Horowicz, 1959) to

$$\psi_D = -\frac{RT}{F} \ln \frac{[K^+]_i + (P_{Na}/P_K)[Na^+]_i}{[K^+]_o + (P_{Na}/P_K)[Na^+]_o} \tag{4}$$

reducing the number of unknowns.

    3. The second of two mechanisms contributing to the membrane potential is an electrogenic pump, and we designate the contribution to the observed membrane potential made by the electrogenic pump as ψ_p. The observed membrane potential is considered the weighted sum of the contributions due to diffusion and to electrogenic pumping,

$$\psi_m = T_D \psi_D + T_p \psi_p \tag{5}$$

where

$$T_D = g_D/(g_D + g_P)$$

and

$$T_P = g_P/(g_D + g_P)$$

the fractions of electrical conductance contributed by current due to the diffusive component and the pump component, respectively.

Electrogenic pumping refers to an energy-expensive ion exchange process in which more ions of a given charge are pumped across the membrane in one direction than in the other. In animal cell membranes, this is a Na^+-K^+ exchange in which more Na^+ is pumped out than K^+ in. There is some uncertainty as to whether the coupling ratio, Na^+_{out}/K^+_{in}, is fixed or modifiable, but in general it seems to be equal to 3/2.

There is no uncertainty that the activity of the pump varies over a great range among different cell types and in the same cell under different conditions. The pump is stimulated by an increase in $[Na^+]_i$. It is inhibited by lowering the temperature, as energy-expensive processes are in general. It is inhibited, relatively specifically, by cardiac glycosides of the digitalis family, particulary strophanthin and ouabain. Dihydroouabain is said to be more specific than ouabain. Advantage has been taken of these inhibitors to study the quantitative contribution of ψ_P to ψ_m.

If one knew exactly how large ψ_D was supposed to be, one could simply measure ψ_m and see if it only equaled ψ_D or exceeded it. However, we do not know how large ψ_D is supposed to be. We can measure ion concentration, but we calculate relative permeabilities P_{Na}/P_K from Equation (4) on the assumption that ψ_D equals the observed ψ_m. It is true that we can measure specific ion electrical conductances, g_{Na} and g_K, that can be reformulated in terms of P_{Na} and P_K, but these measurements require gross changes in ionic composition of bathing solutions that may have other kinds of effects, such as alterations in membrane permeability, membrane surface charge, cell volume and composition, and metabolism.

What is usually done, therefore, is to try to eliminate the contribution of ψ_P in Equation (5) by ouabain or related compounds. Reported experiments of this sort are not all above reproach, when very large concentrations of ouabain are used for a sufficiently long time, there is not only elimination of ψ_P, owing to the desired complete blockade of electrogenic Na : K exchange, but there is time to produce changes in intracellular ionic concentration, increasing $[Na^+]_i$ at the expense of $[K^+]_i$ and so decreasing the absolute magnitude of ψ_D. There is even evidence that P_{Na} may be increased, which further contributes to depolarizing reduction in ψ_D.

Thus, if one is not careful about these possibilities, a ouabain induced reduction in absolute magnitude of observed ψ_m may be due to reduced ψ_D as well as to elimination of ψ_P, and the size of ψ_P prior to exhibition of ouabain will be overestimated. These matters, as well as differences among cell and species types, may account for different reports of estimated ψ_P.

Under conditions in which it is likely that ψ_P is eliminated or at least inhibited by more than 50% and in which intracellular ion concentrations had not yet changed significantly, ouabain does not alter ψ_m of rat caudofemoralis muscle (Zierler and Rogus, 1981b). The likelihood is that in this muscle at 25°C, at rest, ψ_P does not account for more than -1 mV of the approximately -78 mV observed ψ_m. More than 98% of the resting membrane potential in this rat skeletal muscle. at room temperature not at body temperature, is accounted for by the diffusive component expressed quantitatively by Equation (4). Not everyone agrees with this. Moore and Rabovsky (1979) report depolarization by only a few millivolts when frog skeletal muscle is treated with larger doses of ouabain for longer periods, conditions in which ψ_D might also be affected.

There is what appears, in the light of present knowledge, to be an absolute criterion that ψ_P is contributing to ψ_m, although in the absence of this evidence it cannot be said that ψ_P is not contributing. The criterion is this. If observed ψ_m exceeds the maximum theoretical ψ_D in absolute magnitude, then, from Equation (5), there must be a contribution by an electrogenic pump. From Equation (4) we see that for given intra- and extracellular concentration of K^+ and Na^+, ψ_D has its greatest negative value when there is no permeability to Na^+; P_{Na} is zero. Equation (4) then becomes Equation (1), the Nernst potential for K^+.

It is convenient to reexpress Equation (4) in terms of $\log_{10}$ instead of natural logarithms. In that transformation $-(RT/F)\ln x = -2.3(RT/F)\log x$, and, at 25°C, $-2.3\,RT/F$ is approximately -59 mV. Equation (4) becomes, approximately,

$$\psi_D = -59 \log \frac{[K^+]_i + (P_{Na}/P_K)[Na^+]_i}{[K^+]_o + (P_{Na}/P_K)[Na^+]_o} \tag{6}$$

When $P_{Na} = 0$, given $[K^+]_o = 2.5$ mEq/liter for frogs, the ratio $[K^+]_i/[K^+]_o$ is about 40/1 and $\psi_D = -95$ mV, and given $[K^+]_o = 4.8$ mEq/liter for rats, the ratio $[K^+]_i/[K^+]_o$ is about 30/1 and $\psi_D = -88$ mV. Observed ψ_m is frog muscle ranges from about -90 to -95 mV, close to E_N for K^+, but not greater than it, and, in rat muscles, ψ_m ranges from about -75 to -80 mV, somewhat less than predicted for E_N for K^+. Observed values are easily accounted for by assuming $\psi_D = \psi_m$ and assigning a small value to P_{Na}/P_K, usually between 0.01 and 0.05 for skeletal muscle.

III. THE IMMEDIATE MECHANISM OF INSULIN-INDUCED HYPERPOLARIZATION

A. Does Insulin Hyperpolarize by Increasing the Absolute Magnitude of the Electrogenic Pump Component, ψ_P?

Let us first look at evidence for and against insulin stimulation of ψ_P. First, there are no reports that insulin hyperpolarizes to a level in excess of the predicted Nernst potential for K^+, about −95 mV in frogs and −90 mV in rats. There is lacking, therefore, what would be un-equivocal evidence of stimulation of ψ_P.

Second, it is unresolved whether insulin has any effect on the $Na^+–K^+$-activated ATPase that is the molecular basis of the electro-genic pump. We reported no insulin effect on rat skeletal muscle $Na^+–K^+$-ATPase activity (Rogus et al., 1969). Subsequently, in frog muscle, using conditions designed to produce submaximal activity, on the grounds that if assay activity were already "maximum" insulin could not be expected to stimulate it further, Moore (Gavryck et al., 1975) reported insulin stimulation. This seems a reasonable argument. However, unfortunately, under conditions in which Na^+ and K^+ concen-trations in the assay system do not produce maximum activity, one does not know that one is measuring the $Na^+–K^+$-activated ATPase and not some other ATPase that may have no relation to the electro-genic pump. We have duplicated Moore's assay conditions in unpub-lished studies on rat muscle and failed to find insulin stimulation, so that there is a difference between rat and frog muscle in this regard. Erlij and Grinstein (1976) interpret their studies to mean that insulin increases the number of ouabain-binding sites, presumably by increas-ing the available number of $Na^+–K^+$ exchange transporters, that is, by bringing to the surface latent transporters.

Third, there is little doubt that insulin decreases Na^+ content of skeletal muscle if that Na^+ content was previously high or that it pre-vents Na^+ content from increasing under conditions in which, in the absence of insulin, it would increase. Creese (1968) was the first to show this, and reported further than insulin increased efflux of labeled sodium from muscle.

The ratio of passive unidirectional fluxes of a given cation is

$$\frac{M_o}{M_i} = \exp\left(\frac{-(E_N - \psi_m)F}{RT}\right) \tag{7}$$

where M_o is passive efflux and M_i is passive influx of the ion whose Nernst potential is E_N. For an anion, the left-hand side of Equation (7) is inverted. When, as is the case for Cl^-, $E_N = \psi_m$, the ratio (often called the Ussing ratio) is unity.

In the steady state, the concentration of every ion inside the cell is constant. Therefore, total influx (the sum of passive and active influx) must equal total efflux (the sum of passive and active efflux). If passive fluxes are equal, then, in the steady state, there can be no net contribution to flux by an active, energy-expensive mechanism.

In rat skeletal muscle, because E_N for Na^+, which we will write as E_{Na}, and ψ_m are large and of opposite sign, the driving potential for Na^+, $(E_{Na} - \psi_m)$, is very large. $(M_o)_{Na}$ is very small compared to $(M_i)_{Na}$, only ~1/1800. Because total Na^+ efflux must equal total Na^+ influx, the active component of efflux must be nearly the total efflux (about 1799 parts out of 1800).

For K^+, its Nernst potential is only a few millivolts greater (more negative) than ψ_m in frog skeletal muscle and only about 10 mV greater in the rat. $(M_o)_K$ is less than three times $(M_i)_K$ in frog muscle in the steady state at room temperature.

To return to Creese's observation, because Na^+ efflux from muscle is, within about 1 part in 1800, an active process, an increase in Na efflux, accompanied by decreased $[Na^+]_i$ is almost certainly due to stimulation of an active process. This does not require that the increased active Na efflux must be due to stimulation of an electrogenic Na^+-K^+ exchange pump, although it may imply the likelihood.

Fourth, to continue with the evidence for and against insulin stimulation of ψ_P, it is unresolved whether insulin-induced hyperpolarization is prevented or reversed by ouabain under conditions in which the action of ouabain is limited to reducing ψ_P without affecting ψ_D [Equation (4)]. Moore and Rabovsky (1979), in frog muscle, and Flatman and Clausen (1979), in rat soleus muscle, reported ouabain prevention or reversal of insulin-induced hyperpolarization. There is uncertainty about the specificity of the results because the ouabain concentrations were large and the incubation times long, so that unwanted ouabain effects on ψ_D were not ruled out. Furthermore, it is not clear in one case (Flatman and Clausen, 1979) whether the reported change with ouabain was statistically significant because data were analyzed on a per fiber, rather than on a per muscle, basis, a practice that may underestimate standard errors because it uses far too many degrees of freedom. LaManna and Ferrier (1981) did use small concentrations of acetylstrophanthidin on dog and kitten heart muscles, but they did not add insulin "until effects characteristics of digitalis intoxication appears," which took at least 20 min. In dog heart, this included an 11 mV depolarization prior to addition of insulin, so that there may also have been effects on ψ_D.

Fifth, Otsuka and Ohtsuki (1965) in rat diaphragm, Lantz et al. (1980) in cultured chick heart cells, and Zierler and Rogus (1981b) did not find that ouabain prevented insulin-induced hyperpolarization. Our own studies were designed to use ouabain under conditions that did prevent stimulation of the electrogenic pump without altering the diffusive component of membrane potential. We took advantage of the fact that β-adrenergic agonists do stimulate the electrogenic pump in skeletal muscle and do hyperpolarize by that mechanism. A concentration of ouabain exhibited over a long enough time to prevent β-adrenergic stimulus of ψ_P did not prevent insulin-induced hyperpolarization. Ouabain inhibition of β-adrenergic hyperpolarization was concentration-dependent, but there was no effect of ouabain on insulin-induced hyperpolarization over concentration ranges up to ten times greater than that which totally blocked β-adrenergic hyperpolarization.

We concluded that, at least in rat skeletal muscle, insulin does not hyperpolarize by increasing activity of an electrogenic pump.

B. Does Insulin Hyperpolarize by Increasing the Contribution of the Diffusive Component?

We are left with the conclusion that, at least in rat skeletal muscle, insulin hyperpolarizes by increasing the absolute magnitude of the diffusive component ψ_D. How can ψ_D be increased in absolute magnitude?

Equation (4) gives the possibilities, repeated here for ease of pursuit:

$$\psi_D = -\frac{RT}{F} \ln \frac{[K^+]_i + P_{Na}/P_K [Na^+]_i}{[K^+]_o + P_{Na}/P_K [Na^+]_o}$$

The gas constant R and the Faraday are immutable. Raising the temperature will do it, by about 3.7% for 10°C rise, but heat was not the cause of insulin-induced hyperpolarization.

We turn to the logarithmic factor. Anything that (a) increases the numerator or decreases the denominator, (b) increases the numerator more than it increases the denominator, or (c) decreases the denominator more than it decreases the numerator will increase ψ_D.

Could any of these be accomplished by some insulin-induced alteration of ion concentration? It has been known for more than 50 years that insulin, administered to an animal, not only reduces blood glucose concentration but also reduces serum K concentration. Clearly, this could cause hyperpolarization. In mammals, the total amount of K^+ in extracellular fluid is only about 2% of total body K^+. Insulin causes a net shift of K^+ from extracellular fluid to intracellular fluid of insulin-sensitive cells. So large is the intracellular K^+ pool, that to increase it by 1% requires shift of half the extracellular K^+. Skeletal and heart muscle and adipose cells have been demonstrated to respond in this fashion.

In experiments on excised tissues or cell suspensions, the relative K contents are reversed; there is far more extracellular than intracellular K. It is extracellular $[K^+]$ that is held constant experimentally. If insulin-induced hyperpolarization is caused by net shift of K^+ from outside to inside, the numerator of the logarithmic term must have increased; $[K^+]_i$ must have been the cause. However, measurement of the time course of $[K^+]_i$ changes in rat skeletal muscle in response to insulin showed that there was no detectable increase in $[K^+]_i$ at a time when insulin caused hyperpolarization, and at a time when the theoretical increase, on the assumption that only $[K^+]_i$ changed in Equation (4), was so great it could have been detected easily. Over a period of several hours, there was a small increase in $[K^+]_i$, less than theoretical, in response to hyperpolarization (Zierler, 1959a).

Thus, the hyperpolarization produced by insulin is the cause of net shift of K^+ from extracellular to intracellular space, not a result of that shift. No amount of decrease in $[Na^+]_i$, even down to zero, can account for the size of insulin-induced hyperpolarization.

If there are no changes in ion concentration to account for increased absolute ψ_D, then there is nothing left but decreased ratio of P_{Na}/P_K. This could occur by any mechanism that decreased P_{Na} to a greater extent than it decreased P_K or that increased P_K to a greater extent than it increased P_{Na}.

One approach to estimate a permeability coefficient is based on its quantitative relationship to unidirectional diffusive flow of the ion.

With the reasonable assumption that ^{42}K efflux is only passive, one can measure washout of ^{42}K from muscle, previously loaded with ^{42}K, under conditions in which intracellular ^{42}K exchanges for the abundant isotope, stable K, of the bathing solution. Over a period of several hours, ^{42}K washout from rat muscle at room temperature appears to be described by a single exponential. This does not prove that there is only one exponential term or that ^{42}K washout from muscle is governed by a law based on some exponential distribution. If washout is exponential, the time constant for ^{42}K efflux from rat muscle is about 6 hr, so that only about 30% of intracellular ^{42}K is washed out in 2 hr, too small to give much confidence that the process would contiue at that rate. Nevertheless, with these reservations, we make the assumption that ^{42}K efflux from rat muscle is exponential. The rate constant, k, was decreased by up to 45% by insulin, in a concentration-dependent fashion, from a control of 0.16/hr to a minimum of 0.09/hr (Fig. 3). This efflux rate for K, k_K is related to the permeability coefficient, P_K, by the following (Keynes, 1951):

$$P_K = \lambda_K \frac{RT}{\psi F} \left[\exp\left(\frac{\psi F}{RT} \right) - 1 \right] \tag{8}$$

where ψ stands exactly for ψ_D and approximately for ψ_m for rat skeletal muscle, as we discussed earlier, and $\lambda_K = k_K$ divided by the surface—volume ratio of a muscle fiber, which is, for a cylinder, 2/fiber radius.

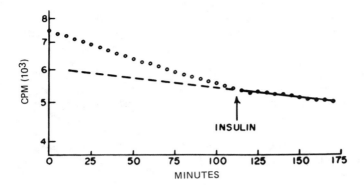

Figure 3 Effect of insulin on ^{42}K efflux from rat extensor digitorum longus muscle. Semilogarithmic plot of ^{42}K remaining in a preloaded muscle. At arrow insulin was added to the bathing solution. The slope of the line is the negative of the rate constant for ^{42}K efflux. Insulin decreased it. The dashed line extrapolated back from the line during exposure to insulin is to emphasize comparison with the control slope. (From Zierler, 1960).

From Eq. (8) with measured ψ_m and ^{42}K efflux, P_K was calculated. It was 1.16×10^{-7} cm sec^{-1} without insulin and only 0.87 with maximum concentration of insulin.

We solve Equation (4) explicitly for the ratio P_{Na}/P_K,

$$\frac{P_{Na}}{P_K} = \frac{[K^+]_i - [K^+]_o e^V}{[Na^+]_o e^V - [Na^+]_i} \tag{9}$$

where $e^V = \exp(\psi F/RT)$.

From measured concentrations of ψ_m, the permeability ratios were calculated in the presence and absence of insulin in muscles from normal and from hypophysectomized rats (Hazlewood and Zierler, 1967). Insulin decreased the ratio from 0.064 to 0.040 in muscles from normal rats and from 0.053 to 0.027 in hypophysectomized rats.

Absolute values of P_{Na} were obtained by combining the calculated ratios [Eq. (9)] with values of P_K from ^{42}K efflux studies [Eq. (8)]. Insulin decreased P_{Na} in muscles from normal rats, from 0.068×10^{-7} cm sec^{-1} to 0.043, and in muscles from hypophysectomized rats from 0.066 to 0.030.

Thus, by these calculations in rat muscle, insulin decreased membrane permeability to both Na$^+$ and K$^+$, but it decreased P_{Na} to a greater extent, thus causing hyperpolarization. These calculations rest on the assumption that equations that hold literally only for the diffusive component ψ_D can be applied to observed ψ_m, ψ_P is negligible for these purposes. Richard Moore has reminded us, correctly, in principle, that the calculations were based on the assumption that ψ_P is zero and not on experiments in which ouabain inhibition assured that it was zero. We have shown in other experiments in rat muscle that with ouabain in concentrations and over times that completely inhibited the electrogenic pump stimulation by β-adrenergic agents, ψ_P is indistinguishable from zero in both insulin-treated and untreated muscle. Therefore, the assumption that $\psi_D = \psi_m$ in rat muscle at rest is reasonable.

Membrane potentials can be expressed in terms of electrical conductances to permeant ions. The contribution to electrical current density (amp cm^{-2}) through the membrane made by the jth species of ion is

$$I_j = g_j(\psi_m - E_j)$$

where E_j is the Nernst equilibrium potential of the jth species of ion and g_j is membrane conductance for that kind of ion. Sum for all the kinds of permeant ions contributing to the total, and set total net membrane current at zero:

$$\psi_m = \Sigma(\bar{g}_j E_j) \qquad (10)$$

where $\bar{g}_j = g_j/\Sigma g_j$, the partial conductance with respect to the jth kind of ion. Equation (10) is analogous to Equation (4). It is the formal statement of an electrical model of parallel units, each consisting of a power supply, E_j, and a resistance. Obviously, there is conceptual resemblance between a permeability coefficient of Equation (4) and a partial conductance of Equation (10).

De Mello (1967) found that insulin hyperpolarized frog sartorius muscle. Insulin also decreased total membrane conductance. It did so by only 23% when muscles were in normal Ringer solution, but by 83% when it was in isotonic K_2SO_4 (including 8 mM $CaSO_4$). In the latter solution, the membrane is depolarized by the high $[K^+]_0$, but also all $[Cl^-]_0$ is removed. Because $\bar{g}_{Cl}$ is about 2 $\bar{g}_K$, and because insulin decreased $\bar{g}_K$, the effect of insulin on total conductance was not impressive until the shunting effect of Cl^- was removed.

There are, then, two pieces of information, one by measuring K efflux rate constants and calculating P_K for rat muscle, the other by measuring total conductance under conditions in which it is all g_K in frog muscle. Both agree that insulin decreases movement of K^+ across the membrane.

However, in cultures of chick embryonic heart cell aggregates, Lantz et al. (1980) interpreted their studies to mean that insulin caused hyperpolarization by increasing conductance to K^+. First, they found a slowly increasing hyperpolarization, peaking at -10 to -12 mV in about 5 min. It was unaffected by ouabain.

Lantz et al. calculated conductance (or its reciprocal, resistance) by a device called current clamping, in which a current is passed through the membrane and maintained constant. The responding change in membrane potential is measured. From a series of such measurements at different levels of clamping, current-voltage curves are generated. For biomembranes, these are not linear, that is, the slope, which is the conductance, is not constant.

Lantz et al. interpreted their current-voltage curves to mean that insulin increased (rather than decreased, as de Mello had said) K^+ conductance, and so, according to Equation (4), caused hyperpolarization. This is a reasonable interpretation of their data, but it is not the only reasonable interpretation. The pair of published current-voltage curves seem to be linearly displaced, so that the slopes in vector space appear almost unchanged. This is compatible with de Mello's finding that Cl^- masks the conductance change and with our studies on rat muscle in which the major cause is assigned to decreased P_{Na}/P_K ratio, with absolute decrease in both. Decreased Na^+ conductance would not be detected by current clamp experiments under conditions in which Na^+ conductance is very small to begin with.

In Figure 4, on the millivolt scale are represented approximate Nernst equilibrium potentials for Na^+ and K^+ for rat caudofemoralis muscle. Observed membrane potentials considered to be only diffusive are indicated in the absence (control) and presence of insulin. They may be considered as weighted sums of E_{Na} and E_K. The approximations are

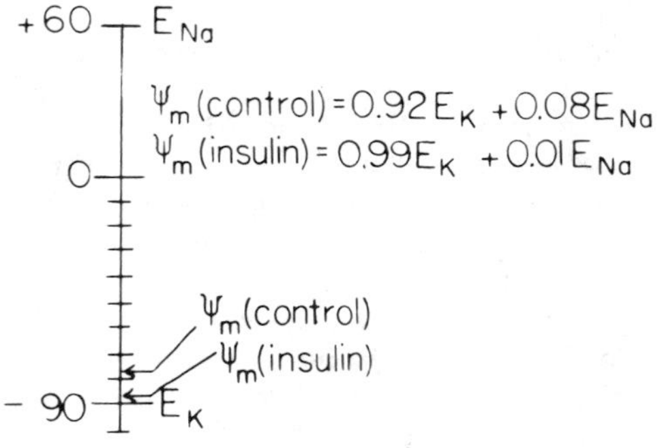

$$+60 \quad E_{Na}$$
$$\Psi_m(control) = 0.92 E_K + 0.08 E_{Na}$$
$$\Psi_m(insulin) = 0.99 E_K + 0.01 E_{Na}$$
$$0$$
$$\Psi_m(control)$$
$$\Psi_m(insulin)$$
$$-90 \quad E_K$$

Figure 4 The relationship between resting membrane potentials with and without insulin, and Nernst equilibrium potentials for Na^+ and K^+.

ψ_m (control) $\cong 0.92 \, E_K + 0.08 \, E_{Na}$

ψ_m (insulin) $\cong 0.99 \, E_K + 0.01 \, E_{Na}$

The evidence from studies of rat caudofemoralis is that insulin causes hyperpolarization by reducing the contribution of E_{Na}.

IV. WHY DOES INSULIN HYPERPOLARIZE SKELETAL MUSCLE, MYOCARDIUM, AND ADIPOSE TISSUE?

I suggested (Zierler, 1972) that hyperpolarization might be a signal, acting by way of its spatially orienting force, to activate or inactivate membrane-associated transport and enzyme systems. Insulin-induced hyperpolarization may be an event in the set interposed between association of insulin with its cell surface receptor and those responses, such as accelerated D-glucose transport. The totality of these responses have come to be regarded as characteristic of insulin. This unknown series of events is the answer to the question, when insulin and its receptor recognize one another, how does the cell know what it is supposed to do? We designate this series the transduction chain.

If insulin-induced hyperpolarization is a transducer, it must satisfy three requirements.

1. Insulin-induced hyperpolarization must occur sooner than those characteristic responses, such as D-glucose uptake.
2. A way must be found to bypass insulin to hyperpolarize a muscle in the absence of insulin, and this hyperpolarization must produce insulinlike responses.
3. A way must be found to intervene between the insulin-receptor complex and hyperpolarization in order to prevent hyperpolarization without preventing binding. When this occurs, characteristic insulin responses, such as D-glucose uptake, must also not occur.

1. Speed of Hyperpolarization

We (Zierler and Rogus, 1981a) injected nanoliters of a solution of insulin, by pressure, from a micropipette on to the surface of a rat muscle fiber impaled with a microelectrode. The injecting micropipette was brought to the surface of the fiber and then backed off, probably about 50 μm. It was 40–100 μm from the probe microelectrode. In 21 of 32 injections, hyperpolarization occurred within 1 sec, sometimes as an abrupt step, sometimes more slowly (Fig. 5). Average hyperpolarization was −8.5 mV, similar to the maximum response in rat caudofemoralis muscle when the bathing solution is changed to one containing insulin.

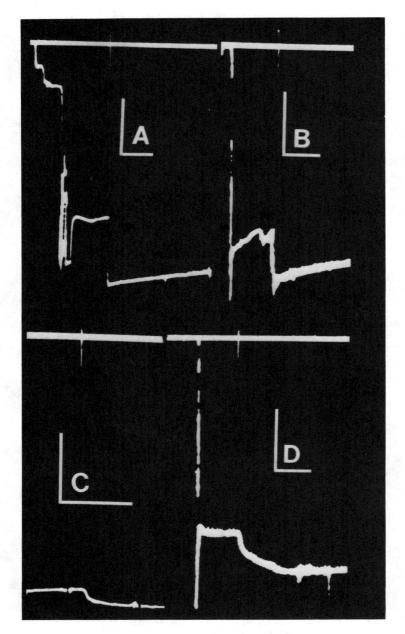

Figure 5 Hyperpolarizing response to insulin injection. Calibration: Vertical, 20 mV; horizontal, 5 sec. Upper line in each tracing is 0 mV; insulin injection indicated by marker. (A) and (B) Step response to maximum hyperpolarization. (C) and (D) Rapid onset of response with slower increase to maximum. The initial downward deflection in (A), (B), and (D) occurred when the electrode tip was on a fiber's surface.

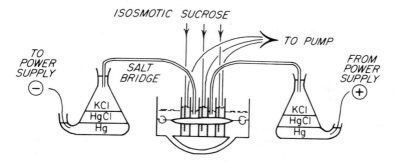

Figure 6 Muscle chamber and electrodes for triple sucrose gap experiments. See text. (From K. Zierler and E. M. Rogus (1980).

In some of those that did not respond within 1 sec, there was hyperpolarization within 15 sec. In others there was no hyperpolarization within 1 min. We attributed one-third of the cases in which the delay was greater than 1 sec to diffusion delay, even to diffusion of the insulin bolus away from the fiber. The injectate bolus had a different refractive index than the bathing solution, and it could be seen to rise from the tip of the pipette to the surface of the bathing solution, so that it may never have reached a fiber if the pipette was not sufficiently close to the fiber surface. Control injections (same volume, pH, and Zn content as insulin injectate, but no protein) never changed membrane potentials.

The most rapid response to insulin with respect to stimulated glucose uptake is about 45 sec.

2. By-passing Insulin: Insulinlike Effect of Electrically-Produced Hyperpolarization and Receptor Antiserum

We (Zierler and Rogus, 1981b) succeeded in developing a method, a triple sucrose gap, by which a segment of a whole muscle was hyperpolarized. The principle is illustrated in Fig. 6. A muscle, in this case, rat caudofemoralis, having parallel fibers from one tendon to the other is passed through three silastic pouches that form snug watertight seals. One pouch is at the middle of the muscle; the other are 4 mm on either side of the first. Through the three pouches isosmolal

---

In (C) the impalement occurred a few seconds before the portion of the trace reproduced here. In (B), (C), and (D) the electrode was in a surface fiber. In (A) the electrode passed through a surface fiber and possibly through the second fiber; the record at the time of injection was from a second or third fiber from the surface. From Zierler and Rogus (1981a).

sucrose solution flows, unrecirculated. The two chambers between the pouches and the two end chambers contain a Krebs-Ringer solution, and the two end chambers are electrically shorted through a Krebs-Ringer bridge. Electrodes are placed in the two central Krebs-Ringer compartments. When sucrose has displaced all the interstitial fluid from the muscle segments in the pouches, a voltage difference is impressed upon the pair of electrodes by way of very poorly polarizable massive Hg-HgCl half-cells.

The circuit cannot be completed between the electrodes except by current passing through the interior of muscle fibers in the sucrose gaps because extracellular paths have been rendered nonconductive by sucrose. There are two current paths, one passing centrally through the middle sucrose gap. The other passing peripherally through the outer sucrose gaps and the Krebs-Ringer bridge.

Current moves inward (into the muscle) beneath one electrode, through fiber interiors and outward across muscle membranes beneath the other electrode. The muscle segment beneath the anode is hyperpolarized; that beneath the cathode is depolarized a like amount.

The D-glucose analogue, 2-deoxy-D-glucose, (2-DG), radiolabeled, was added to the anodal and cathodal compartments. The hyperpolarized segment took up nearly 40% more 2-DG than the neighboring segment. This was not because depolarization decreased 2-DG uptake; there was no difference between unpaired controls not subjected to applied potentials and depolarized segments. Nor was this nonspecific. L-Glucose uptake was not affected, either by the small hyperpolarization or the depolarization.

The effect was small, but it was 40% of the maximum effect of insulin on muscles in this chamber, even though the mean hyperpolarization over the length of the hyperpolarized segment was less than 40% of that produced maximally by insulin.

Hyperpolarization of rat skeletal muscle has been produced by antibodies to insulin receptors (Zierler and Rogus, 1983a) [rabbit antibodies to rat liver receptors, made by Jacobs et al. (1978)]. These antisera were effective in high dilution, and hyperpolarization was concentration dependent. However, maximum effect, a little more than −4 mV, was only about half as great as maximum hyperpolarization by insulin. Maximum stimulation of glucose uptake by antiserum to insulin receptors, however, was also less than that in response to insulin by rat caudofemoralis muscle.

3. Can Insulin-Induced Hyperpolarization Be Blocked without Preventing Insulin Binding, and Does This Also Prevent Stimulation of Glucose Uptake?

There are no published data directed at this question. We (Zierler and Rogus, 1983a) have completed and analyzed a series of experiments in which effects of insulin on rat caudofemoralis muscle were studied when external K concentrations $[K^+]_0$ was varied over ranges greater than normal. It was suspected that increased $[K^+]_0$ might be a condition suitable to test the question because there is a report (Otsuka and Ohtsuki, 1965) that in diaphragm from nutritionally K-deficient rats, insulin did not cause hyperpolarization when $[K^+]_0$ was raised to about 50 mM, and because there are a number of other reports (for example, Kipnis and Parrish, 1965; Kohn and Clausen, 1972; Bihler and Sawh, 1971) that insulin stimulation of transport of glucose or its analogue is decreased as $[K^+]_0$ is increased. We asked if attenuation of the two insulin effects proceeded in a correlated fashion and if high $[K^+]_0$ interfered with specific insulin binding.

We found no effect of $[K^+]_0$, over the range from normal 4.8 mM to about eight times that level, on specific binding of insulin to rat caudofemoralis muscle.

Insulin, 100 µU/ml, produces about half-maximum hyperpolarization of rat caudofemoralis in normal $[K^+]_0$. Increasing $[K^+]_0$ causes

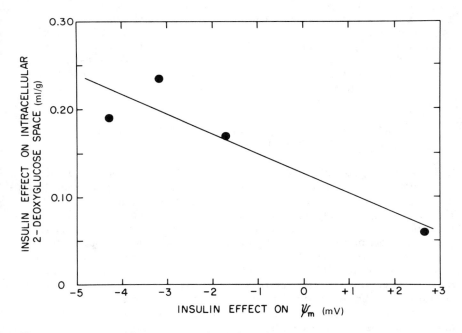

Figure 7 Correlation between insulin-stimulated 2-deoxyglucose uptake and insulin-induced hyperpolarization in rat caudofemoralis muscle when both effects are diminished by increasing K^+ concentration of bathing solution by equimolar substitution of KCl for NaCl. Correlation coefficient was 0.92. From K. Zierler and E. M. Rogus (unpublished).

depolarization in the absence of insulin. Insulin-induced hyperpolarization decreases as $[K^+]_o$ increases and disappears at about 36 mM $[K^+]_o$. The insulin effect on 2-DG uptake also decreased as $[K^+]_o$ increased, but there remained a small, but significantly nonzero, effect at the highest $[K^+]_o$. The decrease in insulin-stimulated 2-DG uptake correlated with the decreased insulin-induced hyperpolarization (Fig. 7). The residual insulin effect on 2-DG uptake in the absence of hyperpolarization argues that (a) the hypothesis is wrong that hyperpolarization is a transducer of insulin-stimulated glucose uptake or (b) there is a small insulin-stimulated glucose uptake independent of membrane potential, or (c) the two sets of experiments were not comparable. The last is true. Membrane potentials were measured only in the outer layer of fibers, or at most the outer few layers, on the upper surface of a muscle containing several thousand fibers. 2-Deoxy-D-glucose uptake was measured in the whole muscle. It is possible that the environment of deeper fibers differed from that of superficial fibers. When $[K^+]_o$ is increased, as it was in these studies, by equimolar substitution of KCl for NaCl, there is net transfer of water from interstitial fluid to cells and there is increased intracellular K^+ at the expense of Na^+, much of which (but not all) is likely to occur in sarcoplasmic reticulum rather than in sarcoplasm. These intracellular-extracellular adjustments are likely to take longer to reach a steady state in deeper fibers because gradients between deep interstitial fluid and the bathing solution are likely to persist longer than those between the outer few layers and the bathing solution due to diffusion delays.

V. HOW MIGHT HYPERPOLARIZATION ALTER METABOLIC OR TRANSPORT PROPERTIES OF CELL MEMBRANES?

The electrical potential difference across cell membranes is exerted only over the membrane itself. Both of the surrounding aqueous phases are isopotential. The electrical potential gradient begins at one interface between membrane and aqueous phase, traverses the membrane, and ends at the opposite interface. As I noted earlier, a membrane potential from perhaps −40 and −70 mV in inexcitable cells and up to −92 mV in excitable cells across a 70−100 Å membrane is at a gradient of the order of 100,000 V/cm. This gradient is $d\psi/dx$, where x is distance from one of the membrane-aqueous phase interfaces inside the membrane in the direction normal to the membrane surface.

If the interfaces were a pair of parallel plates of infinite surface area, the lines of the electrical field through the gaps between the plates would all be straight, parallel to each other, and perpendicular to the plane of the plates. In this circumstance, the gradient $d\psi/dx$ is constant. No matter where a charged particle is placed in the gap between the plates, no matter how close to one plate or the other, the electrical potential gradient is the same and is simply equal to the potential difference between the two plates divided by the distance between them. The constant gradient, or constant field strength, was basic to derivation of the Goldman-Hodgkin-Katz formulation of membrane potential [Eq. (4)].

Electrical field strength E is synonymous with electrical potential gradient. However, we will be using different notation, E, for electrical field strength to indicate that the dimensions are in electrostatic units in the cgs system, whereas we use $d\psi/dx$ in dimensions of volts/cm.

When a charged particle or a dipole is placed in the gap between the two plates, the electrical field strength tends to orient the charged particle or dipole so that the positive charge of the particle faces the negatively charged plate. If the particle has a net charge, it tends to move toward the plate, the tendency depending on the field strength, the dielectric filling the gap, the net charge density (charge per unit mass) of the particle, and, for a dipole, the dipole moment.

Proteins have substantial dipole moments, from 200–300 Debye units for albumin, to 600 Debye units or more for lactoglobulin, to more than 1000 Debye units (1 Debye unit = 10^{-18} esu cm). Every CONH group is a dipole. The CONH dipoles of membrane proteins are subjected to the powerful orienting force of membrane proteins are subjected to the powerful orienting force of 10^5 V/cm. Let us see if we can quantitate effects of the electrical field on membrane protein dipoles. The following treatment is based on, and is a small extension of, one used by Debye (1929).

Figure 8A reviews the concept of dipole moments and dipole angles. As electrical field strength increases, dipoles tend to orient increasingly in the direction of the field; dipole angles decrease.

The electrical work done in rotating a dipole is calculated as follows. First, orient the xy coordinates so that the x-axis coincides with the axis of the dipole (Fig. 8B). Let the lines of the field form an angle θ with the dipole. Lay out the electrical force vector $F = qE$ along angle θ. The x component of F is $F_x = qE \cos \theta$. F_x is an axial force, matched, and cancelled out by an equal and opposite $-F_x$, so that the pair of axial components plays no role. The y component of F is $F_y = qE \sin \theta$. This is tangential to the dipole, tending to rotate it toward the field. Its companion $-F_y$, acting on the negative end of the dipole, tends to rotate the dipole to the same degree and in the same direction. The total tangential force tending to rotate the dipole toward the direction of the field (decreasing dipole angle θ) is $2qE \sin \theta$.

When the dipole rotates, in response to the tangential force, to decrease θ to $\theta-d\theta$, the distance over which the tangential force is exerted is the arc $ad\theta$. The element of electrical work done in rotating the dipole is

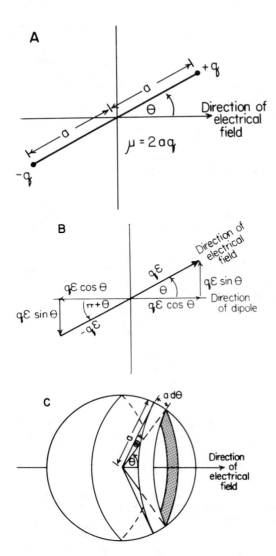

Figure 8 (A) Elements of a dipole moment and dipole angle. Dipole moment μ (dimensions of electrical charge × length) is the product of length 2a and quantity of charge, q. The angle found between the dipole and the direction of the electrical field is the dipole angle θ. (B) The components of force acting on a dipole. Unlike (A) the x axis is now aligned with the dipole, not with the direction of the electrical field. The electrical field strength is a vector at an angle θ from the dipole. The x components of the vector are axial forces operating in opposite directions along the dipole and cancel out. The y components of the vector are tangential forces operating together to rotate the dipole toward the direction of the electrical field. The work that must be done to obtain dipole angle θ in opposition to the effect of electrical field strength on the position of the dipole is calculated by permitting

dW = −2aq$E$ sin θ dθ = −μE sin θ dθ

The electrical work done in rotation from θ = 0 to θ is

$$W(\theta) = \int_0^\theta \mu E \sin \theta \, d\theta = \mu E(1 - \cos \theta)$$

From this we find the probability that, given a dipole moment μ and a field strength E, a dipole angle lies between some specified θ and θ + dθ; that is, we find the probability density function, h(θ), where h(θ)dθ is the fraction of the population of dipoles, with moment μ, lying in an electrical field of strength E, that has dipole angles between θ and θ + dθ.

Two elements enter into the expression f(θ)dθ from which we shall find the density h(θ).

The first element is simply the Boltzmann factor relating electrical energy spent in work to thermal energy,

exp(−W/kT) = exp[−μE(1 − cos θ)/kT]

which we write as $e^{-B}e^{B \cos \theta}$, where k is the Boltzmann constant and B is the energy ratio μE/kT.

The second element is a weighting factor. The dipole charges lie on an annular fraction of a spherical surface, of width adθ and of length 2πa sin θ. Its area is 2πa^2 sin θ dθ. This area is a fraction, (sin θ dθ)/2, of the total surface of the sphere of radius a.

These two elements give the function

$$f(\theta)d(\theta) = (e^{-B}/2)e^{B \cos \theta} \sin \theta \, d\theta$$

where 0 ⩽ θ ⩽ π and B is unrestricted.

---

the tangential forces to act over a distance given by the length of the arc of an angle θ of a circle with radius half the length of the dipole. (C) the spherical surface formed by rotation of a dipole. The electrical field is in the x direction. Any dipole at some angle between a given θ and (θ + dθ) to the x direction may lie in the yz plane formed by rotation of θ about the x axis. The locus of dipole charges lies on a ribbon of spherical surface, of width adθ, where a is half the dipole length, and circumference 2πa sin θ. (It is this symmetry of dipole angle around the x axis that limits θ to the range 0 ⩽ θ ⩽ π rad.) Given a particular dipole moment and a particular electrical field strength, the probability that a dipole angle lies within a specified θ and (θ + dθ) is proportional to the product of the area of the ribbon (as a fraction of total surface of the sphere) and the Boltzmann distribution.

The integral of $f(\theta)$ over the total interval from 0 to π is

$$F(\pi) = (e^B - e^{-B})e^{-B}/2B$$

where $B \neq 0$. For $B = 0$, $F(\pi) = 1$.
The desired probability density is $f(\theta)d\theta/F(\pi)$,

$$h(\theta)d\theta = \begin{cases} \frac{1}{2}\sin\theta\,d\theta, & \text{as B approaches 0} \\ \dfrac{B}{e^B - e^{-B}}e^{B\cos\theta}\sin\theta\,d\theta, & B \neq 0 \end{cases}$$

It is assumed that when there is no electrical field (i.e., when $B = 0$) θ is distributed randomly.

Families of $h(\theta)$ are plotted in Figure 9 for various values of B corresponding to the product of dipole moments of known proteins and field strengths equivalent to 10^5 V cm^{-1}. Notice that as B

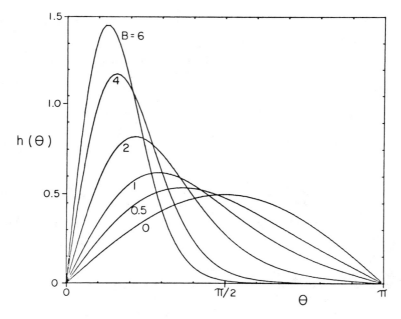

Figure 9 A probability density function, $h(\theta)$, that, given μ and E, a dipole angle will lie between θ and $(\theta + d\theta)$, is plotted as a function of θ. A family of such functions for different values of B (where $B = \mu E/kT$) demonstrate that as B increases, the density function shifts toward $\theta = 0$ and becomes increasingly skewed.

increases, h(θ) becomes more skewed and a larger part of h(θ) is
squeezed into a smaller range of θ. This means that even though it
may take relatively larger changes in B than we are concerned with
to cause substantial shifts in the peak value of h(θ,B), a small change,
by only 5 or 10%, can shift a substantial fraction of the population of
dipole angles.

A region of interest with respect to membrane proteins is for
values of B between 4 and 6. These numbers mean that electrical
work available for rotation is 4 and 6 times thermal energy; that is,
the result is likely to be realized. The midpoint of this region is occupied, for example, by proteins with dipole moments of about 600 Debye units under field strengths equivalent to 10^5 V cm^{-1}. At 25°C,
kT is 4.1×10^{-21} J (or 4.1×10^{-14} statvolt-statcoulomb), and μE is
4.9 times greater than kT at the values given above.

These considerations of effects of electrical field strength on dipole rotation may have important implications for membrane protein
structure and function, although we cannot yet justify transfer of
this simplified development of the situation from a model system with
uniform dielectric and constant field to the more complicated biomembrane. Nevertheless, there does exist this powerful field through
membranes that must be one of the factors placing restraints on the
position and shape of membrane proteins.

Indeed, many of us have wondered for a long time why inexcitable
cells went to the burdensome expense of maintaining large electrical
field strengths, estimated, with various specific outcomes, to account
for a substantial fraction of the cell's total energy dissipation. I have
proposed that the electrical field may be necessary to keep membrane
proteins in a certain desired configuration, a process I called electrometamorphosis (Fig. 10).

A change in field strength can then alter protein configuration by
one of several ways. Depolarization (reduced field strength) permits
dipole angles to increase toward the random distribution. Hyperpolarization decreases dipole angles. In either case, a new stress is imposed
upon the protein spine. It is possible that new dipole-dipole interactions may occur. If the protein has multistable configurations, the
stress of altered field strength may flip the protein from one state to
another in which its function is at a different level. It is not necessary to flip every member of that protein population from state A to
state B to have a functional effect, so that, as Fig. 9 suggests, a small
change in field strength may produce a change in function of membrane
proteins. We have called this effect of altered field strength electro-
morphogenesis.

Specificity can be brought into the picture in several ways. First,
although all proteins in a given membrane lie in the same electric field,
they may have diverse dipole moments. Second, the response of a
given protein to the stress of altered field may differ from that of

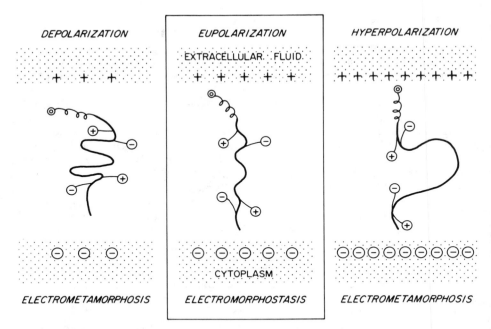

DEPOLARIZATION   EUPOLARIZATION   HYPERPOLARIZATION

EXTRACELLULAR FLUID

CYTOPLASM

ELECTROMETAMORPHOSIS   ELECTROMORPHOSTASIS   ELECTROMETAMORPHOSIS

Figure 10 Representation of possible effects of electrical field on configuration of membrane protein. Middle panel: Shape in normal field.
Dipole angles tend to lie between 0 and $\pi/2$ rad, not randomly. Thus,
the field participates in maintenance of some configuration differing
from that which the protein has in free solution in the absence of the
field. This effect of the normal field in maintaining shape is electromorphostasis. Left-hand panel: With depolarization, dipole angles
tend to be more randomly distributed; the shape of the protein tends
to resemble that which it might have, for example, if inserted into
liposome membranes across which there was no charge. Right-hand
panel: With hyperpolarization, dipole angles tend toward zero. New
dipole-dipole interactions may occur. With either de- or hyperpolarization, as angles change there are different stresses on the spine of
the protein. If the protein has multistable configurations, either stress
may flip it from one stable configuration to another. The change in
shape produced the change in electrical field strength is electrometamorphosis. From K. Zierler and E. M. Rogus (1981c).

another protein with similar dipole moment because there are other constraints on the proteins, because they differ in the likelihood of forming new dipole-dipole interactions at a given field, and because their structures are different and do not permit them to flip configurations at the same value of the electric field strength.

Insulin is not the only peptide hormone reported to alter membrane potentials. Some peptide hormones depolarize, and some hyperpolarize (Table 1). Adrenergic agents, both α and β agonists, alter membrane potentials (Table 2). Many of these studies deserve reinvestigation with more specific agents and with intent to sort out underlying mechanisms. Nevertheless, they suggest that a change in membrane potential may be a widely used mechanism for modulating membrane function.

There are other examples. Secretagogues alter membrane potential (Douglas, 1975; Petersen, 1976), sometimes in cyclic fashion as distinct from the steady-state change produced by insulin.

There is an increasing number of observations in a variety of disciplines in which altered membrane potentials have been reported to occur during the course of cell functions, or in which alterations in membrane potential have altered cell functions. The idea goes back to Eyring et al. (1949) and to Polissar (1956).

These early notions largely went without further development until electrophysiologists began to think in more detail about voltage-dependent ion conductances through membranes of excitable cells and began to ask just what might be the mechanism of gating, by which ions were admitted or excluded from complete passage through the membrane. Many contributed to the development of concepts in this field, particularly Hille in a number of thoughtful articles (for example, Hille, 1979). An ion gate is an energy barrier or perhaps a series of barriers. Molecularly, it is likely to be part of a membrane protein, and because it is voltage dependent, it must be charged or a dipole, whose position in space is altered when the electric field strength is altered.

Changes in membrane potential, occurring rapidly in response to some stimulus, have been reported in fertilization of sea urchin eggs (following entry of the first sperm) (Epel, 1978) and with surface stimulation of neutrophils (Korchak and Weissmann, 1978).

Most of the recent biochemical literature treating membrane potentials considers them only in the thermodynamic Mitchell chemiosmotic fashion, as a component in energy balance. This is not at all the role we are considering. Interestingly, Page and West (1981), in a Mitchellian consideration of β-galactoside transport in *E. coli* speculated that, independently of the thermodynamic effects, "an electric field could cause a conformational change resulting in an increase of affinity for the external substrate(s)," which is in agreement with the notions advanced here.

Table 1 Peptide Hormones That Alter Membrane Potential[a]

Hormone	Tissue depolarized	Hormone	Tissue hyperpolarized
Oxytocin	Myometrium	Insulin	Muscle, fat, etc.
Parathormone	Osteoclasts	Calcitonin	Osteoclasts
ACTH	Adrenocortical cells	Glucagon	Hepatocytes
Thyrotropin-releasing hormone	Pituitary	Vasopressin	Bladder
		Thyrotropin	Thyroid
		Thyrotropin-releasing hormone	Pituitary

[a]See K. Zierler and E. M. Rogus (1981a) for references.

Table 2 Tissues Whose Membrane Potential Is Altered by Adrenergic Agents[a]

Depolarization	Response	Hyperpolarization	Response
Brown fat	β, ?α	Liver slices	α, β
White fat	β	Perfused liver	β
Ehrlich ascites cells	?β	Cockroach salivary gland	α
Fused glioma-neuroblastoma	α	Myometrium	β
		Taenia coli	α
		Parotid acinar cells	α.
		Renal juxtaglomer-ulus	β
		Rat soleus	β

[a]See K. Zierler and E. M. Rogus (1981a) for references.

Berry (1981) has carried the conjectures a step further by including in his thinking all the internal membranes of a cell. By invoking inhomogeneities in membranes with localized separation of charge, Berry proposed that all sorts of reactions, thought of as occurring in cytoplasm, are occurring close to some internal membrane and are influenced by fields and by local currents.

VI. UNRESOLVED PROBLEMS

A. Mechanisms of Insulin-Induced Hyperpolarization

1. Immediate

Three mechanisms have been proposed: stimulation of a ouabain-inhibitable Na^+-K^+ electrogenic pump, absolute increase in K^+ conductance, and decreased Na^+/K^+ permeability ratio with absolute decrease in K^+ permeability. Evidence for the second of these mechanisms comes from studies of aggregates of cultured chick heart cells. Evidence for the other two comes from studies of skeletal muscle. The matter needs to be resolved. If there is an effect on Na^+ conductance, it might be revealed unequivocally by studies specifically directed toward that, such as voltage clamp experiments on patches of cell membrane in which Cl^- and K^+ conductances are blocked.

2. Remote

No matter what the immediate mechanism by which cell membranes hyperpolarize in response to insulin, even though hyperpolarization is demonstrable in less than 1 sec, it is unlikely that the insulin-receptor complex acts directly on the immediate agent (ion channels or Na^+-K^+ ATPase). Direct action implies one-to-one coupling between the insulin-receptor complex and the immediate hyperpolarization process. Although this is conceivable for the case of stimulation of Na^+-K^+ ATPase, it seems unlikely for the cases of ion channels, for there are probably too many of them. Even for the case of Na^+-K^+ ATPase, one-to-one coupling may not be satisfactory because there may be too little amplification of the initial event in such a system; that is, there would be only one molecule of insulin bound to one receptor stimulating one Na^+-K^+ ATPase. The gain would come solely from the speed with which one Na^+-K^+ ATPase separated charges across the membrane. We do not have enough data to make the calculations necessary to see if this could or could not account quantitatively for the observed hyperpolarization.

It seems more likely that at least one amplification step is interposed between the receptor and the immediate mechanism of hyperpolarization. There are several possibilities, all likely to be related to some configurational change in the receptor as a consequence of insulin binding. There is already evidence that the receptor phosphorylates itself (Kasuga et al., 1982). It might also, in the absence of insulin, bind Ca, and lose its affinity for Ca when insulin binds. The Ca^{2+} released might then bind to nearby Na^+ and K^+ channels, decreasing conductance, but blocking Na^+ conductance to a relatively greater extent if there were greater affinity for Na^+ channels.

B. Why Are All Hyperpolarizing Agents Not Insulinomimetic?

For example, in skeletal muscle, β-adrenergic agents hyperpolarize. There is general agreement that they do so by stimulation of a ouabin-inhibitable electrogenic Na^+-K^+ ATPase pump. Some effects of β-adrenergic agonists may resemble some of those of insulin. It has never been clear what these agents do to muscle glucose uptake; there are reports of increase, decrease, and no change. Both insulin and β-adrenergic agonists stimulate net K^+ uptake, which is an expected response to hyperpolarization, but for which there may be additional mechanisms. β-Adrenergic agonists stimulate adenylate cyclase activity, but insulin's effect on this enzyme is unsettled. There are experiments in which insulin stimulates this cyclase, even above the level of activity in the presence of a β-adrenergic agonist. Once we pass the cell membrane, however, there are well-established differences, such as on glycogen synthase and phosphorylase activities.

This question will need to be answered eventually. It is possible that there are parallel transduction series, and the difference between insulin and, for example, β-adrenergic agents, may begin with differences in the first link between the receptor and the transduction chains. The β-adrenergic receptor may be linked to an adenylate cyclase, and this may lead, probably with at least one interposed step, to stimulation of a Na^+-K^+ ATPase (Rogus et al., 1977). It is clearly that increased cAMP in skeletal muscle plays a major role in β-adrenergic responses, but not in insulin responses.

C. If Insulin-Induced Hyperpolarization Is Part of the Transduction Chain, Why Does It Not Occur in All Other Cells?

Hepatic cells respond differently to insulin than do skeletal muscle, heart, and fat cells. The hallmark of insulin effect on muscle has been its stimulation of D-glucose uptake, which does not occur in the liver. Hepatic cells, at least in the whole liver, are electrically coupled (Penn, 1966), but skeletal muscle fibers and adipocytes are not. The aggregates of cultured chick heart cells are, of course, coupled. Until very recently, it had been reported only that insulin had no effect on liver membrane potentials. But in cultured cells, insulin produced a slow depolarization, accompanied by increased input resistance (Wondergem, 1983). [Input resistance is measured by the displacement of the membrane potential produced by passing a known current through the probe electrode. It is a function of all resistances between the probe electrode, not just the membrane resistance. However, when it is changed substantially by an agent that does not produce substantial changes in axial resistance (as by grossly altered water or electrolyte activites), it is fair to attribute the change to altered membrane resistance.] This is concordant with the effect of insulin on skeletal muscle, but in one case there is associated hyperpolarization and in the other depolarization. The mechanism of insulin-induced depolarization on cultured hepatic cells remains to be studied, and it is not known to what extent it may play a role in other hepatic responses to insulin. However, Friedmann and Damback (1980) found a strong correlation between membrane potentials in the perfused rat liver and gluconeogenesis, when membrane potentials were altered, over a range from −20 to −60 mV, by glucagon, valinomycin, tetracaine, or altered ionic concentrations in the bathing solution. In this case, insulin's inhibition of glucagon-induced hyperpolarization was accompanied also by insulin's inhibition of cyclic AMP-induced hyperpolarization and with reduced gluconeogenesis normally associated with these agents.

It is too soon to know yet whether the report by Williams et al. (1982) is in a different category. Williams et al. studied two kinds of preparations of pancreatic acinar cells from mice made diabetic by streptozotocin. It is known that pancreatic acini are depolarized by

secretagogues, and it is also known that at least one of these, chole-
systokinin, stimulates glucose uptake via a mechanism inhibited by
cyclic guanosine monophosphate (cGMP). Williams et al. measured
membrane potentials in fragments of the pancreas and measured uptake
of the glucose analogue 2-deoxyglucose and 3-O-methylglucose in suspensions of acinar cells dissociated from pancreases. Insulin, in
physiological concentrations, stimulated uptake of the glucose analogues about as much as in isolated muscle but less than in adipose
tissue, but the effect was not blocked by cGMP. In the other preparation of acini, membrane potentials were nearly −40 mV, the same as in
pancreatic acini from normal mice, were reduced (depolarized) by
carbachol, and were unaffected by insulin whether or not carbachol
was present.

The experiments by Williams et al. seem to place insulin responsiveness of pancreatic acinar cells in a category that is different from
those tissues that insulin hyperpolarizes and different from liver.
There is the possibility that, because glucose uptake was calculated
in one kind of preparation and membrane potential in another, a relationship between insulin-stimulated glucose uptake and a possible electrical effect might have been found that had it been possible to carry
out the experiment in the same kind of preparation. (Obviously, the
metabolic studies were most effectively carried out in relatively pure
suspensions of acini in order to be sure that one was not misled by
possible effects on nonacinar cells, and electrical measurements, by
electrodes, had to be carried out in the whole pancreas in order to
immobilize the cells.)

VII. CONCLUSION

Insulin hyperpolarizes skeletal and heart muscle, adipose cells, and
some other tissues, but not liver (which it depolarizes in culture) or
pancreatic acini. It hyperpolarizes skeletal muscle within 1 sec.
Electrically produced hyperpolarization, in the absence of insulin,
stimulates specific D-glucose uptake. It is possible then that hyperpolarization may be one of the events in the transduction process between the insulin-receptor complex and classic effector responses to
insulin. The immediate mechanism by which insulin hyperpolarizes is
unsettled. Some experiments have been interpreted to mean that insulin stimulates a ouabain-inhibitable electrogenic Na^+-K^+ exchange
pump, but others claim that it does not. Other experiments are interpreted to mean that insulin causes hyperpolarization by increasing
K^+ conductance, while still others are interpreted to mean that insulin
decreases K^+ conductance. Our own experiments on rat skeletal
muscle show that insulin-induced hyperpolarization is not mediated by
way of a ouabain-inhibitable electrogenic pump and that insulin decreases

permeability of the cell membrane to K^+. On the basis of measured potentials and ion concentration, we calculate that the ratio of Na^+/K^+ permeability is decreased, accounting for observed hyperpolarization.

A mechanism is proposed by which hyperpolarization might produce changes in membrane function. The mechanism is general, including a proposal for the role of membrane potential (considered in the format of electrical field strength) in maintaining configuration of protein dipoles in the membrane (*electromorphostasis*), and of altered potentials (either depolarization or hyperpolarization) in changing dipole angles in the membrane, stressing protein configurations to an extent at which multistable proteins may flip to a new configuration at which there is altered function (*electrometamorphosis*).

ACKNOWLEDGMENTS

Dr. Zierler's research has been supported by grants from the National Institutes of Health, currently, AM 17574, awarded by the National Institute of Arthritis, Diabetes, Digestive and Kidney Diseases, and by the Muscular Dystrophy Association, Inc.

LIST OF SYMBOLS

a	Half the distance between charges of a dipole (dimension, cm).
g_j	Electrical conductance of the jth kind of ion (dimension, Siemen).
$\bar{g}_j$	Partial conductance with respect to the jth kind of ion ($\bar{g}_j = g_j/\Sigma g_j$).
h, h(θ)	A probability density function of the dipole angle θ, the fraction of all dipole angles that lie between some specified θ and $\theta + d\theta$.
k	Boltzmann's constant, thermal energy per molecule per degree.
q	Quantity of electrical charge. For dipoles, this is given in electrostatic units (dimension, esu or statcoulomb).
B	Ratio of electrical potential energy (of a system consisting of a dipole in an electrical field) to thermal energy ($B = \mu E/kT$).
E_N, E_j	The Nernst electrical potential difference of the jth kind of ion; the contribution to the electrical

	potential difference across a membrane made by the jth kind of ion in solution or on the two sides of the membrane when there is no electrochemical potential difference (i.e., there is thermodynamic equilibrium) with respect to that ion (dimension, volt).
E	Electrical field strength (see $d\psi/dx$) (dimensions, statvolt cm^{-1}).
F	Faraday constant, 96,500 coulombs $mole^{-1}$.
I_j	Electrical current density (dimensions, amp cm^{-2}).
M_o, M_i	Unidirectional efflux or influx, respectively, of a specified ion across a specified membrane (dimensions, mole sec^{-1}).
P_{Cl}, P_K, P_{Na}	Permeability constants; index of permeability of a specified membrane to the ion indicated by the subscript (dimensions, cm sec^{-1}).
R	The gas constant, thermal energy per mole per degree (can be in any energy unit; in electrical units, 8.3×10^3 joule $mole^{-1}$ $degree^{-1}$).
T	Temperature, degrees Celsius.
λ_K	Modified rate constant for unidirectional K^+ efflux (dimensions, cm sec^{-1}).
μ	Dipole moment (dimensions, Debye units, 10^{-18} esu or statcoulomb cm).
θ	Dipole angle.
ψ	Electrical potential difference (dimension, volt).
ψ_D, ψ_m, ψ_P	Diffusive component (contribution to membrane potential by chemical potential difference across membrane) of ψ_m, the observed electrical potential difference across the membrane, and the pump component (contribution to ψ_m due to electrogenic Na^+-K^+ exchange), respectively.
$d\psi/dx$	Gradient of electrical potential through the membrane in the x direction perpendicular to the plane of the membrane.

REFERENCES

Armstrong, W. McD. and Garcia-Diaz, J. F. (1981). In *Epithelial Ion and Water Transport*. (A. D. C. MacKnight and J. P. Leader, eds.). Raven, New York.

Beigelman, P. M. and Hollander, P. B. (1962). *Proc. Soc. Exp. Biol. Med. 110*:590.

Berry, M. N. (1981). *FEBS Lett. 134*:133.

Bihler, I. and Sawh, P. C. (1971). *Biochim. Biophys. Acta 241*:302.

Bolte, H.-D. and Lüderitz, B. (1968). *Pflügers Archiv. 301*:254.

Cheng, K., Groarke, J., Osotimehin, B., Haspel, H. C., and Sonenberg, M. (1981). *J. Biol. Chem. 256*:649.

Crabbé, J. (1969). In *Protein and Polypeptide Hormones* (M. Margoulies, ed.), Excerpta Medica Foundation, Amsterdam, p. 260.

Creese, R. (1968). *J. Physiol. (London) 197*:255.

Davis, R. J., Brand, M. D., and Martin, B. R. (1981). *Biochem. J. 196*:133.

Debye, P. (1929). *Polar Molecules*, The Chemical Catalog Company, New York.

De Mello, W. C. (1967). *Life Sci. 6*:959.

Douglas, W. W. (1975). In *Handbook of Physiology, Endocrinology*, American Physiological Society, Washington, Vol. VI, p. 367.

Epel, D. (1978). *Curr. Top. Dev. Biol. 12*:185.

Erlij, D. and Grinstein, S. (1976). *J. Physiol. (London) 259*:13.

Eyring, H., Lumry, R., and Woodbury, J. W. (1949). *Record Chem. Prog. 10*:100.

Flatman, J. A. and Clausen, T. (1979). *Nature (London) 281*:580.

Friedmann, N. and Dambach, G. (1980). *Biochim. Biophys. Acta 596*: 180.

Friedmann, N., Somlyo, A. V., and Somlyo, A. P. (1971). *Science 171*:400.

Gavryck, W. A., Moore, R. D., and Thompson, R. C. (1975). *J. Physiol. (London) 252*:43.

Goldman, D. E. (1943). *J. Gen. Physiol. 27*:37.

Hazlewood, C. F. and Zierler, K. L. (1967). *Johns Hopkins Med. J. 121*:188.

Hille, B. (1979). In *Membrane Transport Processes* (C. F. Stevens and R. W. Tsien, eds.), Raven, New York, Vol. 3.

Hodgkin, A. L. and Horowics, P. (1959). *J. Physiol. (London) 148*: 127.

Hodgkin, A. L. and Katz, B. (1949). *J. Physiol. (London) 108*:37.

Jacobs, S., Chang, K.-J., and Cuatrecasas, P. (1978). *Science 200*:1283.

Kasuga, M., Karlsson, F. A., and Kahn, C. R. (1982). *Science 215*:185.

Keynes, R. D. (1951). *J. Physiol. (London) 114*:119.

Kipnis, D. M. and Parrish, J. E. (1965). *Fed. Proc. 24*:1051.

Kohn, P. G. and Clausen, T. (1972). *Biochim. Biophys. Acta 255*:798.

Korchak, H. M. and Weissmann, G. (1978). *Proc. Natl. Acad. Sci. USA 75*:3818.

LaManna, V. R. and Ferrier, G. R. (1981). *Am. J. Physiol. 240*:H636.

Lantz, R. C., Elsas, L. J., and DeHaan, R. L. (1980). *Proc. Natl. Acad. Sci. USA* 77:3062.

Leader, J. P. (1981). In *Epithelial Ion and Water Transport,* (A.D.C. MacKnight and J. P. Leader eds.), Raven, New York.

Malinow, M. R. (1958). *Acta Physiol. Latinoam.* 8:125.

Miller, J. E. and Constant, M. A. (1960). *Am. J. Ophthalmol.* 50:855.

Moore, R. D. and Rabovsky, J. L. (1979). *Am. J. Physiol.* 236:C249.

Otsuka, M., and Ohtsuki, I. (1965). *Nature (London)* 207:300.

Pace, C. S., Matschinsky, F. M., Lacy, P. E., and Conant, S. (1977). *Biochim. Biophys. Acta* 497:408.

Page, M. G. P., and West, I. C. (1981). *Biochem. J.* 196:721.

Penn, R. D. (1966). *J. Cell Biol.* 29:171.

Petersen, O. H. (1976). *Phys. Rev.* 56:535.

Petrozzo, P., and Zierler, K. (1976). *Fed. Proc.* 35:602.

Polissar, M. J. (1956). In *The Kinetic Basis of Molecular Biology* (F. M. Johnson, H. Eyring, and M. J. Polissar, eds.), Wiley, New York, p. 691.

Rehm, W., Schumann, H., and Heinz, E. (1961). *Fed. Proc.* 20:193.

Rogus, E. M., Cheng, L. C., and Zierler, K. (1977). *Biochim. Biophys. Acta* 464:347.

Rogus, E., Price, T., and Zierler, K. (1969). *J. Gen. Physiol.* 54:188.

Stark, R. J. and O'Doherty, J. (1982). *Am. J. Physiol.* 242:E193.

Stark, R. J., Read, P. D., and O'Doherty, J. (1980). *Diabetes* 29:1040.

Takameri, M., Ide, Y., and Tsujihata M. (1981). *J. Neurol. Sci.* 50:89.

Williams, J. A., Bailey, A. C., Preissler, M., and Goldfine, I. D. (1982). *Diabetes* 31:674.

Wondergem, R. (1983). *Am. J. Physiol.* 244:C17.

Zemkova, H., Teisinger, J., and Vyskocil, F. (1982). *Biochim. Biophys. Acta* 720:405.

Zierler, K. L. (1957). *Science* 126:1067.

Zierler, K. L. (1959a). *Am. J. Physiol.* 197:515.

Zierler, K. L. (1959b). *Am. J. Physiol.* 197:524.

Zierler, K. L (1968). *Am. J. Physiol.* 198:1066.

Zierler, K. L. (1972). In *Handbook of Physiology, Endocrinology I,* American Physiological Society, Washington, Chap. 22.

Zierler, K. and Rogus, E. M. (1980). *Am. J. Physiol.* 239:E21.

Zierler, K. and Rogus, E. M. (1981a). *Biochim. Biophys. Acta* 640:687.

Zierler, K. and Rogus, E. M. (1981b). *Am. J Physiol.* 241:C145.

Zierler, K. and Rogus, E. M. (1981c). *Fed. Proc.* 40:122.

Zierler, K. and Rogus, E. M. (1983a). *Am. J. Physiol.* 244:C58.

Zierler, K. and Rogus, E. M. (1983b). *Trans. Assoc. Am. Physicians* 96:203.

BIBLIOGRAPHY

For critique of microelectrodes

Armstrong, W. McD. and Garcia-Diaz, J. F. (1981). Criteria for the use of microelectrodes to measure membrane potentials in epithelial cells. In *Epithelial Ion and Water Transport*, (A. D. C. MacKnight and J. P. Leader, eds.), Raven, New York.

For reviews of effects of insulin on membrane potentials and/or on cell Na^+ and K^+

Zierler, K. L. (1972). Insulin, ions, and membrane potentials. In *Handbook of Physiology, Endocrinology 1*, American Physiological Society, Washington, Chap. 22.

Zierler, K. and Rogus, E. M. (1981). Effects of peptide hormones and adrenergic agents on membrane potentials of target cells. *Fed. Proc. 40*:121.

Moore, R. D. (1983). Effects of insulin upon ion transport. *Biochim. Biophys. Acta Reviews on Biomembranes 737*:1.

9

The Molecular Basis of Insulin Action: Membrane-Associated Reactions and Intracellular Mediators

FREDERICK L. KIECHLE   *William Beaumont Hospital, Royal Oak, Michigan*

LEONARD JARETT   *University of Pennsylvania School of Medicine, Philadelphia, Pennsylvania*

I. INTRODUCTION

Insulin was discovered 60 years ago, and the main effects of insulin on the cellular metabolism of carbohydrates, fats, and proteins have been established for 20 years. More recently, the receptor for insulin binding has been characterized. However, the molecular events that occur following the binding of insulin to its receptor and initiate intracellular metabolic responses remain unknown. This subject has been discussed in several recent reviews (see Bibliography). As alluded to briefly in Chapters 6 and 7, insulin stimulates three major types of reactions on target tissues: (a) rapid membrane reactions and responses, which occur within seconds; (b) intracellular responses, which occur within minutes; and (c) stimulation of growth, which occurs within hours (Fig. 1). This chapter will review these three reactions initiated by insulin and will discuss their relationship to insulin-sensitive mediators recently characterized in intact cells and subcellular systems.

II. MEMBRANE REACTIONS AND RESPONSES

Several membrane reactions and responses occur within seconds following the binding of insulin to its plasma membrane receptor. These events occur within the plasma membrane of most insulin-sensitive tissues and include covalent modification of the insulin receptor, stimulation of cell surface transport, hyperpolarization of membranes, and alteration in membrane fluidity. The following sections will summarize data relating to some of these membrane reactions and responses.

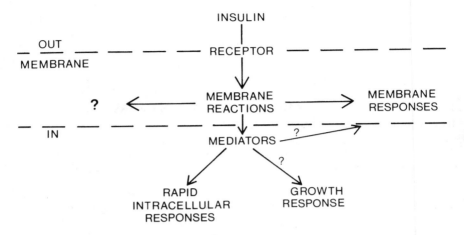

Figure 1 Schematic representation of the mechanism of insulin action. The interaction of the insulin with its receptor on the plasma membrane elicits a series of biochemical reactions within the membrane. These reactions can result directly in membrane responses such as alterations in transport, generation of chemical mediators for insulin action, or initiation of other undefined responses. The mediators or second messengers of insulin action are known to activate a number of the rapid intracellular metabolic responses related to insulin action, but it is not known if these mediators play a role in the longer-term growth effects of insulin or in the short-term membrane responses.

A. Insulin Receptor Phosphorylation

The insulin receptor is a glycoprotein thought to be composed of two principal α and β subunits linked together by disulfide bonds. The molecular models of the receptor are discussed in Chapters 3 and 4. As heralded by the work of Kahn and colleagues (Kasuga et al., 1982), and observed by a number of investigators (Zick et al., 1983a; van Obberghen et al., 1983; Petruzzelli et al., 1982, Shia and Pilch, 1983; Machicao et al., 1982) in subcellular systems from a variety of tissues, the binding of insulin to its receptor stimulates a cAMP-independent tyrosine-specific protein kinase located in the β subunit which phosphorylates itself. The insulin receptor may possess a phosphatase, as well (Machicao et al., 1982). The insulin receptor kinase phosphorylates other substrates at tyrosine residues in a manner similar to the protein kinase produced by Rous sarcoma virus, pp 60v-src. To date, however, insulin treatment of intact cells or tissues has not been shown to cause the same rapid phosphorylation exclusively of tyrosine residues on the receptor or in other substrates. Recently, Zick et al. (1983b) have demonstrated that insulin stimulates the phosphorylation of serine residues in partially purified insulin receptors derived from human hepatoma cells. Insulin stimulates two kinases in this system: a tyrosine kinase and a serine kinase. It is not known whether the serine kinase is an integral part of the insulin receptor, like the tyrosine kinase. Several mitogenic peptide growth factors have also been shown to stimulate tyrosine-specific kinase activity, including epidermal growth factor, platelet-derived growth factor, and insulinlike growth factor I (see Chap. 5). The epidermal growth factor receptor was the first hormone receptor demonstrated to be a protein kinase that catalyzes a self-phosphorylation reaction involving tyrosine residues (Cassel et al., 1983; Cohen et al., 1980). In contrast, the receptor in rat brain for tumor-promoting phorbol diesters copurifies with a Ca^{2+}-dependent, phospholipid-sensitive protein kinase C that does not autophosphorylate the receptor (Neidel et al., 1983). Some receptors that participate in phosphorylation reactions do not possess intrinsic kinase activity, but are phosphorylated by a kinase that is not a structural component of the receptor. For example, two subunits of the nicotinic acetylcholine receptor are phosphorylated by a cAMP-dependent protein kinase located within the membrane (Huganir and Greengard, 1983). The physiological role of receptor phosphorylation by a kinase located within or adjacent to the receptor is unknown. The activation of a receptor kinase by ligand binding may phosphorylate regulatory proteins and thereby alter other membrane reactions and intracellular metabolism. The exact role of ligand-modulated phosphorylation reactions in controlling cell function has not yet been determined.

Since some of the insulin-stimulated intracellular responses are phosphorylation events, it has been proposed by Denton and co-workers (1981) [see Bibliography and Houslay (1981)] that activation of a membrane-associated insulin-dependent protein kinase may be an important early event in metabolic regulation by insulin. The role that the insulin receptor kinase plays in metabolic regulation is unknown. Phosphotyrosine bonds are relatively uncommon; however, the activation of this insulin receptor kinase could initiate a cascade of phosphorylations sufficient to alter intracellular metabolism. This kinase may also play a role in the regulation of insulin-mediated effects on growth and membrane responses. Protein kinase C is another unique kinase whose physiological role is yet to be explained but has the potential for regulating membrane and intracellular metabolic events. Recent evidence indicates that insulin alters phospholipid metabolism in a manner that could lead to the stimulation of kinase C (Farese et al., 1983b). Thus, the role of this kinase in insulin action must be investigated. In summary, kinase reactions, triggered by the interaction of insulin with its receptor, may represent critical biochemical reactions that are involved in generating a cellular response.

B. Stimulation of Cell Surface Transport

Insulin stimulates the transport of sugars, amino acids, ions, and fatty acids across the plasma membranes of certain target tissues. Numerous investigations have been conducted in an effort to determine if the stimulation of membrane transport leads to modulations of the numerous intracellular processes regulated by insulin. At this time, no change in membrane transport can explain all the effects of insulin on target cells. The mechanisms by which insulin increases each of the transport processes are unresolved.

C. Hyperpolarization of Membranes

As discussed in detail in Chapter 8, insulin hyperpolarizes the plasma membranes of two target tissues, rat skeletal muscle and adipose tissue, but not liver. Recently, insulin-dependent depolarization of adipocyte mitochondria has been reported (Davis et al., 1981). These mitochondrial changes in polarization are not initiated by flux of potassium into the cell; their physiological role remains unknown.

D. Membrane Fluidity

Membrane fluidity is determined by at least four major factors: (a) cholesterol/phospholipid ratio; (b) degree of phospholipid acyl chain unsaturation; (c) phospholipid polar head group composition; and (d) phospholipid methylation. An increase in membrane fluidity would result in greater mobility of protein membrane components within the phospholipid bilayer. Alterations in membrane fluidity have been reported following the binding of insulin to red blood cells, liver plasma membranes, and fat cells (Luly and Shinitzky, 1979; Armatruda and Finch, 1979). Also, insulin-responsive membrane functions, including glucose transport (Amatruda and Finch, 1979; Melchoir and Czech, 1979), enzyme activity (Holloway and Garfield, 1981), and insulin binding to its receptor (McCaleb and Donner, 1981; Gould et al., 1982) have been shown to be modulated by the physical characteristics of membrane lipids. The ability of insulin to increase membrane fluidity, even in a local environment, may lead to microaggregation of occupied insulin receptors (see Chaps. 6 and 7). However, until recently, there was very limited formation on the effects of insulin on phospholipids.

1. Phospholipid Phase Transition

The insulin-mimetic effects of phospholipase C or A suggested to Rodbell et al. (1968) that insulin may cause a change in the disposition of

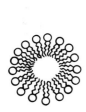 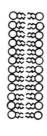

ISOTROPIC   BILAYER   HEXAGONAL

Figure 2 Schematic representation of the phase transitions of phospholipids within the membrane. Phospholipids in membranes are usually aligned in a bilayer configuration. This bilayer can change to an isotropic configuration with polar head groups facing outward and a hydrophobic center. Alternatively, the bilayer can be converted to a hexagonal arrangement with the head groups in the center and hydrophobic regions external.

phospholipids in fat cell membrane from a bilayer to an isotropic configuration (Fig. 2). Recently, Larner et al. (1982, 1983) has hypothesized that insulin induces a rapid reversible hexagonal phase change within the plasma membrane near the insulin receptor. Phosphorus-31 nuclear magnetic resonance (NMR) of membranes provide a signal that represents the average orientation of the phosphodiester head group of the phospholipids. This signal is unique for the bilayer, isotropic, or hexagonal phase (Cullis and de Kruijff, 1979). This technique was used to determine if insulin induced an irreversible phase transition in adipocyte membranes (Leo et al., 1983). Phosphorus-31 NMR studies were conducted on plasma membranes and microsomes prepared from insulin-treated or untreated rat adipocytes and on rat adipocyte plasma membranes untreated or treated with insulin following partial purification. No significant difference was observed when ^{31}P NMR spectra of insulin-treated adipocyte membranes were compared to untreated adipocyte membranes. These data suggest that insulin does not induce a significant irreversible phase transition in adipocyte membranes. However, rapid reversible phase transition cannot be ruled out.

2. Phospholipid Metabolism

Some studies have shown insulin to alter the metabolism of phospholipids and/or their derivatives. It has been suggested that these alterations could be involved in the mechanism of insulin action. Farese et al. (1982) showed that insulin treatment of adipose tissue increased the concentration of phosphatidylserine, phosphatidic acid,

phosphatidylinositol, and phosphatidylinositol 4-phosphate, as measured
by analysis of thin-layer chromatograms for phospholipid phosphorus.

Our laboratory has investigated the direct effect of insulin on adipocyte plasma membrane phospholipids. Insulin treatment of intact
adipocytes has been reported to increase the ^{32}P-labeled ATP pool of
the adipocyte, thereby making it difficult to interpret increases in
labeled phospholipid (Stein and Hales, 1974). To avoid this possible
complication, adipocytes were uniformly labeled with ^{32}P for 2 hr in
the absence of insulin. the ^{32}P-labeled plasma membranes were partially purified, divided in half, and incubated with or without 100 μU
insulin/ml. After 5 min, the membranes and supernatant were separated by centrifugation and extracted with chloroform-methanol, and
the phospholipids were separated by thin-layer chromatography. The
following results were obtained. (a) The total counts in the organic
extract of the supernatant or plasma membranes from the insulin-
treated set exceeded that from controls. (b) The radioactivity associated with phosphatidylcholine was significantly increased, while that
associated with phosphatidylinositol 4-phosphate was significantly decreased in the organic extract of the supernatant and plasma membranes
from the insulin-treated set compared to the control. (c) Kinetic
studies revealed that there was a breakdown of several phospholipids
in control membranes within 1 min that was blocked by the interaction
of insulin with the membrane. In contrast, insulin stimulated the
breakdown of phosphatidic acid. These data suggest that insulin
does alter phospholipid metabolism by at least two different pathways:
(a) inhibiting or stimulating specific phospholipase activities and (b)
stimulating phospholipid methylation with the conversion of phosphatidylethanolamine to phosphatidylcholine.

3. *Phospholipid Methylation*

The conversion by methylation of phosphatidylethanolamine to phosphatidylcholine (Fig. 3) was first reported in rat liver microsomes by
Bremer and Greenberg (1961). This reaction is catalyzed by two
methyltransferases that utilize S-adenosylmethionine as a methyl donor
(Hirata and Axelrod, 1980; Mato and Alemany, 1983). These two enzymes facilitate the translocation of phosphatidylethanolamine from the
cytoplasmic side of the membrane to the outer surface following the
conversion of phosphatidylcholine. This vectorial rearrangement has
been shown to increase membrane fluidity, as mentioned above. The
two methyltransferases are widely distributed in mammalian tissues.
The highest specific activity has been found in the plasma membrane
and microsomal fractions of cells.

Several investigators have examined the possibility that enzymatic
methylation of phospholipids plays a role in the transduction of
receptor-mediated signals through the membranes of a variety of cells.

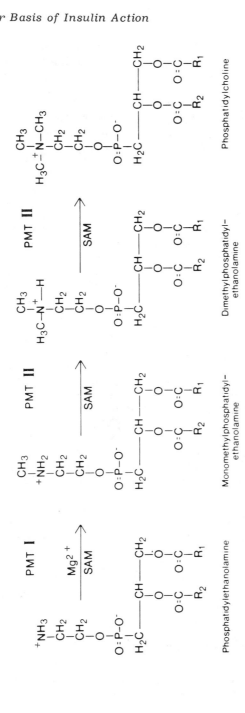

Figure 3 Schematic representation of the enzymatic conversion of phosphatidylethanolamine to phosphatidylcholine. Two enzymes are involved in the conversion, phospholipid methyltransferase I (PMT I) and phospholipid methyltransferase II (PMT II). The methyl groups are donated from the substrate S-adenosylmethionine (SAM).

Hirata and Axelrod (1980) demonstrated a dose-dependent increase in [^{3}H]methyl incorporation into phospholipids following treatment of rat reticulocyte ghosts with the β-adrenergic agonist, L-isoproterenol. Experimental evidence suggested that increased phospholipid methylation following the binding of isoproterenol to the β-adrenergic receptor resulted in increased membrane fluidity in the vicinity of the receptor and facilitated lateral mobility of the β-adrenergic receptor to interact and activate adenylate cyclase. This mechanism may have cellular specificity since it has not been reproduced in isolated hepatocytes (Ogreid et al., 1982).

Other receptor mediated events (Hirata and Axelrod, 1980; Mato and Alemany, 1983) have been linked to an alteration in phospholipid methylation, including the actions of concanavalin A, chemotactic peptide, benzodiazepine, and IgE antibody. Several peptide hormones alter phospholipid methylation including glucagon (Castano et al., 1980), vasopressin (Prasad and Edwards, 1981; Alemany et al., 1981), angiotensin (Alemany et al., 1981), and nerve growth factor (Pfenninger and Johnson, 1980). The increase in phospholipid methylation induced by these hormones was rapid, and in several cases this effect was noted with physiological concentrations of the hormone. The methylation reaction appeared to demonstrate an appropriate specificity with respect to biologically active and inactive peptide analogues.

The activity of phospholipid methyltransferase I and methyltransferase II in liver microsomes of rats made insulin-deficient with alloxan is reduced by 49 to 48%, respectively, compared to control (Hoffman et al., 1981). Therefore, insulin would appear to be required to maintain the increased phospholipid methylation observed in nondiabetic animals. We have used partially purified plasma membranes from rat adipocytes to determine the effect of insulin on phospholipid methylation of membrane phospholipids (Kelly et al., 1984). Insulin increased the incorporation of [^{3}H]methyl from [^{3}H-methyl]-S-adenosylmethionine (SAM) into total phospholipid extracts. Thin-layer chromatographic separation of the three methylated species, phosphatidyl-N-monomethylethanolamine, phosphatidyl-N,N-dimethylethanolamine, and phosphatidylcholine, demonstrated that insulin increased the [^{3}H]methyl incorporation into all methylated products. The effects of insulin were rapid and apparently occurred as early as 15 sec after insulin addition. The effects continued for at least 20 min. It remains to be determined if there is a link between insulin-induced changes in phospholipid methylation or in other aspects of phospholipid metabolism and the mediation of insulin action.

III. INTRACELLULAR RESPONSES

Following the binding of insulin to its receptor, several intracellular responses take place within minutes, including alterations in the activity of cytoplasmic and membrane-bound enzymes that regulate carbohydrate, lipid, and protein metabolism. The rapidity of these intracellular responses have suggested to many investigators that a mediator or second messenger is generated following the insulin-receptor interaction. A number of substances have been suggested as mediators, including cyclic adenosine 3',5'-monophosphate (cAMP), cyclic guanosine 3',5'-monophosphate (cGMP), calcium, and hydrogen peroxide. However, none of these compounds appear to exhibit all of the characteristics required of a true "second messenger" (see Bibliography). If insulin does cause the generation of a second messenger or mediator from the plasma membrane, then it should be possible to generate such a material from a plasma membrane preparation in which the structural and functional integrity necessary to produce the mediator is retained.

A series of studies from various laboratories have shown that the interaction of insulin with the plasma membrane from a variety of insulin-sensitive tissues has generated a low molecular weight (1000–3000) substance that can alter the activity of a variety of enzymes that regulate various insulin-sensitive metabolic pathways. The following section will review the adipocyte subcellular system in which the mediator was discovered, the plasma membranes and intact cells from which the mediator has been obtained, the insulin-sensitive enzymes on which the mediator acts, the experimental evidence that supports the existence of more than one mediator, and the known physical and chemical properties of the mediator (3). These data suggest that these mediators fulfill the roll of a second messenger for at least some of the short-term intracellular effects of insulin.

A. Subcellular System

Initial studies from our laboratory showed that the addition of physiological concentrations of insulin to a subcellular system composed of adipocyte plasma membranes and mitochondria generated a mediator from the plasma membrane that dephosphorylated the α subunit of mitochondrial pyruvate dehydrogenase with activation of the enzyme complex (Jarett et al., 1981, 1983; Seals et al., 1979; Seals and Jarett, 1980). The addition of insulin-mimetic agents, concanavalin A and anti-insulin receptor antibody, to the subcellular system also activated pyruvate dehydrogenase, eliminating the concept that a piece of the insulin molecule could be the mediator. These effects were observed only when the plasma membranes were present.

At the time these studies were performed, Larner et al. (1979, 1982, 1983) reported a low molecular weight (1000–1500), acid-stable mediator generated by insulin in rabbit skeletal muscle that stimulated glycogen synthase phosphatase and inhibited the cAMP-dependent protein kinase. This same material isolated from insulin-treated muscle also stimulated pyruvate dehydrogenase in adipocyte mitochondria

(Jarett and Seals, 1979). The insulin-sensitive mediator from adipocyte plasma membranes has been characterized further by two laboratories (Kiechle et al., 1981; Seals and Czech, 1981). Spontaneous partial release of the mediator as assessed in the pyruvate dehydrogenase assay can occur without hormonal stimulation. Repeated centrifugation followed by washing with phosphate buffer could deplete the mediator from the plasma membrane. Gel filtration of this material revealed a fraction in the M.W. range of 1000−1500 that stimulated pyruvate dehydrogenase. This same low M.W. fraction from the supernatant of insulin-treated membranes contained a greater quantity or activity of mediator than did control samples. Thus, this low M.W. material released from the plasma membranes appears to represent the mediator whose existence was suggested in the earlier studies using the subcellular system.

Table 1 summarizes the various plasma membrane preparations used to generate the low molecular weight mediator during insulin treatment. Tepperman's laboratory (Begum et al., 1982a,b, 1983a,b) has shown that diet affects the insulin-dependent generation of the mediator from adipocyte and liver plasma membranes. The adipocyte or liver plasma membranes from rats fed high fat diets failed to generate the mediator in response to insulin. This phenomenon may be related to structural variation of these membranes attributable to the high fat in the diet. Differences in the amount of cholesterol, phosphatidylserine, and phosphatidylinositol as well as the distribution of fatty acid moieties attached

Table 1 Plasma Membranes Used to Demonstrate that Insulin Alters the Amount or Activity of the Mediator Which Modulates the Activity of Pyruvate Dehydrogenase

Plasma membranes tested	Response to insulin treatment
1. Adipocyte plasma membranes	
rats fed regular diet	Increase
2. Adipocyte or liver plasma membranes	
rats fed high carbohydrate diet	Increase
rats fed high fat diet	No increase
3. Liver plasma membranes	
ethanol-insoluble stimulator	Increase
ethanol-soluble inhibitor	Decrease
rats fasted for 60 hr	No increase
diabetic rats	No increase
4. Placental plasma membranes	Increase

to membrane phospholipids have been reported in liver plasma membranes from carbohydrate and fat fed rats (Sun et al., 1979) but not for adipocyte plasma membranes. Marked variations in these fatty acid constituents will alter membrane fluidity, membrane responsiveness, and insulin binding. A similar low molecular weight mediator has been generated from liver plasma membranes that stimulated pyruvate dehydrogenase in adipocyte and liver mitochondria. Saltiel et al. (1981, 1982, 1983) have shown that ethanol precipitation of this material separates the material into an ethanol-insoluble residue that contains a pyruvate dehydrogenase stimulatory substance and an ethanol-soluble fraction that inhibits pyruvate dehydrogenase. Additional data indicating the existence of more than one mediator of insulin action will be presented below. Amatruda and Chang (1983) have shown that, following incubation with insulin, hepatocyte plasma membranes from diabetic or fasted animals failed to release the mediator that stimulated pyruvate dehydrogenase. Treatment of the diabetic rats or refeeding the fasted animals restored the ability of insulin to release the mediator from plasma membranes. The binding of insulin to hepatocyte membranes is normal or increased in these altered states. Therefore, these studies suggest that alterations at the plasma membrane may be responsible for or accompany the insulin resistance of liver in fasted or diabetic rats. Insulin treatment of human placental membranes has been shown recently to generate a mediator that activates pyruvate dehydrogenase (Sakamoto et al., 1982).

Additional experimental evidence is required to substantiate further that these materials represent the mediators of insulin action. First, the mediator should be generated following the treatment of intact cells with insulin. Second, the mediator should alter the activity of a variety of enzymes in the same manner as the addition of insulin to intact cells.

B. Studies with Intact Cells

An intracellular mediator of insulin action should have a fairly ubiquitous distribution among various target tissues, and its concentration should be altered by insulin in a manner that is consistent with the known effect of insulin on that cell type. The ability of insulin to alter the amount of activity of the mediator in various cell types is indicated in Table 2. Larner et al. (1979) were the first to identify this low molecular weight, acid-stable material in intact cells. Insulin treatment of rabbits increased the amount or activity of this mediator in skeletal muscle. Kiechle et al. (1980) have shown that treatment of adipocytes with insulin increases the amount or activity of an acid-stable, low molecular weight material that activated pyruvate dehydrogenase. Thus, it appears that the material responsible for insulin's effect on the subcellular system is the same insulin-sensitive material isolated from adipocytes and skeletal muscle.

Table 2 Intact Cellular Systems That Have Been
Tested for the Presence of the Mediator of Insulin Action and the Ability of Insulin to Alter
the Amount or Activity of the Mediator

Intact cell tested	Response to insulin treatment
1. Skeletal muscle	Increase
2. Adipocytes	Increase
3. IM-9 lymphocytes	Decrease
4. H_4 hepatoma cells	Increase

A human cell line, the IM-9 lymphocyte, was selected as a control
cell for study. There have been no reports of a biological response of
this cell to insulin, although the plasma membrane is rich in insulin receptors. A low molecular weight mediator has been extracted from
IM-9 lymphocytes that stimulated pyruvate dehydrogenase (Jarett et al.,
1980). However, in contrast to all other intact cells studied, insulin
treatment of IM-9 lymphocytes significantly reduced the amount or
activity of the material that stimulated pyruvate dehydrogenase. In
this cell, insulin could hypothetically reduce the production of the
material, increase its degradation, or produce another mediator or
antimediator that competes with the stimulator of pyruvate dehydrogenase activity.
     Liver represents another target tissue for insulin action. The
mediator has been shown to be generated from liver plasma membranes
(Saltiel, et al., 1981, 1982, 1983; Jarett and Kiechle, 1981; Begum et al.,
1983a,b). Studies with insulin-sensitive H_4 hepatoma cells have shown
that insulin treatment produced a substantial increase in the mediator
(Parker et al., 1982). Our laboratory has now extracted the mediator
from the liver of insulin-treated rats. In conclusion, insulin increased
the amount or activity of the mediator in three major target tissues for
insulin action: skeletal muscle, adipocytes, and liver. Insulin decreased
the activity or amount of the mediator in IM-9 lymphocytes. These
insulin-induced variations of the generation of mediator are consistent
with the biological responses of these cells to insulin treatment.

C. Insulin-Sensitive Enzymes

The insulin-sensitive mediator modulates several enzyme systems in a
manner analogous to that observed following insulin treatment of whole
cells (see Table 3). The enzymes studied included those that modulate

insulin-sensitive intracellular processes, such as glucose and lipid metabolism and calcium transport. The activity of these enzymes was altered by insulin in intact cells or by the mediator of insulin action by phosphorylation (acetyl-CoA carboxylase), dephosphorylation (pyruvate dehydrogenase, glycogen synthase), or some other mechanism (low K_m cAMP phosphodiesterase). For example, acetyl-CoA carboxylase is activated by insulin via phosphorylation by a cAMP-independent protein kinase (Witters, 1981; Brownsey and Denton, 1982). This kinase phosphorylates sites that are distinct from those phosphorylated by a cAMP-dependent kinase activated by glucagon or epinephrine; cAMP-dependent phosphorylation leads to an inhibition of enzyme activity. In contrast, the activity of the pyruvate dehydrogenase enzyme complex is regulated by a cAMP-independent kinase and a phosphoprotein phosphatase (Denton and Hughes, 1978) (see Fig. 4).

Table 3 Enzyme Systems That Have Been Tested for Response to the Insulin-sensitive Mediator

Enzyme	Alteration in activity
1. cAMP-dependent protein kinase	Decrease
2. Glycogen synthase phosphoprotein phosphatase	Increase
3. cAMP-independent protein kinase	No effect
4. Pyruvate dehydrogenase	Increase
cAMP-independent kinase	No effect
phosphatase	Increase
5. Low K_m cAMP phosphodiesterase	Increase
6. High K_m cAMP phosphodiesterase	No effect
7. $(Ca^{2+} + Mg^{2+})$ ATPase (adipocyte plasma membrane)	Increase
8. Acetyl-CoA carboxylase	Increase[a] Decrease[b]
9. Adenylate cyclase	No effect[a] Decrease[b]
Pyruvate dehydrogenase	Increase[a] Decrease[b]

[a]Ethanol-insoluble residue from insulin-treated liver plasma membranes.
[b]Ethanol-soluble material from insulin-treated liver plasma membranes.

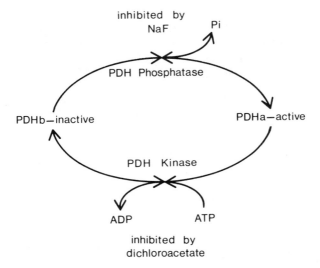

Figure 4 Schematic representation of the activation and inactivation of pyruvate dehydrogenase complex by dephosphorylation and phosphorylation, respectively. The pyruvate dehydrogenase (PDH) phosphatase, which controls dephosphorylation, is inhibited by NaF. The PDH cAMP-independent protein kinase that controls phosphorylation is inhibited by dichloroacetate.

Phosphorylation of the α subunit inactivates the enzyme complex, whereas, dephosphorylation of the α subunit activates it. The mediator of insulin action could alter pyruvate dehydrogenase activity through changes in phosphorylation of the α subunit by increasing phosphatase activity, by decreasing kinase activity, or by both. A series of studies were performed in the presence and absence of ATP, sodium fluoride (a known inhibitor of the pyruvate dehydrogenase phosphatase), and dichloroacetic acid (an inhibitor of the kinase). These studies utilized the mediator derived from several sources; identical results were obtained (Jarett et al., 1981, 1983). The increase in pyruvate dehydrogenase activity was attributable to activation of the pyruvate dehydrogenase phosphatase and not to any alteration of the pyruvate dehydrogenase kinase (Popp et al., 1980). The mechanism by which the mediator activates the phosphatase is unknown.

Insulin treatment of hepatocytes (Loten et al., 1978) or adipocytes (Loten and Sneyd, 1970; Makino and Kono, 1980) increased the activity of the low K_m cAMP phosphodiesterase present in the microsomal fraction. This enzyme is also activated by insulin in the plasma membranes of adipocytes (Macaulay et al., 1983a). The enzyme system, as it exists in the microsomal membrane fraction of the adipocyte, was stimulated by the addition of the mediator from several sources (Parker et al., 1982; Kiechle and Jarett, 1981). The mediator increased the V_{max} of the enzyme and had no effect on the K_m. The low K_m cAMP phosphodiesterase in liver plasma membranes has been reported to be activated by phosphorylation (Marchmont and Houslay, 1981). Our laboratory has been unable to demonstrate control of the adipocyte microsomal or plasma membrane enzyme by phosphorylation. Therefore, at this time, low K_m cAMP phosphodiesterase from adipocytes appears to be regulated by a mechanism other than phosphorylation. The mediator from various sources had no affect on the high K_m cAMP phosphodiesterase in the adipocytes microsomes. This finding is consistent with the insensitivity of the enzyme to insulin in intact cellular systems (Loten et al., 1978; Loten and Sneyd, 1970).

D. How Many Mediators?

Present evidence suggests that insulin generates more than one mediator from the plasma membrane (Jarett et al., 1983; Larner, 1983; Smith and Rosen, 1983). For example, biphasic or bell-shaped responses have been detected in some test systems to increasing concentrations of insulin and insulin-mimetic agents. Turakulov et al. (1977) first reported that the insulin treatment of rats resulted in an increase in a low molecular weight material in the cytosol of liver, which produced a biphasic response in calcium uptake by mitochondria. Mediators from various sources have been reported to alter the activity of certain enzymes in a biphasic dose-response relationship with respect to the addition of insulin or insulin-mimetic ligands (Table 4). In H4

Table 4 Sources From Which Increasing Concentrations of Insulin or Other Ligands Produce a Biphasic Response in Generation of the Insulin Mediator as Tested on Various Enzymes

Mediator source	Enzyme assayed	Ligands
Skeletal muscle	Glycogen synthase phosphatase	Insulin
Adipocyte subcellular system	Pyruvate dehydrogenase	Insulin Concanavalin A Anti-insulin receptor antibody
Liver plasma membranes	Pyruvate dehydrogenase Acetyl-CoA carboxylase Adenylate cyclase	Insulin

hepatoma cells, insulin did not produce a biphasic curve, but simply increased mediator activity to a maximum, even at high insulin concentrations, suggesting that only an activating material was generated (Parker et al., 1982). One possible explanation of the biphasic response data could be the existence of two mediators, one having a high affinity for certain enzyme systems and the other a lower affinity for these systems. When the mediator with a lower affinity for these systems is at high concentrations, it may interfere with the action of the first mediator. This second mediator might possess a higher affinity for other enzyme systems, thus reversing the role of the two mediators.

More direct proof of the existence of two mediators has been provided by Chen et al. (1980) and by Saltiel et al. (1981, 1982, 1983). Chen et al. (1980) have separated the muscle mediator into two fractions by electrophoresis, one that activates enzymes and another that inhibits the same enzymes. The biphasic response disappeared with this separation. Saltiel et al. (1981, 1982, 1983) have shown a similar separation of activities using ethanol precipitation of the mediator generated from liver plasma membranes (see Table 3).

E. Physical and Chemical Characteristics of the Mediators

The insulin mediators have yet to be purified and chemically identified. The mediators from various tissues have several common characteristics including: low molecular weight (1000–3000), acid stability, thermostability, isoelectric point of 4.0–5.0, and elution from anion exchange resins at high salt concentration. Since the mediators are derived from plasma membranes, they must be generated from membrane components or their derivatives, such as proteins, glycoproteins, glycolipids, phospholipids, proteolipids, fatty acids, prostaglandins, or leukotrienes.

Early studies suggested that the mediators might be peptides (Larner et al., 1979, 1982; Kiechle et al., 1980, 1981). This observation was based on the fact that the mediator copurified with a peak of absorbance at 230 nm and is ninhydrin positive. There was no correlation between the amount or activity of the mediator and the absorbance, attributable to the impure nature of the material. Some investigators have been able to destroy mediator activity with protease (trypsin) digestion (Sakamoto et al., 1982; Seals and Czech, 1980); other workers have seen no effect or only partial inactivation following protease digestion (Jarett et al., 1983; Larner et al., 1983). Several investigators report that the addition of inhibitors of arginine-specific proteases to plasma membranes prevents the generation of the mediator by insulin. Seals and Czech (1980) have proposed that after insulin binds to its receptor a membrane bond protease is activated that cleaves the mediator at an arginine residue. Muchmore et al. (1982) have shown that the effects of most proteolytic inhibitors on the effects of insulin on adipocytes may be secondary to decreased cellular ATP. Originally, our laboratory had been unable to confirm that peptide bonds were necessary for biological activity of the mediator based on studies involving proteolytic enzymes, dansylation, treatment with fluorescamine, and high-pressure liquid chromatography. Recently, with the mediator from the skeletal muscle of insulin-treated rats, we have found trypsin to have little effect on mediator activity, whereas chymotrypsin had a greater effect and pepsin had the greatest effect on activity. Complete inactivation was not obtained. These data indicated that the mediator contains amino acids but that the biological activity was not totally dependent on their presence. Furthermore, we could not substantiate that common sugars or amino sugars were part of the mediator structure, since the material did not bind to a variety of immobilized lectins. However, Begum et al. (1983a) have shown that both neuraminidase and β-D-galactosidase treatment inactivates the mediator generated by liver plasma membranes. The presence or absence of carbohydrate and amino acid residues in the mediator have been assessed by their requirement for biological activity. Certainly, when greater quantities of purified mediator are available, direct chemical analytical techniques will be employed to substantiate these data.

The above data led us to consider other membrane components, such as phospholipids and their derivatives as potential mediators. The existence of a phospholipid-sensitive, calcium-dependent protein kinase (protein kinase C) with a wide tissue distribution (Kaibuchi et al., 1981; Wrenn et al., 1980; Kuo et al., 1980) suggests a direct relationship between phospholipid release and protein phosphorylation. Farese, et al. (1982) showed that insulin treatment of adipocytes increased the content of several phospholipids. Walaas et al. (1981) reported that insulin increased the phosphorylation of a muscle sarcolemmal proteolipid with a molecular weight of 3600. Wasner (1981) found that insulin increased the amount of a low molecular weight compound called cyclic AMP antagonist, which may contain PGE_1 as a structural component. This compound inhibits adenylate cyclase and protein kinases and activates phosphoprotein phosphatases and pyruvate dehydrogenase. A preliminary report from Begum et al. (1983b) demonstrates that indomethacin, an inhibitor of prostaglandin synthesis, prevented mediator generation from liver plasma membrane by insulin. This inhibitory effect of indomethacin was reversed by the addition of prostaglandin E_2. Perhaps, the mediator is generated following activation of a membrane-bound phospholipase A_1 or A_2 as suggested by others (Bereziat et al., 1978; Dietze, 1982).

We have investigated the role of phospholipids and related compounds in insulin action. The mediator preparation from adipocyte plasma membranes before and after gel filtration contains at least ten phospholipids. The addition of aqueous dispersions of these phospholipids

to assays for pyruvate dehydrogenase and low K_m cAMP phosphodiesterase demonstrated specific effects. Phosphatidylserine and
phosphatidylinositol 4-phosphate were found to stimulate and inhibit specifically, respectively, pyruvate dehydrogenase activity,
while other phospholipids had no effect (Kiechle and Jarett, 1983).
Similarly, phosphatidylserine and phosphatidylcholine stimulated and
phosphatidylinositol 4-phosphate inhibited the low K_m cAMP phosphodiesterase activity of adipocyte microsomal (endoplasmic reticulum) and plasma membrane preparations (Macaulay et al., 1983a,b).
The high K_m enzyme was unaffected by these same phospholipids.
These initial studies suggest that phosphatidylserine and phosphatidylinositol 4-phosphate could have a counterregulatory role that
could be of physiological importance in regulating enzyme activity.
Although Farese et al. (1983a,b) have shown that the insulin-
induced increase in phosphatidylserine in adipose tissue precedes
the activation of pyruvate dehydrogenase (a temporal relationship
required for a second messenger), it seems unlikely that phosphatidylserine alone represents the mediator for insulin action. However, phospholipids may be involved in an alternative regulatory
role for certain insulin-sensitive enzymes, such as pyruvate dehydrogenase and low K_m cyclic AMP phosphodiesterase.

IV. OTHER SYSTEMS IN WHICH SIMILAR MEDIATORS ARE GENERATED AND THEIR RELATIONSHIP TO GROWTH EFFECTS

Does the insulin mediator alter cell growth through effects on macromolecular synthesis? Horvat (1980) has described an insulin-
induced factor from perfused liver with a molecular weight of less
than 1000 that stimulated the synthesis of RNA when added to isolated nuclei. Liver nuclei possess insulin receptors. Recently, it
has been shown that the direct addition of insulin to these nuclei
results in the stimulation of mRNA efflux from intact nuclei (Schumm
and Webb, 1981) and the stimulation of nucleoside triphophatase
activity (Purrello et al., 1982), the enzyme that regulates mRNA
efflux. Both effects demonstrate a biphasic response with respect
to insulin concentration. Therefore, the regulation of mRNA synthesis in these nuclei may be controlled by intact insulin and/or
low molecular weight degradation product of insulin or a metabolite
generated by insulin action.
    The addition of ligands to other membrane systems may generate
mediators similar to the insulin mediators. The interaction of two
mitogenic lectins, concanavalin A or phytohemagglutinin, with

lymphocyte plasma membranes activated lymphocyte and adipocyte pyruvate dehydrogenase (Beachy et al., 1981). Growth hormone fragments with insulinlike (Heng et al., 1982) or insulin-antagonistic (Ng et al., 1982) activities generated a low molecular weight material that either activated or inhibited, respectively, pyruvate dehydrogenase and acetyl-CoA carboxylase. Oxytocin has been reported to have insulinlike activity and activates pyruvate dehydrogenase in adipocytes (Hanif et al., 1982). It may also generate a similar low molecular weight mediator.

V. SUMMARY

In this chapter, we have reviewed the three major types of reactions that insulin stimulates on target tissues and the relationship of these reactions to the low molecular weight mediators of insulin action. The relationship between the mediator(s) and insulin stimulation of rapid membrane reactions and responses and stimulation of growth are unknown. The binding of insulin to its plasma membrane receptor must induce specific reactions that led to mediator generation. The nature of these reactions requires further study.

There may not be a single mediator. Only a systematic study of its presence and its structure in many insulin-sensitive cell types will resolve this question. The mediators of insulin action have been detected in several intact cells and subcellular systems composed of plasma membrane and other cellular components. The mediators alter the activity of a variety of enzymes in the same manner as the addition of insulin to intact cells. The chemical structure of these mediators remains unknown. The availability of greater quantities of this material will permit the purification required prior to chemical analysis. The finding of low molecular weight mediators in systems sensitive to other hormones suggests that these compounds may represent a new group of regulatory molecules that are perhaps structurally related. These initial observations concerning the low molecular weight mediators of insulin action provide a new avenue for research in diabetes mellitus. Some patients with insulin resistance may have a deficiency in the quantity or an abnormality in the structure of the mediators of insulin action. Similar defects may be determined in other hormone-resistant states in which these compounds function as mediators of hormone action. If deficiencies in the production of these low molecular weight compounds are related to resistant states, then it may be feasible to develop chemotherapy to reestablish a normal pattern of production.

ACKNOWLEDGMENTS

This work was supported in part by U.S. Public Health Service Grant AM-28144-02 (L.J.) and Grant BRSG SO7-05415-21 (F.L.K.) awarded by the Biomedical Research Support Grant Program, Division of Research Resources, National Institute of Health. F.L.K. was a Hartford Fellow.

REFERENCES

Alemany, S., Verela, I., and Mato, J. M. (1981). FEBS Lett. 135:111.
Amatruda, J. M. and Chang, C. L. (1983). Biochem. Biophys. Res. Commun. 112:35.
Amatruda, J. M. and Finch, E. D. (1979). J. Biol. Chem. 254:2619.
Beachy, J. C., Goldman, D., and Czech, M. P. (1981). Proc. Natl. Acad. Sci. USA 78:6256.
Begum, N., Tepperman, H. M., and Tepperman, J. (1982a). Endocrinology 110:1914.
Begum, N., Tepperman, H. M., and Tepperman, J. (1982b). Endocrinology 111:1491.
Begum, N., Tepperman, H. M., and Tepperman, J. (1983a). Endocrinology 112:50.
Begum, N., Tepperman, H. M., and Tepperman, J (1983b). Diabetes 32 (Suppl. 1):34A.
Bereziat, G., Wolf, C., Colard, O., and Polonovski, J. (1978). Adv. Expt. Biol. Med. 101:191.
Bremer, J. and Greenberg, D. M. (1961). Biochim. Biophys. Acta. 46:205.
Brownsey, R. W. and Denton, R. M. (1982). Biochem. J. 202:77.
Cassel, D., Pike, L. J., Grant, G. A., Krebs, E. G., and Glaser, L. (1983). J. Biol. Chem. 258:2945.
Castano, J. G., Alemany, S. Nieto, A., and Mato, J. M. (1980). J. Biol. Chem. 255:9041.
Chen, K., Galasko, G., Huang, L., Kellogg, J., and Larner, J. (1980). Diabetes 29:659.
Cohen, S., Carpenter, G. and King, L. Jr. (1980). J. Biol. Chem. 255:4834.
Cullis, P. R. and de Kruijff, B. (1979). Biochim. Biophys. Acta 559:399.

Davis, R. J., Brand, M. D., and Martin, B. R. (1981). *Biochem. J.* 196:133.

Denton, R. M. and Hughes, W. A. (1978). *Int. J. Biochem.* 9:545.

Denton, R. M., Brownsey, R. W. and Belshaz, G. J. (1981). *Diabetologica* 21:347.

Dietze, G. J. (1982). *Mol. Cell. Endocrinol.* 25:127.

Farese, R. V., Larson, R E., and Sabir, M. A. (1982). *J. Biol. Chem.* 257:4042.

Farese, R. V., Farese, R. V., Jr., Sabir, M. A., and Trudeau, W. L. (1983a). *Clin. Res.* 30:877a.

Farese, R. V., Sabir, M. A., Larson, R. E. and Trudeau, W. L. (1983b). *Biochim. Biophys. Acta* 750:200.

Gould, R. J., Ginsberg, B. H., and Spector, A. A. (1982). *J. Biol. Chem.* 257:477.

Hanif, K., Lederis, K., Hollenberg, M. D., and Goren, H. J. (1982). *Science* 216:1010.

Heng, D. L. F., Ng, F. M., and Bornstein, J. (1982). *12th Intl. Cong. Biochem. Abst.* 001–188, 138.

Hirata, F. and Axelrod, J. (1980). *Science* 209:1082.

Hoffman, D. R., Hanig, J. A., and Cornatzer, W. E. (1981). *Proc. Expt. Biol. Med.* 167:143.

Holloway, C. T. and Garfield, S. A. (1981). *Lipids* 16:525.

Horvat, A. (1980). *Nature (London)* 286:906,

Houslay, M. D. (1981). *Biosci. Rep.* 1:19.

Huganir, R. L. and Greengard, P. (1983). *Proc. Natl. Acad. Sci. USA* 80:1130.

Jarett, L. and Kiechle, F. L. (1981). *Current Views on Insulin Receptors (Serono Sumposium No. 41)*, (D. Andreani, R. DePirro, R. Lauro, J. Olefsky, and J. Roth, eds.), Academic Press, New York, pp. 245–253.

Jarett, L. and Seals, J. R. (1979). *Science* 206:1407.

Jarett, L., Kiechle, F. L., Popp, D. A., Kotagal, N., and Gavin, J. R., III (1980). *Biochem. Biophys. Res. Commun.* 96:735.

Jarett, L., Kiechle, F. L., Popp, D. A., and Kotagal, N. (1981). *Cold Spring Harbor Conference on Cell Proliferation*, Cold Spring Harbor Laboratory, Cold Spring Harbor, New York, Vol. 8, pp. 715–726.

Jarett, L., Kiechle, F. L., Parker, J. C., and Macaulay, S. L. (1983). *Am. J. Med.* 74(1A):31.

Kaibuchi, K., Takai, Y., and Nishizuka, Y. (1981). *J. Biol. Chem.* 256:7146.

Kelly, K. L., Kiechle, F. L., and Jarett, L. (1984). *Proc. Natl. Acad. Sci. USA* 81:1089.

Kiechle, F. L. and Jarett, L. (1981). *FEBS Lett.* 133:279.

Kiechle, F. L. and Jarett, L. (1983). *Mol. Cell. Biochem.* 56:99.

Kiechle, F. L., Jarett, L., Popp, D., and Kotagal, N. (1980). *Diabetes* 29:852.

Kiechle, F. L., Jarett, L., Popp, D. A., and Kotagal, N. (1981). *J. Biol. Chem.* 256:2945.

Kuo, J. F., Anderson, R. G. G., Wise, B. C., Mackerlova, L., Salomonsson, I., Brackett, N. L., Katoh, N., Shoji, M., and Wrenn, R. W. (1980). *Proc. Natl. Acad. Sci. USA* 77:7039.

Larner, J (1983). *Am. J. Med.* 74(1A):38.

Larner, J., Galasko, G., Cheng, K., DePaoli-Roach, A. A., Huang, L., Daggy, P., and Kellog, J. (1979). *Science* 206:1408,

Larner, J., Cheng, K., Schwartz, C. K., Kuchi, K., Tamura, S., Creacy, S., Dubler, R. Galasko, G., Pullin, C., and Katz, M. (1982). *Rec. Prog. Horm. Res.* 38:511.

Leo, G. C., Kiechle, F. L., and Opella, S. J. (1983). *Clin. Res.* 31:390A.

Loten, E. G. and Sneyd, J. G (1970). *Biochem J.* 120:187.

Loten, E. G. Assimacopoulos-Jeannet, F. D., Exton, J. H., and Park, C. R. (1978). *J. Biol. Chem.* 253:746.

Luly, P. and Shinitzky, M. (1979). *Biochemistry* 18:445.

Macaulay, S. L., Kiechle, F. L., and Jarett, L. (1983a). *Arch. Biochem. Biophys.* 225:130.

Macaulay, S. L., Kiechle, F. L., and Jarett, L. (1983b). *Biochim. Biophys. Acta* 760:293.

Machicao, F., Urumow, T., and Wieland, O. H. (1982). *FEBS Letters* 149:96.

Makino, H. and Kono, T. (1980). *J. Biol. Chem.* 255:7850.

Marchmont, R. J. and Houslay, M. D. (1981). *Biochem. J.* 195:653

Mato, J. U. and Alemany, S. (1983). *Biochem. J.* 213:1.

McCaleb, M. L. and Donner, D. B. (1981). *J. Biol. Chem.* 256:11051.

Melchoir, D. L. and Czech, M. P. (1979). *J. Biol. Chem.* 254:8744.

Muchmore, D. B., Raess, B. U., Bergstrom, R. W., and DeHaen, C. (1982). *Diabetes* 31:976.

Niedel, J. E., Kuhn, L. J., and Vandenbark, G. R. (1983). *Proc. Natl. Acad. Sci. USA* 80:36.

Ng, F. M., Blaskett, E., Larsen-Disney, P., and Bornstein, J. (1982). *12th Intl. Cong. Biochem. Abst.* 001-187, 138.

Ogreid, J. S. S., Doskeland, S. O., Refanes, M., Sand, T. F., Yeland, P. M., and Christofferson, T. (1982). *FEBS Lett.* 138:167.

Parker, J. C., Kiechle, F. L., and Jarett, L. (1982). *Arch. Biochim. Biophys.* 215:339.

Petruzzelli, L. M., Ganguly, S., Smith, C. J., Cobb, M. H., Rubin, C. S., and Rosen, O. M. (1982). *Proc. Natl. Acad. Sci. USA* 79:6792.

Pfenninger, K. H. and Johnson, M. P. (1980). *Proc. Natl. Acad. Sci. USA* 78:7797.

Popp, D., Kiechle, F. L., Kotagal, N., and Jarett, L. (1980). *J. Biol. Chem.* 255:7540.

Prasad, C. and Edwards, R. M. (1981). *Biochem. Biophys. Res. Commun.* 103:559.

Purrello, F., Vigneri, R., Clawson, G. A., and Goldfine, I. D. (1982). *Science* 216:1005

Rodbell, M., Jones, A. B., Chiappe de Cingolani, G. E., and Birnbaumer, L. (1968). *Rec. Prog. Horm. Res.* 24:215.

Sakamoto, Y., Kuzuya, T., and Sato, J. (1982). *Biomed. Res.* 3:599.

Saltiel, A., Jacobs, S., Siegel, M., and Cuatrecases, P. (1981). *Biochem. Biophys. Res. Commun.* 102:1041.

Saltiel, A. R., Sigel, M. I., Jacobs, S., and Cuatrecasas, P. (1982). *Proc. Natl. Acad. Sci. USA* 79:3513.

Saltiel, A. R., Doble, A., Jacobs, S., and Cuatrecasas, P. (1983). *Biochem. Biophys. Res. Commun.* 110:789

Schumm, D. E. and Webb, T. E. (1981). *Arch. Biochem. Biophys.* 210:275.

Seals, J. R. and Czech, M. P. (1980). *J. Biol. Chem.* 255:6529.

Seals, J. R. and Czech, M. P. (1981). *J. Biol. Chem.* 256:2894.

Seals, J. R. and Jarett, L. (1980). *Proc. Natl. Acad. Sci. USA* 77:77.

Seals, J. R., McDonald, J. M., and Jarett, L. (1979). *J. Biol. Chem.* 254:6997.

Shia, M. A. and Pilch, P. F. (1983). *Biochemistry* 22:717.

Smith, C. J. and Rosen, O. M. (1983). *Diabetes Mellitus: Theory and Practice* (M. Ellenberg and H. Rifkin, eds.), Medical Examination Publ., New Hyde Park, New York, pp. 89–96.

Stein, I. M. and Hales, C. N. (1974). *Biochim. Biophys. Acta.* 337:41.

Sun, J. V., Tepperman, H. M., and Tepperman, J. (1979). *J. Nutr.* 109:193.

Turakulov, H. K., Gainutdinov, M. D., Lavina, J. I., and Akhmatou, M. D. (1977). *Rep. Acad. Sci. USSR* 234:1471 (Russ).

Van Obberghen, E., Rossi, B., Kowalski, A., Gazzano, H., and Ponzio, G. (1983). *Proc. Natl. Acad. Sci. USA* 80:945.

Walaas, O., Sletten, K., Horn, R.S., Lystad, E., Adler, A., and Alertsen, A. R. (1981). *FEBS Lett.* 128:137.

Wasner, H. K. (1981). *FEBS Lett.* 133:260.

Witters, L. A. (1981). *Biochem. Biophys. Res. Commun.* 100:872.

Wrenn, R. W., Katoh, N., Wise, B. C., and Kuo, J. F. (1980). *J. Biol. Chem.* 255:12042.

Zick, Y., Kasuga, M., Kahn, C. R., and Roth, J. (1983a). *J. Biol. Chem.* 258:75.

Zick, Y., Grunberger, G., Podskalny, J. M., Moncada, V., Taylor,
    S. I., Gorden, P., and Roth, J. (1983b). *Biochem. Biophys. Res.
    Commun. 116*:1129.

BIBLIOGRAPHY

Czech, M. P. (1977). Molecular basis of insulin action. *Ann. Rev.
    Biochem. 46*:359—384.
Czech, M. P. (ed.) 1985. *Molecular basis of insulin action*. Plenum,
    New York.
Denton, R. M., Brownsey, R. W. and Belsham, G. J. (1981). A par-
    tial view of the mechanism of insulin action. *Diabetologica 21*:347—362.
Houslay, M. D. (1981). Membrane phosphorylation: A crucial role in
    the action of insulin, EGF, and pp60^{src}? *Biosci. Rep. 1*:19—34.
Houslay, M. D. and Heyworth, C. M. (1983). Insulin: In search of a
    mechanism. *Trends Biochem. Sci. 8*:449—452.
Jarett, L., Kiechle, F. L., Popp, D. D., and Kotagal, N. (1981).
    The role of a chemical mediator of insulin action in the control of
    phosphorylation. *In Cold Spring Harbor Conference on Cell
    Proliferation*. Vol. 8, *Protein Phosphorylation*, Cold Spring
    Harbor Laboratory, Cold Spring Harbor, New York, pp. 715—726.
Jarett, L., Kiechle, F. L., Parker, J. C., and Macaulay, S. L.
    (1983). The chemical mediators of insulin action: Possible tar-
    gets for postreceptor defects. *Am. J. Med. 74*(1A):31—37.
Larner, J., Cheng, K., Schwartz, C., Kikuchi, K., Tamura, S.,
    Creacy, S., Dubler, R., Galasko, G., Pullin, C., and Katz, M.
    (1982). Insulin mediators and their control of metabolism through
    protein phosphorylation. *Rec. Prog. Horm. Res. 38*:511—556.
Larner, J. (1983). Mediators of postreceptor action of insulin. *Am. J.
    Med. 74*(1A):38—51.
Smith, C. J. and Rosen, O. M. (1983). Mechanism of action of insulin.
    In Diabetes Mellitus: Theory, and Practice (M. Ellenberg and
    H. Rifkin, eds.), Medical E0amination Publ. Co., New Hyde Park,
    New York, pp. 89—96.
Walaas, O. and Horn, R. S. (1981). The controversial problem of in-
    sulin action. *Trends Pharmacol. Sci. 2*:196—198.

10

Receptors in the Central Nervous System for Insulin and Other Circulating Peptide Hormones

MARK VAN HOUTEN* and BARRY I. POSNER *McGill University Clinic and Royal Victoria Hospital, Montreal, Quebec, Canada*

I. INTRODUCTION

The endocrine and nervous sytems are the two major integrators of mammalian physiology. Together they coordinate both rapid homeostatic responses to stress and prolonged adaptations to growth and reproduction, which determine the survival of the individual and the species. Investigations into the integration of the two systems have focused classically on the effector role of the nervous system in the control of endocrine secretion. Recently, the importance of peptide hormone feedback regulation of CNS function has been increasingly recognized.

It appears that certain circulating peptide hormones, notably prolactin (Höhn and Wuttke, 1978; Perkins et al., 1979) and growth hormone (Müller, 1973; Tannenbaum, 1980; Berelowitz et al., 1981) and perhaps lutenizing hormone (LH) and follicle-stimulating hormone (FSH) (Sawyer, 1975; Sanghera et al., 1978) influence endocrine control centers that regulate their own secretion. Insulin (Woods and Porte, 1978; Woods et al., 1979), cholecystokinin (CCK) (Saito et al., 1981), and calcitonin seem to act directly on central feeding centers, angiotensin II directly stimulates central systems that modulate drinking, blood pressure, and antidiuresis (Simpson, 1981); neurotensin and bombesin influence central thermoregulation (Mason et al., 1980); and corticotropin facilitates learning and memory (de Wied, 1978).

Evidence for a direct action of blood-borne peptide hormones on the brain appear to be contradicted by the inability of polypeptides to

Present affiliation: Department of Neurology, University of California at Los Angeles, School of Medicine, Los Angeles, California

traverse the blood-brain barrier (Reese and Karnovsky, 1967; Ramsay and Reid, 1975; Cornford et al., 1978). The issue could be resolved, if it were possible to locate the hormone receptors that are responsible for the initial recognition phase of peptide hormone action (Posner, 1975). Grossly regional localization of receptors in brain, using classic in vitro competitive binding methods, has been achieved for a variety of peptide hormones, including insulin (Havrankova et al., 1977), Angiotensin II (Sirret et al., 1977), calcitonin (Rizzo and Goltzman, 1981); CCK (Saito et al., 1981) vasoactive intestinal polypeptide (VIP) (Taylor and Pert, 1979), neurotensin (Uhl et al., 1977), Bombesin (Moody et al., 1978), prolactin (DiCarlo and Muccioli, 1981 ; Posner et al., 1982), and opoid peptides (Pert and Snyder, 1973; Snyder and Simantov, 1977). However, this approach fails to differentiate between receptors for endogenous brain peptides and those that interact with blood-borne peptides, nor does the approach permit a precise identification of the structures bearing the peptide hormone receptors.

We have attempted to visualize receptors in the central nervous system for blood-borne peptide hormones by utilizing light and electron microscopic approaches (Bergeron and Posner, 1979). According to our procedures, ^{125}I-labeled peptide hormones with high specific activity and biological activity are injected into the arterial circulation of experimental rats either alone or in combination with graded amounts of unlabeled peptides, analogues, or structurally dissimilar peptides. Moments later, unbound radioactivity remaining in the circulation and within interstitial spaces is flushed out by systemic perfusion, first with a buffered isotonic solution and then with an appropriate protein fixative to retain receptor-bound radioactivity for radioautographic visualization. The intensity of the radioautographic reaction over brain tissue sections, which is an accurate reflection of the amount of bound radioactivity (Junger, 1978), is quantitatively analyzed by grain counting. Comparison of data from treatments with unlabelled peptides yields conclusions regarding the specificity as well as the location of the binding sites.

The purpose of this chapter is to summarize our observations concerning peptide hormone feedback on the brain. These observations are obtained by the application of the radioautographic approach to the elucidation of in vivo binding interactions.

II. THE UNIQUE PROPERTIES OF THE CIRCUMVENTRICULAR ORGANS

The four circumventricular organs (CVO) are phylogentically old regions of the midline periventricular brain (Hofer, 1958; Weindl, 1973). The most well-known of these specialized regions is the median eminence, which spans the third ventricle to unite the basal halves of the hypothalamus. The lesser known circumventricular organs include the organum vasculosum of the lamina terminalis (OVLT), which is located in the ventral wall of the rostral third ventricle; the subfornical organ (SFO), which protrudes into the dorsal third ventricle where it is suspended from the ventral hippocampal commissure; and the area postrema, which bulges dorsally into the fourth ventricle at the level of the motor and sensory subdivisions of the vagal nuclei.

The specialized vasculature of the circumventricular organs is unique in the central nervous system. Microvessel endothelia in these regions are fenestrated to permit rapid equilibration of polypeptides between blood and adjacent nervous tissue (Weindl, 1973; Broadwell and Brightman, 1976). In the median eminence and OVLT, the adjacent nervous tissue consists primarily of abundant nerve terminals (LeBeaux, 1972). The SFO (Dellman and Simpson 1976) and area postrema (Klara and Brizzee, 1977) contain neuronal perikarya as well. It has been speculated repeatedly that the unique permeability of the circumventricular organs permits the adjacent nervous tissue to interact directly with the systemic circulation in either a sensory, absorptive, or secretory capacity (Koella and Sutin, 1967). Neurosecretion is the well-recognized role of the median eminence, which represents the proximal segment of the hypophyseal infundibulum and is linked to the adenohypophysis via a direct portal circulation. The other circumventricular organs are not directly linked to a target gland and hence are not likely to be neurosecretory in function. Nonetheless, all of the circumventricular organs permit rapid and direct interaction of the adjacent nervous tissue with circulating peptides, whereas all other regions of the brain are shielded from circulating peptides by an impermeable blood-brain barrier. Our radioautographic studies with numerous systemically injected iodopeptide hormones (van Houten et al., 1979; 1980a; 1981a,b; van Houten and Posner, 1981b,c) indicate that the circumventricular organs are the major if not the exclusive mediators of a direct interaction between blood-borne peptide hormones and the brain.

III. THE CIRCUMVENTRICULAR ORGANS POSSESS SPECIFIC RECEPTORS FOR BLOOD-BORNE PEPTIDE HORMONES

Mere diffusion of blood-borne peptide hormones into the CVOs would have little functional significance, if cellular elements in the adjacent nervous tissue did not possess specific receptors for these peptides. We analyzed quantitatively the radioautographic pattern of peptide binding to the CVOs of rats under conditions of competitive binding, and we found that cellular elements in the circumventricular organs can recognize blood-borne peptide hormones and bind them with specificity. Thus, for a variety of polypeptide hormones, including insulin (van Houten et al., 1979), angiotensin II (van Houten et al., 1980b), lactogen (van Houten et al., 1980c), adrenocorticotropin (van Houten et al.,

1981a), and calcitonin (van Houten et al., 1982b), the binding of the radioiodinated polypeptide to the circumventricular organs was blocked by coinjected unlabeled polypeptides of the same or structurally homologous species, but not by structurally dissimilar peptides.

In the case of adrenocorticotropin, the specificity of the receptor site probably reflects its function. We have observed that both the hypothalamic median eminence and the adrenal zona fasciculata bind blood-borne [^{125}I]ACTH with specificity (van Houten et al., 1981a). However, α- and β-MSH, which represent a small peptide sequence contained with the N-terminal region of the ACTH 1−24 polypeptide (Kreiger and Martin, 1981), blocked the binding of [^{125}I]ACTH to the median eminence but not to the adrenal (van Houton et al., 1981b). The differential peptide specificity of the median eminence and adrenal binding site is consistent with previous studies, which have shown that the N-terminal ACTH 4−10 region influences memory function (de Wied, 1977), whereas the C-terminal region of the polypeptide is steroidogenic (Ontjes et al., 1977). The differential specificity of these binding sites and the close correlation between binding specificity and functional activity constitutes strong evidence of the biological importance of the circumventricular receptor system.

IV. NEURONAL MEDIATION OF CIRCUMVENTRICULAR RECEPTIVITY

The circumventricular receptor system may represent the link between endocrine effectors and central neuronal networks that regulate endocrine secretion, autonomic outflow, and behavior. We have attempted to identify the cellular elements in the CVOs that could mediate the hormone-receptor interaction.

In the median eminence, specific binding sites for blood-borne [^{125}I]insulin have been localized to nerve terminals (Fig. 1) and in the adjacent hypothalamic arcuate nucleus (Fig. 2) to synaptic terminals (van Houten et al., 1980a). These axonal receptors may be hypophysiotropic terminals involved in mediating insulin effects on the secretion of growth hormone (Pecile et al., 1971) or gonodotropin (Rossi and Bestetti, 1981). In addition, insulin-receptive nerve terminals may play a more complex role in mediating insulin effects on hypothalamic electrical activity (Oomura, 1976), catecholamine turnover (McCaleb et al., 1979), and limbic functions related to glucose homeostasis (Storlien et al., 1979; Szabo and Szabo, 1975; Iguchi et al., 1981), caloric balance, and satiety (Hatfield et al., 1974; Strubbe and Mein, 1977; Woods et al., 1979).

The neuronal circuitry to which these axons belong has been elucidated recently by combined application of surgical ablation and radioautography (van Houten et al., 1983). These studies show that

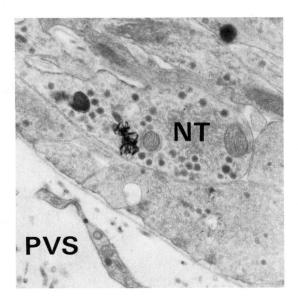

Figure 1 Electron microscope radioautograph illustrating the binding of [125I]insulin to a nerve terminal (NT) in rat median eminence. Blood-borne peptides enter this region by passing through the fenestrated endothelia and the broad perivascular spaces (PVS) that characterize all of the circumventricular organs.

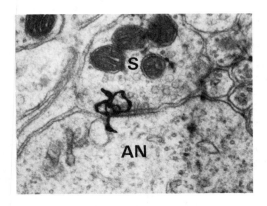

Figure 2 Electron microscope radioautograph illustrating the binding of [125I]insulin to a synaptic terminal (S) on a hypothalamic arcuate neuron (AN). Synaptic receptors for insulin may account for the rapid effects of insulin on hypothalmic electrical activity. (From Oomura, 1976.)

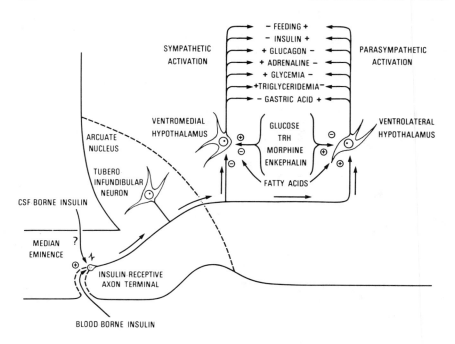

Figure 3 The ventral hypothalamus functions as if it were composed of a medial and lateral component, each of which exerts reciprocally opposite influences over central autonomic outflow. Stimulation of the ventromedial hypothalamus produces sympathetic catabolic activation, i.e., hyperglycemia (Bernardis and Frohman, 1971; Barkai and Allweis, 1972), glycogenolysis (Matsushita and Shimazu, 1980), gluconeogenesis (Shimazu and Ogasawara, 1975), and lipolysis (Bray and Nishizawa, 1978; Texeira et al., 1975), in part by tonically inhibiting insulin secretion (Frohman and Bernardis, 1971; Rohner et al., 1977; Berthoud and Renaud, 1979) and gastric acid secretion (Weingarten and Powley, 1980) while stimulating the secretion of adrenaline (Frohman and Bernardis, 1971; Frohman et al., 1973), glucagon (Frohman and Bernardis, 1971; DeJong et al., 1977; Shimazu and Ishikawa, 1979), and growth hormone (Frohman et al., 1968). Stimulation of the ventrolateral hypothalamus produces parasympathetic anabolic activation, such as increasing basal (DeJong et al., 1977) and glucose-stimulated insulin release (Curry and Joy, 1974) in part by activating pancreatic vagal fibers (Kita et al., 1980), decreasing hepatic glycogen synthesis (Matsushita and Shimazu, 1980), and increasing gastric acid secretion (Carmona and Slagen, 1973). The two regions are reciprocally innervated, are mutually inhibitory, and exhibit reciprocal activation/inhibition under a variety of contrasting metabolic states (Anand et al., 1964; Oomura et al., 1969). Neurons in the ventromedial hypothalamus are inhibited, whereas neurons in the lateral hypothalamus are stimulated by insulin (Oomura, 1976).

insulin-receptive nerve terminals in the median eminence arise from so-called tuberoinfundibular neurons of the hypothalamic arcuate nucleus. Tuberoinfundibular neurons in this region are thought to possess a complexly branched axonal tree that projects into the CNS as well as the median eminence and could permit these neurons to act on the brain and pituitary simultaneously (Renaud and Martin, 1976). Recent studies have shown that blood-borne peptide hormones can electrically activate certain neurosecretory axon terminals (Baertschi et al., 1981), and that electrical signals generated at the neurosecretory terminal can be transmitted "backward" into the brain via the tuberoinfundibular neuron (Renaud and Martin, 1976). We have speculated that the result of insulin binding to its receptor in the median eminence is the production of an electrical signal that is relayed to specific regulatory centers in the brain via the axonal tree of the receptive tuberoinfundibular neuron (Fig. 3). These peptide-receptive neurons could provide the essential anatomic pathway linking endocrine feedback to the appropriate central regulatory centers.

In the area postrema, insulin-specific binding sites have been localized to nerve cell bodies and dendrites (van Houton and Posner, 1981a). These peptide-receptive neurons could provide indirect hormone feedback on parasympathetic and sympathetic neuronal centers via connection with the visceral subdivisions of the nucleus solitarius (Fig. 4).

Moreover, the neuronal relay circuitry may exist for a wide variety of hormonal feedback signals that have receptors in the CVOs. Angiotensin II-receptors (van Houten et al., 1980b) and angiotensin I-responsive neurons (Felix and Akert, 1974) have been identified in the SFO, which mediates the central effects of circulating angiotensin II on drinking, blood pressure, and antidiuresis (Simpson, 1981). Neurons in SFO project to regions of the CNS that are essential to the normal regulation of these functions (Miselis et al., 1979). It may well be that circulating angiotensin II activates specific regulatory centers of the brain via discrete central pathways emanating from angiotensin II-receptive neurons of the SFO.

Insulin-sensitive units are inversely affected by glucose and fatty acids (Oomura, 1976), TRH (Ishibashi et al., 1979), and morphine/enkephalins (Ono et al., 1980). Insulin directly influences hypothalamic centers regulating feeding and body weight (Hatfield et al., 1974; Strubbe and Mein, 1977) and glucostatic reflexes (Storlein et al., 1975; Szabo and Szabo, 1975; Iguchi et al., 1981). We have suggested that blood-borne insulin activates or inhibits specific hypothalamic functions by stimulating directly tuberoinfundibular neurons, which could relay feedback messages by retrograde conduction of electrical inpulses. Interaction of the median eminence receptor with CSF-borne insulin may provide a more sustained uniform regulation of basal activity. (From van Houten and Posner, 1983.)

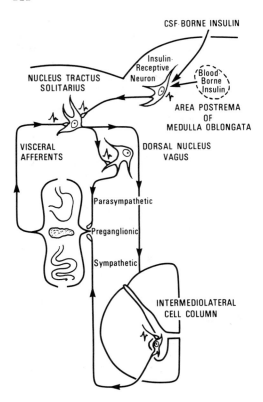

Figure 4 Peptide hormone-receptive neurons in the area postrema represent the first element in a chain that could link peptide hormone feedback signals via central neurons to brainstem and spinal centers that determine autonomic outflow to the gut (Kerr and Preshaw, 1969). Circulating insulin could activate hormone-sensitive neurons in the area postrema, which in turn could modulate visceral afferent input into the nucleus tractus solitarius (Morest, 1967). The net result would determine the appropriate blend of activities among sympathetic and parasympathetic preganglionic neurons in the regulation of gut function.

V. FUNCTIONAL TOPOGRAPHY OF CIRCUMVENTRICULAR RECEPTORS

Peptide hormone receptors in the CVOs show a peptide-specific pattern of regional distribution (Fig. 5). Adrenocorticotropin binding sites occur exclusively in the median eminence, whereas binding sites for other peptides investigated are present in all the CVOs but show regional variation: insulin-binding sites are most dense in the median eminence; angiotensin II-binding sites are most dense in the SFO; and calcitonin binding sites are most dense in the OVLT.

Furthermore, peptide hormone-binding sites show a peptide-specific histological pattern within each CVO, which is well-illustrated in the median eminence (Fig. 6). In this CVO, specific binding sites for insulin and adrenocorticotropin occur broadly across the external zone, and insulin-binding sites continue into the adjacent arcuate nucleus. In contrast, angiotensin II receptors are concentrated in the medial palisade zone, where they are ideally situated possibly to influence vasopressin secretion (Leclerc and Pelletier, 1974). Binding sites for lactogen are concentrated in the lateral palisade zone, a region of median eminence rich in dopamine and luteinizing hormone releasing hormone (LHRH) (Fuxe et al., 1978). Moreover, calcitonin receptors display a uniquely bilateral distribution that overlaps the distribution of somatostatinergic nerve terminals (Baker and Yu, 1976). The essential point is that blood-borne peptide hormones bind with specificity to discrete regions containing concentrations of neurosecretory substances

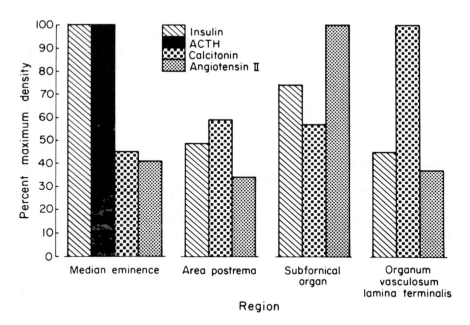

Figure 5 Peptide hormone receptors show a peptide-specific pattern of regional distribution among the various CVOs. The density of receptors for blood-borne peptide hormones is greater in some regions than others, depending upon the peptide. (From van Houten and Posner, 1983.)

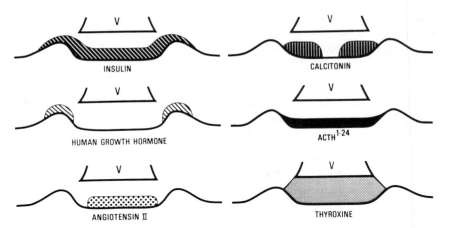

Figure 6 Peptide hormone receptors show a peptide-specific histological pattern of distribution within the median eminence (see text for explanation). From van Houten and Posner (1983).

whose own secretion is thought to be regulated by specific circulating peptide hormones. The implications for the elucidation of peptide hormone regulation of hypophysiotropic function are obvious.

VI. ROLE OF CIRCUMVENTRICULAR RECEPTORS IN ENDOCRINE HEALTH AND DISEASE

What effect would an imbalance in the endocrine milieu have on hormone-sensitive receptors in the brain and on the functions they modulate? It is possible that specific central regulatory centers may malfunction in turn and thereby compound the disorder. Thus, insulin-sensitive hypothalamic functions may malfunction in the insulin-dependent diabetic. Activation of sympathetic autonomic components of the ventromedial hypothalamus produces hyperglycemia, in part by inhibiting insulin secretion (Bernardis and Frohman, 1971; Rohner et al., 1977; Berthoud and Renaud, 1979), stimulating hepatic glucose production (Bernardis and Frohman, 1971; Barkai and Allweis, 1972; Shimazu and Ogasawara, 1975; Matsushita and Shimazu, 1980) and stimulating the secretion of epinephrine (Bernardis and Frohman, 1971; Frohman et al., 1973), glucagon (Bernardis and Frohman, 1971; DeJong et al., 1977; Ishikawa et al., 1982), and growth hormone (Frohman et al., 1968). The presence of insulin in this region of the brain suppresses ventromedial electrical activity (Oomura, 1976) and produces hypoglycemia (Storlien et al., 1975; Szabo and Szabo, 1975), presumably by direct inhibition of the ventromedial center for hyperglycemia. Hence, it may well be that the intrinsic ventromedial autonomic drive for hyperglycemia is chronically unrestrained in the absence of insulin and may contribute to the inappropriate hyperglucagonemia (Gerich et al., 1975; Sherwin et al., 1976), which characterizes and fuels the hyperglycemia of diabetic ketoacidosis.

Morphological studies verify that the medial basal hypothalamus is damaged by the diabetic state (Bestetti and Rossi, 1980). Whether the damage is to insulin-sensitive structures is unclear, because previous studies have reported no change in brain insulin receptors in diabetic rats (Havrankova et al., 1979; Pacold and Blackard, 1979). We have observed, in radioautographic studies (van Houten and Posner, 1983), no change in the insulin-specific binding capacity of the median eminence and area postrema in rats made severely diabetic for 10 days following parenteral exposure to streptozotocin.

Conversely, certain types of obesity may reflect a disorder in hypothalamic function (Jung et al., 1982), possibly due to elevated insulin (Woods and Porte, 1978; Woods et al., 1979). Destruction of the medial basal hypothalamus by surgical (Brobeck et al., 1943; Palka et al., 1971) or chemical techniques (Debons et al., 1970) produces a profound hyperphagia-obesity syndrome in experimental rodents. The presence of insulin in the hypothalamus reduces food intake and body weight in rats (Hatfield et al., 1974), indicating that insulin is capable of regulating hypothalamic satiety functions (Strubbe and Mein, 1977; Woods and Porte, 1978). Recently, we have observed that parenteral treatment of neonatal rats with monosodium L-glutamate (MSG), which produces short, fat adults that are deficient in arcuate hypothalamic neurons, reduces the insulin-specific binding capacity of the median eminence-arcuate region of the hypothalamus (van Houton et al., 1983). We have speculated that the stunting and obesity of the MSG-treated rat may result from the loss of an "insulin-monitoring" function by hormone-receptive arcuate neurons that regulate caloric balance.

Changes in circumventricular receptors have been observed as possible primary defects in endocrine pathophysiology. Calcitonin-specific binding sites are reduced by one-third in the median eminence of homozygous Brattleboro rats (van Houten et al., 1982). Since these rats lack endogenous vasopressin production (Valtin et al., 1975), we replaced vasopressin exogenously; but this did not correct the median eminence binding deficit. It may well be that the calcitonin-binding deficit reflects an intrinsic lesion in the median eminence of these rats.

In contrast, angiotensin II-binding sites are reduced by 50% in all of the CVOs of the homozygous Brattleboro rat (van Houten et al., 1980d). It remains to be seen whether vasopressin replacement will reverse the angiotensin II-binding deficit in these rats. Since vasopressin replacement also normalizes the elevated levels of circulating angiotensin II in these rats (Balment et al., 1975), it may be the case that the angiotensin II-binding deficit in these rats reflects a down-regulation of receptor numbers by angiotensin II itself.

VII. SUMMARY AND CONCLUSIONS

In this chapter we have presented the circumventricular organs as receptor sites that function as the main, if not exclusive, mediators of direct peptide hormone feedback on brain. In addition, we have presented speculations concerning the neural mechanisms whereby information produced by local hormone interaction might be relayed into the CNS, and we have illustrated the possible involvement of CVO receptors in endocrine disorders such as diabetes.

ACKNOWLEDGMENTS

This work was supported by grants from the Juvenile Diabetes Foundation and the Medical Research Council of Canada.

REFERENCES

Anand, B. K., Chhina, G. S., Sharma, K. N., Dua, S., and Singh, B. (1964). *Am. J. Physiol.* 207:1146.
Baertschi, A. J., Zingg, H. H., and Dreifuss, J. J. (1981). *Brain Res.* 220:107.
Baker, B. L. and Yu, Y. Y. (1976). *Anat. Res.* 186:343.
Balment, F. J., Gemderson, I. W., and Oliver, J. A. (1975). *Gen. Comp. Endocrinol.* 26:468.
Barkai, A. and Allweis, C. (1972). *Metabolism* 21:921.
Berelowitz, M., Szabo, M., Frohman, L. A., Firestone, S., Chu, L., and Hintz, R. L. (1981). *Science* 212:1279.
Bergeron, J. J. M. and Posner, B. I. (1979). *J. Histochem. Cytochem.* 27:1512.
Bernardis, L. L. and Frohman, L. A. (1971). *J. Comp. Neurol.* 141:107.
Berthoud, H. R. and Renaud, B. (1979). *Endocrinology* 105:146.
Bestetti, G. and Rossi, G. L. (1980). *Acta Neuropath.* 52:119.
Bray, G. A. and Nishizawa, Y. (1978). *Nature (London)* 274:900.
Brightman, M. W., Prescott, L., and Reese, T. S. (1975). In *Brain-Endocrine Interactions II. The Ventricular System. 2nd Int. Symp. Shizuoka 1974,* K. M. Knigge, D Scott, H. Kobayashi, and S. Ishii, eds.) Karger, Basel, p. 165.
Broadwell, R. D. and Brightman, M. W. (1976). *J. Comp. Neurol,* 166:257.

Brobeck, J. R., Tepperman, J., and Long, C. H. N. (1943). *Yale J. Biol. Med. 15*:831.

Carmona, A. and Slagen, J. (1973). *Physiol. Behav. 10*:657.

Cornford, L. M , Braun, L. D., Crane, P. D., and Oldendorf, W. H. (1978). *Endocrinology 103*:1297.

Curry, D. L. and Joy, R. M. (1974). *Endocrin. Res. Commun. 1*:229.

Debons, A. F., Krimsky, I., and From, A. (1970). *Am. J. Physiol. 219*:938.

DeJong, A., Strubbe, J. H., and Steffens, A. B. (1977). *Am. J. Physiol. 233*:280.

Dellman, H. D. and Simpson, J. B. (1976). *Brain Res. 116*:389.

De Wied, D. (1977). *Ann. N.Y. Acad. Sci. 297*:263.

DeWied, D. (1978). In *Clinical Psychoneuroendocrinology in Repro-duction*. (L. Carenza, ed.), Academic Press, London, p. 15.

DiCarlo, R. and Muccioli, G. (1981). *Life Sci. 28*:2299.

Felix, D. and Akert K. (1974). *Brain Res. 76*:350.

Frohman, L. A., Bernardis, L. L., and Kant, K. J. (1968). *Science 162*:580.

Frohman, L. A., Muller, E. E., and Cocchi, D. (1973). *Horm. Metab. Res. 5*:21.

Fuxe, K., Andersson, K., Hokfelt, T., Agnati, L. F., Ogren, S. O., Eneroth, P., Gustafson, J. A., and Skett, P. (1978). In *Prolactin Physiology and Pathology* (R. Robyn and J. Harters, eds), Elese-vier-North Holland Biomedical Press, Amsterdam, p. 94.

Gerich J. E., Lorenzi, M., Bier, D. M., Schneider, V., Tsaukian, E., Karam, J. H., and Forsham, P. H. (1975). *New England J. Med. 191*:985.

Hatfield, J. S., Millward, W. J., and Smith, C. J. V. (1974). *Pharma-col. Biochem. Behav. 2*:223.

Havrankova, J., Brownstein, M., and Roth, J. (1978). *Nature (London) 272*:827.

Havrankova, J., Roth, J., and Brownstein, M. (1979). *J. Clin. Invest. 64*:636.

Hofer, H. (1958). *Deut. Zool. Ges. Verhandl. 8*:202.

Höhn, H. G. and Wuttke, W. O. (1978). *Brain Res. 156*:241.

Iguchi, A., Burleson, P. D., and Szabo, A. J. (1981). *Am. J. Phy-siol. 240*:E95.

Ishibashi, S., Oomura, Y., and Okajima, T. (1979). *Physiol. Behav. 22*:785.

Ishikawa, K., Suzuki, M., and Shimazu, T. (1982). *Neuroendo-crinology 34*:310.

Jung, R. T., Campbell, R. G., James, W. P. T., and Callingham, B. A. (1982). *Lancet 1*:1043.

Junger, E. (1978). *Cytobiologie 18*:250.

Kerr, F. W. L. and Preshaw, R. M. (1969). *J. Physiol. 205*:405.

Kita, H., Niijima, A., Oomura, Y., Ishizuka, S., Aou, S., Yamabe, K., and Yoshimatsu, H. (1980). *Brain Res. Bull.* 5 (Suppl. 4): 163.

Klara, P. M. and Brizzee, K. R. (1977). *J. Comp. Neurol.* 171:409.

Koella, W. P. and Sutin, J. (1967). *Intern. Rev. Neurobiol.* 10:31.

Kreiger, D. T. and Martin, J. B. (1981). *N. Engl. J. Med.* 304(15): 876.

LeBeaux, Y. J. (1972). *Z. Zeuforsch.* 127:439.

LeClerc, R. and Pelletier, G. (1974). *Am. J. Anat.* 140:583.

Mason, A. G., Nemeroff, C. B., Luttinger, D., Hatley, O. L., and Prange, A. J. (1980). *Regulatory Peptides:* 1:53.

Matsushita, H. and Shimazu, T. (1980). *Brain Res.* 183:79.

Matsushita, H., Ishikawa, K., and Shimazu, T. (1979). *Brain Res.* 163:253.

McCaleb, M. L., Myers, R. D., Singer, G., and Willis, G. (1979). *Am. J. Physiol.* 236:R312.

Miselis, R. R., Shapiro, R. E., and Hand, P. J. (1979). *Science* 205:1022.

Moody, T. W., Pert, C. B., Rivier, J. E., and Brown, M. R. (1978). *Proc. Natl. Acad. Sci. USA* 75:5372.

Morest, D. K. (1967). *J. Comp. Neurol.* 130:377.

Müller, E. E. (1973). *Neuroendocrinology* 11:338.

Olney, J. W., Schwainker, B., and Rhee, V. (1976). In *Hormones, Behaviour and Psychopathology*, (E. J. Sacher, ed.), Raven Press, New York, p. 153.

Ono, T., Oomura, Y., Nishino, H. Sasaki, K., Muramoto, K., and Yano, I. (1980). *Brain Res.* 185:208.

Ontjes, D. A., Ways, D. K., Mahaffee, D. D., Zimmerman, C. F., and Gwynne, J. T. (1977). *Ann. N.Y. Acad. Sci.* 297:295.

Oomura, Y. (1976). In *Hunger: Basic Mechanisms and Clinical Implications*, (D. Ovin, W. Wyrwicka, and G. Bray, eds.), Raven Press, New York, p. 145.

Oomura, Y., Ooyama, T., Naka, F., Yamamoto, T., Ono, T., and Kobayashi, N. (1969). *Ann. N.Y. Acad. Sci.* 157:666.

Pacold, S. T. and Blackard, W. G. (1979). *Endocrinology* 105:1450.

Palka, Y., Liebelt, R. A., and Critchlow, V. (1971). *Physiol. Behav.* 7:187.

Pecile, A., Muller, E. E., Felici, M., and Nett, C. (1971). In *Growth and Growth Hormone*, (A. Pecile and E. E. Muller, eds.), Excerpts Medica, Medica, Amsterdam, p. 261.

Perkins, N. A., Westfall, T. C., Paul, C. V., Macleod, R., and Rogol, A. D. (1979). *Brain Res.* 160:431.

Pert, C. B. and Snyder, S. H. (1973). *Proc. Natl. Acad. Sci. USA* 70:2243.

Posner, B. I. (1975). *Can. J. Physiol. Pharmacol.* 53:689.

Posner, B. I., van Houten, M., and Walsh, R. J. (1982). *Exp. Brain Res. 178*:1.

Ramsey, D. J. and Reid, I. A. (1975). *J. Physiol. Lond. 253*:517.

Reese, T. S. and Karnovsky, M. J. (1967). *J. Cell. Biol. 34*:207.

Renaud, L. P. and Martin, J. B. (1976). *Brain Res. 105*:59.

Rizzo, A. J. and Goltzman, D. (1981). *Endocrinology 108*:1672.

Rohner, F., Dufour, A. C., Karakash, C., LeMarchand, Y., Ruf, K. B., and Jeanrenaud, B. (1977). *Diabetologia 13*:239.

Rossi, G. L. and Bestetti, G. (1981). *Diabetologia 21*:476.

Saito, A., Williams, J. A., and Goldfine, I. D. (1981). *Nature (London) 289*:599.

Sanghera, M., Harris, M. C., and Morgan, R. A. (1978). *Brain Res. 140*:63.

Sawyer, C. H. (1975). *Neuroendocrinology 17*:97.

Sherwin, R. ., Fisher, M., Hendler, R., and Felig, P. (1976). *N. Engl. J. Med. 294*:455

Shimazu, T. and Ishikawa, K. (1979). *Neurosci. Letters Supp. 2*:S50.

Shimazu, T. and Ogasawara, S. (1975). *Am. J. Physiol. 226*:1787.

Simpson, J. D. (1981). *Neuroendocrinology 32*:248.

Sirrett, N. E., McLean, A. S., Bray, J. J., and Hubbard, J. I. (1977). *Brain Res. 122*:299.

Snyder, S. H. and Simantov, R. (1977). *J. Neurochem. 18*:13.

Storlien, L. H., Bellingham, W. P., and Martin, G. M. (1975). *Brain Res. 96*:156.

Strubbe J. H. and Mein, C. G. (1977). *Physiol. Behav. 19*:309.

Sxabo, D. and Szabo, A. J. (1975). *Diabetes 24*:328.

Tannenbaum, G. S. (1980). *Endocrinology 107*:117.

Taylor, D. P. and Pert, C. B. (1979). *Proc. Natl. Acad. Sci. USA 76*:660.

Texeria, V. L., Atunes-Rodriguez, J., and Migliorini, R. H. (1975). *J. Lipid Res. 14*:672.

Uhl, G. R., Bennett, J. P., and Snyder, S. H. (1977). *Brain Res. 130*:299.

Valtin, H., Sohol, H. W., and Sunde, D. (1975). *Rec. Prog. Hormone Res. 31*:447.

van Houten, M. and Posner, B. I. (1979). *Nature (London) 282*:623.

van Houten, M. and Posner, B. I. (1981a). *Endocrinology 109*:853.

van Houten, M. and Posner, B. I. (1981b). *Diabetologia 20*:255.

van Houten, M. and Posner, B. I. (1981c). In *Current Views on Insulin Receptors*, (D. Andreani, R. DePirro, R. Mauro, J. Olefsky, and J. Roth, eds.), Academic Press, London, p. 76.

van Houten, M. and Posner, B. I. (1983). *Advan. Metabol. Disord. 10*:269.

van Houten, M., Posner, B. I., Kopriwa, B. M. and Brawer, J. R. (1979). *Endocrinology 105*:666.

van Houten, M., Posner, B. I., Kopriwa, B. M., and Brawer, J. R. (1980a). *Science 207*:1081.

van Houten, M., Schiffrin, E. L., Mann, J. F. E., Posner, B. I., and Boucher, R. (1980b). *Brain Res. 186*:480.

van Houten, M., Posner, B. I., and Walsh, R. J. (1980c). *Exp. Brain Res. 38*:455.

van Houten, M., Schiffrin, E. L., and Posner, B. I. (1980d). *Soc. Neurosci. Abst. 176*:8.

van Houten, M., Khan, M. N., Khan, R. J., and Posner, B. I. (1981a). *Endocrinology 108*:2385.

van Houten, M., Khan, M. N., Chretien, M., and Posner, B. I. (1981b). *Endoc. Soc. Abstr. 52* and submitted.

van Houten, M., Rizzo, A. J., Goltzman, D., and Posner, B. I. (1982). *Endocrinology 111*:1704.

van Houten, M., Nance, D. M., Gauthier, S., and Posner, B. I. (1983). *Endocrinology 113*:1393.

Weindl, A. (1973). In *Frontiers in Neuroendocrinology*, (W. F. Ganong and L. Martini, eds.), Oxford University Press, New York, p. 1.

Weingarten, H. P. and Powley, T. L. (1980). *Am. J. Physiol. 239*:G221.

Woods, S. C. and Porte, D. Jr. (1978). *Advan. Metabol. Disord. 9*:283.

Woods, S C., Lotter, E. C., McKay, L. D., and Porte, D., Jr. (1979). *Nature (London) 282*:503.

BIBLIOGRAPHY

Debons, A. F., I. Krimsky, and From A. (1970). A direct action of insulin on the hypothalamic satiety center. *Am. J. Physiol. 219*:938–943.

Dellman, H. D. (1979). The subfornical organ. *Intern. Rev. Cytol. 58*:333–421

Krieger, D. T. and J. C. Hughes, *Neuroendocrinology*, Sinauer Assoc. Inc., Sunderland, Massachusettes, 1980.

Simpson, J. D. (1981). The circumventricular organs and the central actions of angiotensin. *Neuroendocrinology 32*:248–256.

Weindl, A. (1973). Neuroendocrine Aspects of the Circumventricular organs. In *Frontiers in Neuroendocrinology* (W. F. Ganong and L. Martini, eds.), Oxford University Press, New York, p. 1–32.

11

Lymphocyte Insulin Receptors

J. HAROLD HELDERMAN *The University of Texas Health Science
Center at Dallas and The Southwestern Medical School, Dallas, Texas*

I. INTRODUCTION

The study of insulin receptors has broadened to include a wide range
of tissues and cells beyond traditional targets for the hormone. Initial
work examining target tissues had two goals: (a) the characterization
of insulin receptors in particular and hormone receptors in general by
direct radioligand-binding studies and (b) to determine at the cellular
level the manner in which peptide hormones such as insulin can instruct
the cell. After these initial studies, in which the basic concepts of receptor chemistry were learned, researchers began to explore the mechanisms that underlie several disorders of carbohydrate metabolism. In order to characterize receptor-related defects in human disease, experimental protocols require a cell or tissue that can be frequently, safely, and
conveniently sampled. The search for such convenient and safely obtained tissues led to the original description of lymphocytes as "mirrors
of metabolism." This chapter will review the insulin receptor on the
T- and B-lymphocyte, one such mirror of metabolism.

The study of the lymphocyte model has led to several new concepts
of receptor regulation, has added information to the general understanding of the insulin receptor for all tissues, and has fostered new
hypotheses of immunobiology. Indeed, lessons learned from the study
of the lymphocyte insulin receptor have been the cornerstone for and
genesis of a new field in immunology, hormonal immunomodulation.
This chapter will begin by reviewing the initial studies of the insulin
receptor on the lymphocyte and by providing the pharmacokinetic
principles that govern this unique receptor. The chapter will then
deal with the concept of the insulin receptor on the lymphocyte as a
marker of the active state of the immunocompetent cell. The discussion

will then turn to an understanding of the manner in which the lymphocyte model may be used to explore receptor regulation and disorders
of carbohydrate metabolism. Lastly, the immunobiologic role of the insulin receptor on a lymphocyte will be discussed.

II. INSULIN RECEPTOR CHARACTERISTICS ON THE
LYMPHOCYTE

Shortly after the pioneering work of Lefkowitz, Roth, and co-workers
and of Cuatrecasas and colleagues detailing the methods by which
hormone receptors may be directly measured by radioligand-binding
techniques, the search for convenient and safely obtainable tissues to
study disease in humans was launched. Insulin receptors were characterized initially on circulating blood cells recovered from the aqueous
interface of density gradients comprised of iodinated complex saccha-
rides (Ficoll-Hypaque) (1). These cells were all mononuclear in morphology and were thought to be lymphocytes [mistakenly, as it later
turned out (2)]. Simultaneously, other investigators recovering these
same mononuclear cell fractions from the density gradient, but further
treating these cells by percolation through nylon wool columns to separate the T-dependent lymphocytes (hereafter called T-cells) from the
monocytes and bursal-dependent lymphocytes (hereafter called B-cells),
failed to find insulin receptors (3). The initial confusion was shortly
settled by an understanding of the nature of the cell type recovered
by each of the two laboratory's separation techniques. Cells recovered
directly from the density gradient were determined to be of the macro-
phage-monocyte lineage rather than of lymphocytic origin. Because
these cells bear receptors in the circulation and are easy to obtain, it
is believed that they may serve as the sought-after model to explore
the role of the insulin receptor in disease. An understanding of the
role of the receptor will lead to a substantial advance in our understanding of pathogenesis of carbohydrate disorders at the cellular level.
    On the other hand, it was clear that "resting" lymphocytes them-
selves do not bear the insulin receptor in the plasma space, but require special treatment in order to generate the capacity to bind the
hormone at the cell membrane. When cells that could be rigorously
characterized as T-lymphocyte in origin are recovered from peripheral
blood of patients or animals and are placed into tissue culture with various mitogens or specific antigens, the insulin receptor will present (4).
I will return to the importance of this observation and its use later in
the chapter. For the purposes of this section, it is sufficient to know
that after mitogen stimulation one may obtain true T-lymphocytes complete with surface insulin receptors available for characterization.
    By direct radioligand-binding studies one could demonstrate that
the insulin binding site on the membrane of the T-lymphocyte shared

common features with the insulin receptor on traditional target tissues
that had previously been described. The site demonstrated saturability
with ligand, highly specific binding, ready reversibility with unlabeled
ligand, heirarchical binding of ligand analogue that correlated with the
physiological capabilities of that analogue, and high affinity. Indeed,
the affinity of the receptor for insulin calculated directly from association or dissociation binding isotherms or from data transformed by
any of the accepted mathematical means (e.g., Scatchard analysis) was
nearly identical to that described for all previous tissues, about 1 nM.
These features, which describe in "classic" terms the properties of insulin receptors are reviewed in Figure 1. In direct radioligand-binding

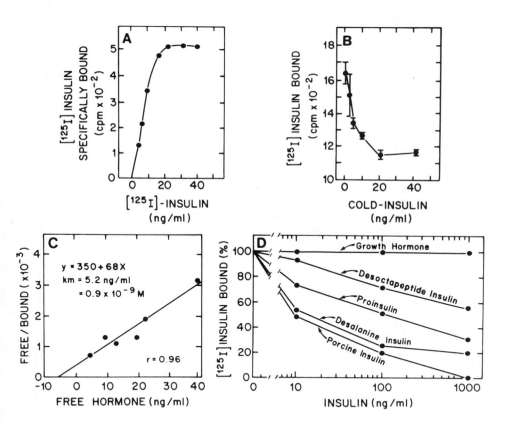

Figure 1 Kinetic properties of the lymphocyte insulin receptor. (A)
Saturable ligand binding. (B) Dissociation with unlabeled ligand.
(C) High affinity with a K_M in the physiologic range for insulin (nM)
(the Hanes plot of the binding data is linear for this cell type). (D)
Recognition by the receptor of analogues of insulin in a pattern reflect-
ing the physiological potency of each analogue.

assays, nonspecific binding varies considerably among model tissue studies. (The binding of radiolabeled insulin to nonreceptor sites is termed "nonspecific." This nonspecific binding of ^{125}I-labeled insulin is observed in the presence of a comparatively high (9.1 μM) concentration of unlabeled insulin.) For the T- or B-lymphocyte insulin receptor, the nonspecific binding is a substantial fraction of the total binding and may be as high as 35—40%. This high nonspecific binding can be a problem for individual experimental protocols and may preclude measuring very small numbers of receptors on cell surface, a problem obviated in circumstances of antigen stimulation in which plentiful receptors appear on lymphocytes. Additionally, the number of insulin receptors on cells varies considerably from tissue to tissue. Most investigators exploring the T-lymphocyte model have observed between 6000 and 8000 receptor sites per activated cell.

New preliminary information on the chemistry of the T-lymphocyte insulin receptor elucidates further similarities with traditional or classic target tissue receptors. It appears that the T-lymphocyte insulin receptor is chemically similar to other insulin receptors in that two subunit structures are present on the lymphocyte cell membrane, one approximately 125,000 M.W. and one of 95,000 M.W., respectively. In the T-lymphocyte, the cellular processing of the ligand-receptor complex proceeds by mechanisms described for traditional "target" tissues (5) (see Chap. 6, Fig. 3). The insulin-receptor complex is internalized into the cytosol and is ultimately taken into a lysosome. Experiments that utilize inhibitors of lysosomal enzymes alter profoundly the binding of insulin to the cell surface in the lymphocyte. Once internalized into the lysosome, the ligand (insulin) is released or degraded and the receptor, in part, is reinserted into the membrane. A cautionary note is important here. Certain other immunocompetent cells, such as cultured immunoblasts (IM-9 cells), do not exhibit this internalization and lysosomal processing of the receptor (e.g., see Chap. 7). Thus, it is likely that these cell lines cannot serve as models for ligand-receptor complex processing or even for the manner by which insulin conveys its intracellular signals. The search for the second messenger for insulin after receptor engagement on the T-cell is a fertile area for research for all cell types. Moreover, since the binding kinetics and chemistry of the receptor in the lymphocyte parallel so closely the receptor properties observed in other cell types, lessons learned from the T-cell model may be widely applicable to other tissues. Useful experimental probes, such as photoaffinity labels, should lead to productive studies in the T-cell and may lead to a deeper understanding of the nature and kinetics of the reinsertion of the receptor into the membrane of these cells.

Thus, the chemical and binding kinetic aspects of the T-lymphocyte insulin receptor, which appears after cell stimulation, indicates that the T-cell model may serve as a mirror of metabolism in order to explore the role of the receptor in certain diseases of carbohydrate metabolism. The lymphocyte, in contrast to most studied tissues, does not bear the insulin receptor in the circulation unless a subject or animal is strongly immunologically perturbed. The lymphocyte will develop the insulin receptor after overwhelming antigenic challenge, as we shall see, or after stimulation in tissue culture. The insulin-binding structure that appears on the lymphocyte cell membrane kinetically resembles in most ways the classically described insulin receptor on a multiplicity of tissues. The rules that govern the metabolism of the ligand-receptor complex and the chemical structure of the receptor also are similar on this cell as in traditional or classic target tissues for insulin. Thus, the T-lymphocyte is a valid model tissue to study aspects of insulin receptor biology.

III. THE LYMPHOCYTE INSULIN RECEPTOR AS A MARKER OF THE ACTIVE STATE

Having concerned ourselves with describing how the lymphocyte insulin receptor is similar to the receptor in other tissues, I want to address the manner in which the lymphocyte model is quite unique. As alluded to in an earlier section, the resting T-lymphocyte does not bear a measurable insulin receptor on its surface as it circulates in normal circumstances. Lymphocyte activation caused specifically by antigen in vivo or in vitro or nonspecifically by biochemical mitogens (e.g., plant lectins) will lead to the appearance in the lymphocyte of measurable insulin receptors on the cell membrane (6). As can be seen in Table 1, a series of different stimulants have been tried, all of which have the capacity to activate the lymphocyte in vivo or in vitro; all lead to the capability of measuring the insulin receptor on the activated lymphocyte. The table further demonstrates that this property of lymphocyte activation is not confined to the T-cell alone. Unique B-cell stimulants also lead to the generation of insulin receptors on B-cells.

The ability of the lymphocyte to generate new insulin receptors upon stimulation allows one to use the measurement of the receptor on the cell as a probe to analyze the lymphocyte active state. Spira and colleagues have been interested in the ontogeny of B-lymphocytes (7). Taking as their point of departure the elegant analysis of surface immunoglobulin isotype present on maturing B-lymphocytes by Vittetta and Uhr, Spira and colleagues (7) probed the state of maturity of various clones of lymphoblasts by looking at surface IgG, IgD, IgM, and the insulin receptor. From their work, it is clear that the insulin receptor appears on primitive lymphocytes near to the point of the IgD to IgM switch. As the cell matures and attains surface IgM and later the surface IgG isotype, the insulin receptor is no longer present on

Table 1 Activation of Rodent Lymphocytes and the Insulin
Receptor

	T-Cells	B-Cells
In vivo[a]		
Transplantation	++	+
Graft-versus-host	++	+
Secondary antigen challenge	++	+
In vitro[b]		
Phytohemagglutinin	++	−
Concanavalin A	++	−
Lipopolysaccharide	−	++
Mixed lymphocyte culture	++	±
Antigen restimulation	+	++

[a]After transplantation, graft-versus-host reaction, or secondary antigenic challenge in vivo, T-cell and B-cell populations were isolated from peripheral blood and the presence of
insulin receptors was determined.
[b]Purified T-cell or B-cell populations isolated from peripheral
blood were stimulated in vitro by plant lectins (phytohemagglutinin and concanavalin A), lipopolysaccharide, mixed lymphocyte culture (cells from noncompatible donors) or by re-
stimulation in vitro with antigen. The presence of insulin receptors in the stimulated cell population was then measured
using a [^{125}I]insulin binding assay.

the cell surface. These stages of maturation are not driven by antigen and are part of the normal maturation of these immunocompetent
cells. Later, under antigenic pressure, clonal expansion will be accompanied by the reappearance of measurable insulin receptors. Thus,
the insulin receptor not only marks the active state of the lymphocyte,
but also can be used to determine the state of maturation of the cell.
    A further, and perhaps more practical, use of the insulin receptor
as a marker of the activated state has been in the realm of tissue typing. A number of observers have demonstrated that vascularized organ transplant success can be well predicted by matching of the class
II HLA antigens. Such matching has been shown to correlate best to
responses in an immunological culture test called the mixed lymphocyte
culture, which reflects variations at the broad D region of the HLA
chromosome. The mixed lymphocyte culture requires 5—7 days of
tissue culture, a time that constrains its clinical utility. In the past

10 years, there has been an assiduous search for alternative and rapid means of tissue typing for the *HLA-D* region. Recently, a serological assay that identifies the unique HLA-DR antigen carried by the B-lymphocyte and macrophage has been in wide use, but its ability to predict transplant outcome accurately is hampered by differences, chemically and immunologically, between HLA-D and HLA-DR. One new approach to HLA-D tissue matching has grown out of the observation that measurable insulin receptor binding that appears within 24 hr of culture can mark alloantigenic responses due to D region disparities (8). Careful family analysis has demonstrated the quantitative and qualitative utility of the lymphocyte insulin receptor as a marker of an active state.

That the insulin receptor can be generated after appropriate cellular stimulation is a unique feature of the T-cell receptor model. Not only can one use this property of the T-cell to probe the lymphocyte active state, one may also use it to analyze time regulation of the insulin receptor per se. Cells have the capacity to synthesize new receptor molecules, an event that is amenable to regulation and thus may relate to the display of receptors on the cell surface (e.g., see Chapter 12). Receptors also move on and off the cell surface through the process of internalization and reinsertion, events which also may be regulated (discussed in Chap. 6). The T-lymphocyte insulin receptor model allows one to study each of these events in an isolated fashion. One can show, using various inhibitors of intracellular synthetic events, that antigenic stimulation of a lymphocyte leads to the synthesis of new glycoproteins that bind insulin (Fig. 2) (9). There is at this time no evidence for preformed, cryptic receptors present in the cytosol of unstimulated T-cells that might move to the membrane by virtue of lymphocyte activation. Indeed, when α-amanitin, an agent that blocks nuclear messenger RNA transcription, is used to pretreat lymphocytes prior to antigenic stimulation, no insulin receptors will appear on the cell surface. One can infer that the most proximal step in the activation-induced appearance of insulin receptors is the translation of message. Blockade of various stages of lymphocyte blast cell transformation, such as the S phase of DNA synthesis or cell division, does not interfere with receptor generation. It can be shown that the synthesis of the insulin receptor is an event that precedes S phase and is a marker for one of the earlier steps in the activation of lymphocytes by antigen. It is this feature that allows one to use the insulin receptor as a probe of cell activation at an early enough step to be clinically useful, such as in the tissue typing example already discussed. This property will also permit now an in-depth analysis of these early stages of antigen activation of cells. It is possible that part of the appearance of insulin receptors after antigen stimulation may be related to insertion of some preformed cryptic receptors and that the de novo synthesis of receptor may not explain the entire story. If this were to be true, then

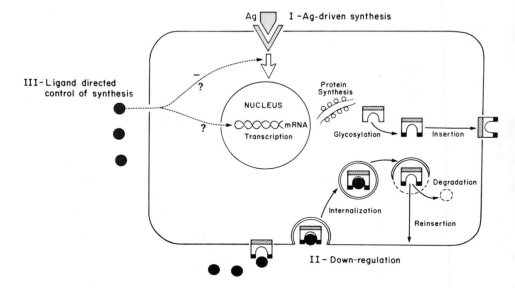

Figure 2 Fine regulation of the T-lymphocyte insulin receptor. The
figure depicts three separate modes by which the insulin receptor can
be regulated. I depicts an all-or-none antigen-driven synthesis of a
new receptor molecule, the first event of which is new synthesis of
messenger RNA followed by glycosylation and insertion of an active
binding moiety into the membrane. II Depicts down-regulation of receptors once in place utilizing internalization into lysosomes followed
by reinsertion of receptor after degradation of ligand. III depicts
ligand-directed control of synthesis on receptor-negative cells representing a negative signal (possibly of monocyte origin) either inter-
rupting the antigen-directed process (arrow) or altering the signal
at the nucleus itself.

elements of the cytoskeleton responsible for the mechanical insertion of
glycopeptides would be important for the appearance of a full complement
of insulin receptors after antigen stimulation. One can show with specific probes that disrupt the cytoskeleton that insertion is not an important feature of this aspect of the lymphocyte insulin receptor display (10). Insertion of cryptic receptors on receptor-negative cells
thus seems to be unimportant.

Certain important biological lessons may be learned from these data
dealing with activation-induced appearance of insulin receptors. The
degree of hormone action is generally a function of the amount of

hormone present at the receptor site, the number of receptors available for binding, and/or the integrity of the postreceptor machinery. In most all systems, it is the concentration of insulin per se and the ability of insulin itself to regulate the receptor that are the major factors governing tissue responsiveness. However, in the T-cell system, the appearance of the insulin receptor depends to a large extent on antigenic stimulation and not on the presence of insulin. Since antigen activation of the cell appears to be an all-or-none effect, and since the ligand, insulin, is governed by the concentration of blood sugar and not a T-cell function, the lymphocyte must govern its capacity to respond to the hormone by the very presence of the receptor or its absence. This novel means of regulation of hormone effect has been first characterized by this model but now can be shown to be extant for a series of cells and ligands. Interestingly, as we will learn below, there can be fine regulation of the number of receptors displayed on the cell so that one may observe two levels of control of the generation of insulin receptors on cell surfaces. The first, antigen dependent, is an all-or-none event that leads to the signal to synthesize de novo insulin receptors on the cell surface. The second, an antigen-independent event, will lead to the fine regulation of the number of receptors that ultimately will be displayed and will be under the control of ligand feedback in a similar fashion as traditional target tissues. This second means of receptor regulation can occur only after the cell has synthesized its complement of receptors, in part, since this mechanism requires ligand receptor binding, internalization, and recycling. More will be said of this second mechanism after a discussion of the use of the T-cell model to explore the genesis of certain disorders of carbohydrate metabolism.

IV. THE T-LYMPHOCYTE INSULIN RECEPTOR AS A MIRROR OF METABOLISM

The special features of the T-lymphocyte model allow one to reanalyze this insulin receptor system as a mirror of metabolism in order to study disorders of carbohydrate metabolism. One could, a priori, assume that the T-lymphocyte model may be able to discern a genetic predisposition for alterations in insulin receptor characteristics, since environmental factors may not play a role in the regulation of the receptor Indeed, if one examines in the fasting state single measurements of insulin binding in lymphocytes from a wide range of patients with disorders of carbohydrate metabolism, one can see that patients with type II diabetes mellitus associated with obesity have a defect in the number of receptors found on the lymphocyte after lectin stimulation (11). This defect is greater than can be accounted for by the degree of obesity of the given patient, since there is an important biological difference

between the number of receptors displayed on cells from obese diabetic patients and the numbers found on the cells of similarly obese
nondiabetics who exhibit normal glucose tolerance. One could conclude that the T-lymphocyte model points to a unique, perhaps genetic,
predisposition for a defect in the number of receptors displayed on
the cells of certain patients who exhibit insulin resistance. On the
other hand, it is possible that in a unique manner the T-lymphocyte
is amenable to receptor regulation by environmental changes. In order
to test whether alterations of the bathing environment of the lymphocyte in vivo may regulate the receptor, patients were perturbed by
protocols designed to raise or lower insulin concentrations subacutely
(12). Curiously, the number of insulin receptors that appear in tissue culture subsequent to lymphocyte activation seem to be governed
by the concentration of insulin that was present in plasma space from
which the lymphocytes were obtained. Although the induction of the
synthesis of receptors by plant lectins is an all-or-none phenomenon,
the fine tuning of this phenomenon can be set and remembered by
lymphocytes based on the environment from which they came. Thus,
one can no longer state categorically that the binding defects observed
by the T-lymphocyte model reflect genetic defects in the ability of
certain patients to synthesize the insulin receptor in the course of
lymphocyte activation. After the insulin receptor appears on the lymphocyte, fine regulation of receptor number can be achieved by the
ligand-directed internalization processes outlined in Chapter 6. This
entire insulin-mediated receptor regulation process can occur only
after the receptor has been synthesized in response to antigen or lectin. This insulin-directed mechanism cannot explain the means by
which environmental changes in ambient plasma insulin in patients may
subsequently modulate receptor display in the cells from these patients,
stimulated in tissue culture; for the lymphocyte present in the plasma
of the patients is not thought to bear a receptor at the time the blood
sample is obtained. One might argue, of course, that there may be
receptors on the circulating lymphocytes, but that these structures
are too few in number to be measured by the direct radioligand binding techniques. This undetectable but hypothetically present number
of receptors might be adequate to signal the cell subsequently to reduce the numbers of insulin receptors after stimulation in vitro. This
explanation requires a religious belief in an unmeasurable quantity.
More attractive is the hypothesis that the lymphocyte is being signaled
as to the concentration of insulin in the plasma space by other cell
types that themselves bear insulin receptors in the circulation (Fig. 2).
We have strong preliminary evidence that this is indeed the case, with
the circulating monocyte serving as the partner in the afferent recognition of the insulin concentration. This function of the monocyte in
monitoring insulin concentration has a parallel in its role in the recognition of antigens (13). One can thus expand our understanding of the

fine regulation of insulin receptor display in lymphocytes, describing three separate levels: (a) an all-or-none signal from antigen that leads to the important first signal to synthesize a complement of insulin receptors; (b) afferent signals relaying the concentration of ambient insulin to the T-cell from the monocyte, in order that the lymphocyte may synthesize, after antigen stimulation, an appropriate number of insulin receptors for full immunoregulating function, without pathologic responses; (c) a final fine tuning of insulin receptor display by virtue of the continued binding of insulin to the receptor in place on the activated lymphocyte cell surface (Fig. 2).

V. THE ROLE OF INSULIN AND ITS RECEPTOR IN IMMUNOREGULATION OF T-CELL FUNCTION

The lessons learned from the T-lymphocyte insulin receptor model have been important in advancing our understanding of receptor biology in general, while teaching us new lessons of immunobiology. What we have discussed so far uses the insulin receptor on lymphocytes more or less as a marker, in a rather mechanical fashion. What makes study of the insulin receptor so much more exciting is that the structure performs an important immunobiological function. That insulin subserves an important function in immunocompetent cells has been known for as long as we have known about insulin receptors on the lymphocyte cell surface. Strom, in his quest to understand various hormonal and neurotransmitter modulations of cytotoxic T-lymphocytes, has shown that insulin, when exposed to sensitized cytotoxic T-cells, has the capacity to enhance the destruction of appropriate target cells (14). It became clear that insulin functions in cytotoxic T-cells by activating the insulin receptor that is synthesized during the alloresponse that leads to the arming of the cytotoxic T-cell. In fact, as Figure 3 shows, there is a tight relationship between the appearance of the insulin receptor on the sensitized T-cell and the capacity of insulin to alter the cell's functions. Insulin modulates the function of the cell only because antigen has initiated the development of a cytotoxic function of the lymphocyte. This is shown well by the fact that the killing capacity of the lymphocyte appears in many systems before or concomitant to the appearance of the insulin receptor and lasts after allosensitization beyond the time that insulin receptors are measurable. However it is only during the period when the insulin receptors are present on the cell membrane that the cytotoxic capacity of the cell can be modulated by insulin itself. Since insulin can serve as a regulator of the immune function of the cell in the early phases of the response to antigen, one can see a time when such stimulation would be helpful in allowing for full immune response. However, insulin's effect is lost at the end of the immune response, when further enhancement

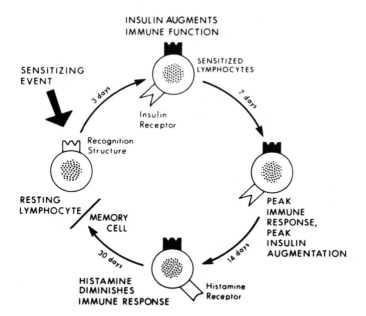

Figure 3 Temporal relationship between the appearance of insulin receptors on antigen-sensitized T-lymphocytes and the insulin effect.
Shown here is the insulin effect on cytotoxic T-cell function. Antigen
induces the synthesis of new insulin receptors prior to which insulin
exerts no biological effect. During the time at which insulin receptor
is present, provision of physiological concentrations of insulin will enhance cytotoxic T-cell destruction of targets bearing the sensitizing
antigen. At a time in the life of the cytotoxic T-cell at which the cell
is still armed but no longer bears the insulin receptor, insulin no longer
can play its physiological role. Other receptors have different time
courses and may play different roles for the ligand related to them.

of cytotoxic capacity might indeed be pathological. This tight time
course relationship between the appearance of receptor and effectiveness of insulin demonstrates an intriguing mechanism for regulating
hormone responsiveness in that the cell responds by regulation of the
binding site rather than by regulation of the hormone level. Further
support for the impact of insulin on cytotoxic T-cells and for the importance of the insulin receptor as the mediator of the insulin effect
has come from cell enrichment experiments. The cell density and shape
characteristics of the allosensitized cell are used to identify cytotoxic
cells and to enrich other cell populations with these armed cells (15).
These enriched populations, bearing an increased concentration of

cells with insulin receptors, are also enriched for insulin responsiveness. We have shown that elimination of the transcription of messenger RNA after antigen challenge not only blocks the synthesis of new insulin receptors, but also abrogates the effect of insulin in these cells. Finally, insulin augmentation of cytotoxic T-cell function is tightly related to receptor binding affinity, such that when a series of insulin analogues with progressively less avid binding for the T-lymphocyte insulin receptor are probed, one observes dose-response curves that are in accord with the relative binding affinities (16).

This immunologically directed effect of insulin is by no means the only role that insulin subserves in the activated lymphocyte. In these cells, insulin also functions in its traditional or classic sense, to enhance intracellular intermediary metabolism. Many investigators have attempted to use the peripheral resting blood lymphocyte as a signal tissue to explore classic insulin-directed effects, such as the stimulation of glucose or amino acid transport, without finding a specific insulin effect. These findings are not surprising in the light of our new understanding of the lymphocyte insulin receptor system, in that the originally studied tissues were collected directly from blood and did not contain activated lymphocytes bearing insulin receptors in this setting. However, if one activates the lymphocyte first with mitogen or antigen, then one can observe that such cells, which now bear insulin receptors, will exhibit an enhancement of glucose transport, amino acid transport, and glucose oxidation in response to insulin. Thus, the activated lymphocyte, a cell that has been transformed from one of the most metabolically quiescent cells to an active cell requiring substantial increases in energy production, attains a structure on the cell surface (the insulin receptor) that permits ambient insulin to meet the increased demands of the cell (17,18). In this fashion, once again, one can see that insulin responsiveness is governed not by the plasma insulin level per se, but by the presence or absence of the receptor. Additionally, insulin through its receptor now serves biological energy economy in permitting maximal response to antigen.

VI. PARALLELS BETWEEN RULES OF IMMUNE CONTROL AND HORMONAL CONTROL

This chapter has centered on the description of, utility of, and the meaning of the T-lymphocyte insulin receptor model. As has been discussed, this model has taught new lessons illustrating certain new aspects of receptor biology. These new aspects have now been confirmed by a number of other laboratories. Recently, we have obtained intriguing evidence' suggesting that certain rules that govern the interaction of subsets of lymphocytes in response to specific antigen may also apply to the cellular cooperation observed among the same cells for the

induction of hormone receptors (18). This exciting possibility grew
out of a paradox noted in several experiments using lectins as stimulants for insulin receptor generation. When lectins that specifically
stimulate T-lymphocytes are used, T-cells but not purified B-cells synthesize insulin receptors. Yet, when a heterogeneous population of
peripheral blood lymphocytes are cultured with the same T-lymphocyte-
specific mitogen, both T- and B-lymphocytes acquire the insulin receptors. This apparent paradox was resolved by showing that T-
lymphocytes, when activated, have the capacity to provide "helper
function" for naive B-lymphocytes so that the B-cells in turn generate insulin receptors. The precise rules that govern T-cell-B-cell
cooperation for T-cell-dependent antigen recognition, apply also to
T-B cooperation for the generation of insulin receptors. In terms of
T-cell-directed production of insulin receptors on B-cells, the part-
ners in the cell-cell cooperation (both T- and B-lymphocytes) must
share surface class II HLA antigens. The T-lymphocyte, which provides help, must bear the helper T-cell surface marker (Lyl + antigen
in rodents or the OKT4 marker in humans). The helper function of
the T-cell may be mediated by a soluble T-cell factor secreted into
the culture medium. Thus, activation of T-cells by antigen will re-
cruit specific clones of cooperating B-lymphocytes into the insulin-
receptor-bearing cell populations. This phenomenon associated with
antigenic activation, permits insulin to subserve the enhancement of
intracellular energy stores for both T- and B-lymphocytes. This
T-cell-B-cell communication, resulting in the appearance of insulin receptors, is an exciting example of the manner in which rules of immune
regulation are involved in the control of response to hormones. Thus,
in summary, prior to T-cell activation, the monocyte appears to communicate to the T-cell a message related to the plasma insulin concentration. This message leads to a fine tuning of the number of T-
cell insulin receptors that appear as a consequence of antigenic stimulation. Additionally, in the course of T-cell activation, the T-cell
sends a message to the B-cell, resulting in the appearance of insulin
receptors on B-cells as well.

VII. SUMMARY

This chapter has characterized the nature of the insulin receptor system on T- and B-lymphocytes. This discussion has demonstrated the
manner in which this model system is quite similar to that on traditional
target cells or tissues and has pointed out the manner in which this
model is unique. The chapter has shown how an understanding of the
unique features of the T-lymphocyte system may permit its use as a
probe of disorders of carbohydrate metabolism and of the fine regulation of insulin receptor display. Moreover, an understanding of this

unique model points to a new way in which cell-cell communication can regulate the appearance of hormone receptors, thereby regulating hormone responsiveness. The interesting parallels and overlaps between the immunological protection of the internal milieu and the regulation of that milieu by hormones has been discussed. Continued intense investigation into this unique insulin receptor model should lead to a more thorough understanding of the interface between hormonal control and the control of the immune response (i.e., hormonal immunomodulation). The biochemical events involved in insulin receptor biosynthesis and turnover will be discussed in Chapter 12.

REFERENCES

1. Gavin, J. R. III, Roth, J., Jen, P., and Freychet, P. (1972). Insulin receptors in human circulating cells and fibroblasts. *Proc. Natl. Acad. Sci. USA* 69:747—751.
2. Schwartz, R. H., Bianco, A. R., Handwerger, B. S., and Kahn, C. R. (1975). Demonstration that monocytes rather than lymphocytes are the insulin-binding cells in preparation of human peripheral blood mononuclear leukocyte. Implications for studies of insulin-resistant states in man. *Proc. Natl. Acad. Sci. USA* 72474—478.
3. Krug, U., Krug, F., and Cuatrecasas, P. (1972). Emergence of insulin receptors on human lymphocytes during in vitro transformation. *Proc. Natl. Acad. Sci. USA* 69:2604—2608.
4. Helderman, J. H. and Strom, T. B. (1977). The emergence of insulin receptors upon alloimmune cells in the rat. *J. Clin. Invest.* 59:338—344.
5. Helderman, J. H. (1984). Cellular processing of the T-lymphocyte insulin receptor. *Clin. Res.* 32:398.
6. Helderman, J. H., Reynolds, T. C., and Strom, T. B. (1978). The insulin receptor as a universal marker of activated lymphocyte. *Eur. J. Immunol.* 8:589—595.
7. Spira G., Aman, G., Koiden, G., Lundin, G., Klein, G., and Hall, A. (1981). Cell surface immunoglobulin and insulin receptor expression in an EBV-negative lymphoma cell line and its EBV-converted sublines. *J. Immunol.* 126:122—126.
8. Helderman, J. H., Strom, T. B., and Garovoy, M. R. (1981). Rapid mixed lymphocyte culture testing by analysis of the insulin receptor on alloactivated T-lymphocyte: Implications for human tissue typing. *J. Clin. Invest.* 67:509—513.
9. Helderman, J. H. and Strom, T. B. (1979). Role of protein and RNA synthesis in the development of insulin binding sites on activated thymus-derived lymphocytes. *J. Biol. Chem.* 254:7203—7207.

10. Helderman, J. H. and Strom, T. B. (1979). Role of the cellular exoskeleton in the emergence of the T-lymphocyte insulin receptor. *Exp. Cell Res. 123*:119—126.

11. Helderman, J. H., and Raskin, R. (1980). The T-lymphocyte insulin receptor in diabetes and obesity: An intrinsic binding defect. *Diabetes 29*:551—557.

12. Helderman, J. H., Pietri, A., and Raskin P. (1983). In vitro control of T-lymphocyte insulin receptors by in vivo modulation of insulin. *Diabetes 32*:712—717.

13. Helderman, J. H. and Raskin, P. (1984). Mechanisms of acute regulation of the T-cell insulin receptors by changes in plasma insulin: Monocyte-T-cell interaction. *Clin. Res. 32*:520.

14. Strom, T. B., Bear, R. A. and Carpenter, C. B. (1975). Insulin-induced augmentation of lymphocyte-mediated cytotoxicity. *Science 187*:1206—1208.

15. Helderman, J. H., Strom, T. B., and Dupuy-d'Angeac, A. (1979). A close relationship between cytotoxic T-lymphocytes generated in the mixed lymphocyte culture and insulin receptor-bearing lymphocytes: Enrichment by density gradient centrifugation. *Cell. Immuno. 46*:247—258.

16. Strom, T. B., and Helderman, J. H. (1980). Comparison of ligand-specific rat allosensitized lymphocyte insulin receptors as assessed in binding and functional (lymphocyte-mediated cytotoxicity) assays. *Cell. Immuno. 53*:382—388.

17. Helderman, J. H. (1981). The role of insulin in the intermediary metabolism of the activated thymic-derived lymphocyte. *J. Clin. Invest. 67*:1636—1642.

18. Helderman, J. H. (1983). T-cell cooperation for the genesis of B-cell insulin receptors. *J. Immunol. 131*:644—650.

12

Life Cycle and Regulation of the Insulin Receptor

M. DANIEL LANE   *The Johns Hopkins University School of Medicine, Baltimore, Maryland*

I. INTRODUCTION

Insulin serves the vital role in higher animals of regulating energy metabolism. Together with glucagon and other counterregulatory hormones (e.g., ACTH and epinephrine), insulin modulates the flux of nutrient-derived metabolites into energy-storage versus energy-mobilizing pathways. Thus, insulin promotes the synthetic phase of energy metabolism by activating glucose uptake, glycogen synthesis, and lipogenesis—the level of the hormone in the blood reflecting the global energy status of the animal.

The first site at which insulin interacts, and thereby alters the metabolism of target cells, is at its specific receptors on the outer face of the plasma membrane. It is through this receptor-insulin interaction that a transmembrane signal is generated that triggers the pleiotropic response to insulin. While the nature of the signal and the molecular properties of the second messenger of insulin have not been established, a number of targets and metabolic responses of insulin action have been identified. These include activation of glucose transport across the plasma membrane, glycogen synthase, fatty acid synthesis, amino acid transport/protein synthesis, pyruvate dehydrogenase, and cAMP phosphodiesterase.

The magnitude of the metabolic response (and presumably the magnitude of the signal) depends not only upon the concentration of insulin to which the cell is exposed, but also upon (a) the number of functional receptors on the cell surface, (b) the affinity of these receptors for insulin, and (c) the extent to which these cell surface receptors are coupled to the response system(s). Most cells have the ability to regulate the number of functional insulin receptors on their cell surfaces in response to specific stimuli and, thereby, to adapt to

changes in physiological state. A number of physiological perturbations have been identified that cause alterations of insulin receptor
level; these are discussed in Section VIII of this chapter. Consequently, insulin receptors are in a dynamic state and subject to either "down-
regulation" or "up-regulation" of their cellular level or their cellular
localization.

As the regulation of receptor level must be exerted at a specific
step(s) in its synthesis, processing, or turnover, it will be instructive to outline the sequence of steps involved. The pathway for insulin receptor metabolism consistent with current knowledge (1) is
shown in Figure 1.

The proreceptor is synthesized in the rough endoplasmic reticulum
(step 1, Fig. 1), but is incapable of binding insulin until further
processing has occurred. The insulin receptor becomes "active", i.e.,
capable of binding insulin, only 1.5 hr after translation has occurred
presumably because posttranslational processing is required to perfect
the structure of the insulin-binding site (step 2, Fig. 1). The receptor appears to be terminally processed in the Golgi apparatus and
is then translocated to the plasma membrane in a Golgi-derived vesicle.
After insertion into the plasma membrane (step 3, Fig. 1) the receptor has a finite lifetime on the plasma membrane during which it can
function in transmembrane signal transmission. Cell surface insulin
receptors periodically cluster and undergo endocytosis (steps 4 and
5, respectively, Fig. 1), but then encounter a branch point in the
intracellular metabolic pathway. At this branch point, the receptor
can either recycle back to the plasma membrane (Step 8, Fig. 1) or
undergo inactivation and entry into the lysosomal degradative pathway (steps 6 and 7, Fig. 1).

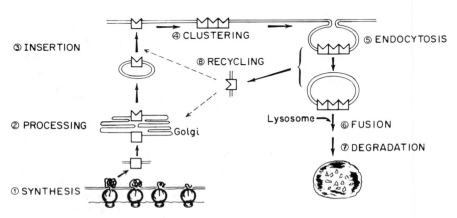

Figure 1 Life cycle of the insulin receptor. ▫, inactive (incapable of
binding insulin) precursor of the insulin receptor; ⋈, active (capable
of binding insulin) insulin receptor. From Krupp and Lane (1).

In this chapter, the metabolic pathways by which functional insulin receptor is formed and then undergoes inactivation and degradation will be discussed. It is through regulation of specific steps in this pathway that the level of functional insulin receptor in the plasma membrane is controlled. The mechanisms and physiological circumstances that lead to alterations in receptor level will also be discussed.

II. STRUCTURE OF THE INSULIN RECEPTOR

The mature insulin receptor is an integral membrane glycoprotein that spans the plasma membrane bilayer of most animal cells. As indicated in Chapters 3 and 4, the receptor contains two types of subunits: a 135,000 M.W. α subunit and a 95,000 M.W. β subunit (2–4). The model of the receptor that has been discussed in Chapter 4 suggests that the receptor exists as an oligomer with an $\alpha_2\beta_2$ composition in which the subunits are covalently linked to one another by α-β and α-α disulfide bonds (3,4) (see Fig. 2) (5). The α subunit houses the insulin-binding site that is located on the outer face of the plasma membrane where it is accessible to extracellular insulin (3). The β subunit possesses a tyrosine protein kinase catalytic site (6,7) that is capable of autophosphorylation (of the β subunit) and of catalyzing the phosphorylation of intracellular protein substrates. Recently, the amino acid sequences of the α- and β-subunits of the receptor were established from the nucleotide sequence of the cDNA which encodes the insulin proreceptor (29,30). The amino acid sequence indicates that the β-subunit possesses a single hydrophobic transmembrane domain consisting of 23 amino acid residues which separate the external one-third of its polypeptide chain from the intracellular two-thirds. The α-subunit, which contains no evident transmembrane sequence, must, therefore, be located entirely external to the plasma membrane. Presumably, the α-subunit and the insulin binding domain it houses are firmly attached to the cell surface through covalent disulfide cross-links to the β-subunit as depicted in Fig. 2. Hence, the kinase catalytic site is disposed on the inner face of the plasma membrane where it has access to intracellular ATP and target protein substrates.

This structure suggests a scenario for transmembrane signaling induced by insulin. The binding of insulin at the "extracellular" ligand-binding site of the receptor presumably induces a conformational change in the α subunit that is transmitted through the membrane bilayer to the tyrosine protein kinase domain of the β-subunit where catalysis is activated. This in turn would allow the receptor to phosphorylate an intracellular target protein(s), thereby initiating the cascade of events leading to the well-known actions of insulin.

The insulin receptor has been shown to be a glycoprotein (8–10) in which the oligosaccharide side chains are N-linked complex structures. These complex carbohydrate side chains are linked to asparagine N in the polypeptide backbone of the receptor and contain *N*-acetylglucosamine, mannose, galactose, fucose, and sialic acid. It

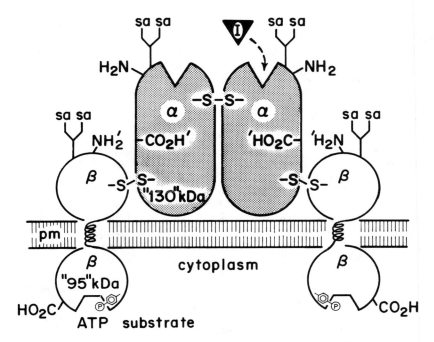

Figure 2 Model of the mature insulin receptor in the plasma membrane.
I, insulin; $\vee$, the insulin-binding site; $\frown$, the tyrosine kinase catalytic
side; $-S-S-$, disulfide bond; Sa, sialic acid; pm, plasma membrane.

is known that glycosylation is a prerequisite for the formation of functional insulin receptor (8,10). The unique structure of the insulin receptor can now be accounted for by events known to occur in its biosynthetic pathway. These events are described in Sections IV and V
of this chapter.

III. DYNAMICS OF INSULIN RECEPTOR SYNTHESIS,
TRANSLOCATION TO THE CELL SURFACE, AND
DEGRADATION

In most cell types, insulin receptors are in a dynamic state. New receptors are continuously being synthesized, while previously synthesized receptors are concurrently undergoing degradation as shown in
Figure 3. The total number of receptors a cell possesses in the steady
state, i.e., when total cellular receptor number is constant, will be
determined by the equation,

$$R = k_S / k_D \tag{1}$$

where R is total receptor number, k_S is the zero-order rate constant for receptor synthesis, and k_D is the first-order rate constant for receptor inactivation/degradation. Receptor synthesis is believed to be dependent upon the cellular concentration of the specific mRNA for the receptor.

The kinetics of receptor synthesis and degradation is most accurately described (11,12) by a more useful form of the equation

$$R_t = (k_S/k_D)(1-e^{-k_Dt}) + R_0 e^{-k_Dt}$$

where receptor level, R_t at time t is described by a constant (zero-order) synthetic rate, k_S, a first-order degradation constant, k_D, and an initial receptor level, R_0, at zero time.

We have made extensive use of the heavy isotope density-shift method to determine the rates of synthesis and inactivation-degradation of the insulin receptor (11,12) and to determine which of these rates is affected by physiological perturbations known to alter cellular insulin receptor level (11,13--17). Density labeling of receptors provides an unambiguous method for distinguishing between both "old" and newly synthesized receptors in the absence of inhibitors of protein synthesis. Some investigators have used inhibitors of protein synthesis, e.g., cycloheximide, to inhibit receptor synthesis and then have followed the rate of receptor degradation through the loss of cell surface or total cellular insulin-binding activity. If receptor synthesis is blocked, k_D can be measured and knowing receptor level, R, in the uninhibited state, k_S can be calculated. This approach was shown to be invalid in many instances, however, since inhibitors of protein synthesis also block the synthesis of a protein(s) necessary for receptor turnover and, thereby, erroneously lengthen the half-life of the insulin receptor (8). The heavy isotope density-shift method does not utilize inhibitors and therefore, does not suffer this disadvantage.

To employ the heavy density-shift method, cells are shifted from a medium containing "light" (^1H, ^{12}C, ^{14}N) amino acids to a medium containing "heavy" (>95% ^2H, ^{13}C, ^{15}N) amino acids. The incorporation of amino acids into receptor protein during its synthesis substantially

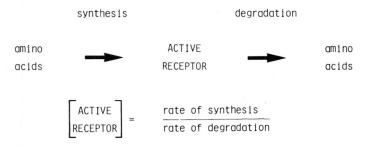

Figure 3 Dynamic state of cellular insulin receptors.

increases the density of the newly synthesized insulin receptor. Hence, new "heavy" and old "light" receptor, solubilized with detergent, can be resolved by isopycnic banding on CsCl density gradients. Light and heavy receptors at the heavy and light positions in the gradients can be quantitated, based on their insulin-binding activity, at various times after the shift to heavy medium (see Fig. 4) (18). From the results obtained, the rate of formation of newly synthesized heavy insulin receptor and the rate of inactivation of old light receptor can be determined concomitantly. It should be stressed that the density-shift method follows the rate at which "active" receptor, i.e., receptor capable of binding insulin, is produced or lost. Thus, the method measures the physiologically relevant rate-limiting step in the formation and inactivation of functional receptor.

As illustrated in Fig. 4, soluble receptor extracted at any time prior to the shift to medium containing heavy amino acids would be composed entirely of light amino acids and when banded isopycnically in a CsCl density gradient, would generate only a single light (L) receptor peak (Fig. 4A). Gradients with receptor extracted from cells after the shift to heavy medium, e.g., beyond day 4, should contain both a heavy (H) peak of newly synthesized receptor and a reduced light peak of receptor synthesized prior to the shift (Fig. 4B). Gradient profiles of soluble receptor obtained after longer periods, e.g., 5–8 days (Fig. 4C),

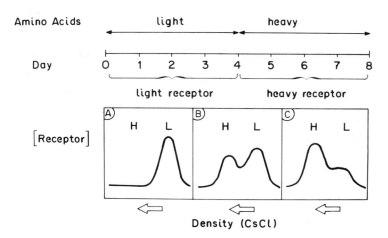

Figure 4 Illustration of the application of the heavy isotope density-shift technique used to follow the synthesis and degradation of cellular insulin receptors. Light and heavy amino acids refer to amino acids containing ^1H, ^{12}C, ^{14}N and >95% ^2H, ^{13}C, ^{15}N, respectively, present in the culture medium. (A), (B), and (C) represent hypothetical isopycnic CsCl density gradients of detergent-solubilized cellular insulin receptors on days 4, 5, and 8, respectively. From Lane et al. (18).

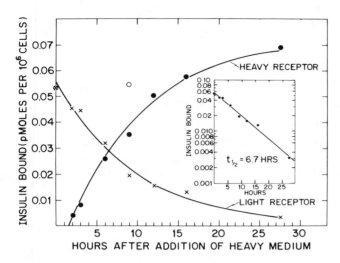

Figure 5 Kinetics of heavy receptor synthesis and light receptor degradation in differentiated 3T3-L1 adipocytes. Inset: semilog plot of light receptor degradation. From Reed and Lane (11).

should show increasing amounts of heavy receptor and decreasing amounts of light receptor. By quantitating the changes in the light and heavy receptor peaks with time after the switch to the "heavy" medium, progress curves for receptor synthesis and degradation can be generated as illustrated in Fig. 5. The example shown is for fully differentiated 3T3-L1 adipocytes (11), which are typical of other cell types. It is evident that within 1 day after the shift to heavy medium, light receptor has almost totally disappeared and has been replaced by heavy receptor.

The exact half-life for light receptor can be obtained by plotting the degradation data for light receptor semilogarithmically as shown in the inset to Fig. 5. In this case, the half-life for the insulin receptor (in the down-regulated state) was shown to be 6.7 hr. From this number the first-order rate constant for receptor decay can be calculated; from R and k_D, the synthetic rate, k_S can be calculated (see Eq. 1 and footnote 1). It will be shown later in this chapter (Section VIII) that during preadipocyte differentiation into adipocytes, the synthetic rate constant, k_S, for receptor formation increases dramatically without a change in k_D. This leads to an increased steady-state level of receptor. On the other hand, insulin-induced down-regulation of receptor level is the result of an increased rate of receptor degradation with no change in the rate of receptor synthesis.

It should also be noted (Fig. 5) that there is a 1.5-hr lag in the first appearance of "active" heavy receptor. This lag is the result of posttranslational processing of inactive insulin proreceptor into active receptor. The basis for this "activation" is discussed below (Sections IV and V).

IV. POSTTRANSLATIONAL ACTIVATION OF THE INSULIN PRORECEPTOR IN TRANSIT TO THE PLASMA MEMBRANE

The insulin receptor is not "active" (capable of binding insulin) immediately upon translation, but requires approximately 1.5 hr for acquisition for insulin-binding activity (11). This was demonstrated in heavy isotope density-shift experiments which showed that 1.5 hr elapse between translation and the first appearance of active "heavy" receptor (see Fig. 5). This posttranslational lag in the activation of newly synthesized receptor has been observed in several cell types including 3T3-L1 preadipocytes, 3T3-C2 fibroblasts, 3T3-L1 adipocytes, and chick hepatocytes (11,13−15,19). This lag correlates with specific events in the processing of the insulin proreceptor (see Section V).

This lag in receptor activation is consistent with the finding that a long time is required, i.e., about 3 hr, for newly translated proreceptor to undergo processing and to become incorporated into the plasma membrane. The time required for newly synthesized receptor to move from its site of synthesis in the rough endoplasmic reticulum to the plasma membrane was determined by combining the heavy isotope density-shift approach with surface labeling of receptor as it becomes incorporated into the plasma membrane (16) (see Fig. 6). The surface labeling procedure involved cooling the cells to 2°C to prevent further exo- or endocytosis, binding of [^{125}I]insulin to cell surface receptors, cross-linking of cell surface [^{125}I]insulin to receptors with the bifunctional cross-linking reagent disuccinimidyl suberate, and then separation and quantitation of heavy and light ^{125}I-labeled receptors by isopycnic banding on CsCl. Thus, when cells are shifted to culture medium containing "heavy" amino acids (>95% ^{13}C, ^{15}N, ^{3}H), heavy receptor will appear at the cell surface where it can be labeled with [^{125}I]insulin, but only after the processing pipeline has first been cleared of "light" receptor (see Fig. 6).

The results using this approach with 3T3-L1 adipocytes showed that only after about 3 hr did newly synthesized "heavy" insulin receptors reach the plasma membrane, at which time additional heavy receptors began to accumulate on the cell surface (16). The decline in the amount of light insulin receptor at the cell surface occurs only 3 hr after the density shift, i.e., when the pipeline of light receptor moving to the cell surface has been cleared. The long time requirement for activation of the receptor, i.e., 1.5 hr, and its translocation

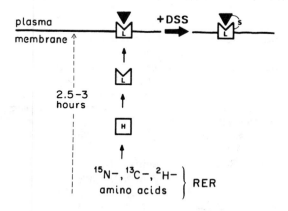

$$\text{DSS}$$
disuccinimidyl suberate

Figure 6 Strategy for determining the time for translocation of newly synthesized heavy receptor from the rough endoplasmic reticulum to the plasma membrane. Cells are shifted to medium containing heavy (>95%, ^{15}N-, ^{13}C-, ^{2}H-containing) amino acids. At intervals following the density-shift, cell monolayers are subjected to a ligand debinding protocol to remove cell-associated insulin and are then cooled at 4°C. At this temperature the processes of exocytosis and endocytosis are blocked. To determine the amounts of heavy and light receptors at the cell surface, [^{125}I]insulin is bound to the cell monolayers at 4°C after which bond insulin is covalently cross-linked to surface receptors with disuccinimidyl suberate (DSS). The [^{125}I]insulin-labeled receptors are then extracted from total cellular membranes with Triton X-100, and the extract is applied to CsCl gradients to resolve and quantitate heavy and light receptors. The gradients are fractionated, and the heavy and light peak fractions subjected to SDS-polyacrylamide gel electrophoresis to quantitate ^{125}I-labeled surface insulin receptor. From Ronnett et al. (16).

to the plasma membrane, i.e., 3 hr, after synthesis correlates well with the long time requirement for newly synthesized receptor to undergo processing and terminal glycosylation.

V. POSTTRANSLATIONAL PROCESSING OF THE PRORECEPTOR TO FORM ACTIVE INSULIN RECEPTOR

The lengthy time requirement for acquisition of insulin-binding activity and for incorporation of the insulin receptor into the plasma membrane suggested that newly synthesized receptor undergoes substantial processing. Considerable progress has been made recently in the identification of intermediates in the pathway by which insulin proreceptor is converted into functional mature form (10,20). To identify and characterize the mature insulin receptor subunits, 3T3-L1 adipocytes were pulsed for 1 hr with either [^{35}S]methionine or [^{3}H]sugars and then were chased for 6 hr with unlabeled methionine or sugars (10). The ^{35}S-labeled receptor polypeptides were then specifically immunoprecipitated with anti-receptor antibody, subjected to SDS-polyacrylamide gel electrophoresis, and the gels were radioautographed. Only the two expected receptor subunits of 135,000 M.W. (α subunit) and 95,000 M.W. (β subunit) were detected on these gels; both were glycosylated.

To identify the early intermediates in the receptor translation-processing pathway, 3T3-L1 adipocytes were incubated for 1 hr in the presence of [^{35}S]methionine, [^{3}H]mannose, or [^{3}H]glucosamine, but without a subsequent unlabeled chase (10). No [^{35}S]polypeptides corresponding to the mature α- or β subunits of the receptor were detected (Fig. 7, lane 1); however, five new polypeptides were observed. Four of these polypeptides (210K, 190K, 125K, and 83K) were subsequently found to be precursors of the insulin receptor in the posttranslational processing pathway. An additional polypeptide (90K—92K), which exhibits properties of an insulin receptor-associated polypeptide, is not on the main receptor processing pathway (10). All these receptor precursors are glycoproteins, as evidenced by their labeling with [^{3}H]mannose or [^{3}H]glucosamine (Fig. 7, lanes 3 and 5, respectively).

To assess the precursor-product relationships among these apparent receptor precursors, pulse-chase experiments were conducted in which 3T3-L1 adipocytes were pulsed for 15 min with [^{35}S]methionine and were then chased with unlabeled methionine for 2—3 hr (10). At various times after the pulse, immunoprecipitable receptor and its precursors were isolated and subjected to SDS-polyacrylamide gel electrophoresis. As shown in Figure 8, three-labeled polypeptides were observed immediately following the 15-min pulse. These were the true receptor precursors of 190 K and 210 K and the 90 K—92 K receptor-associated polypeptide. No labeled receptor subunits were detected at

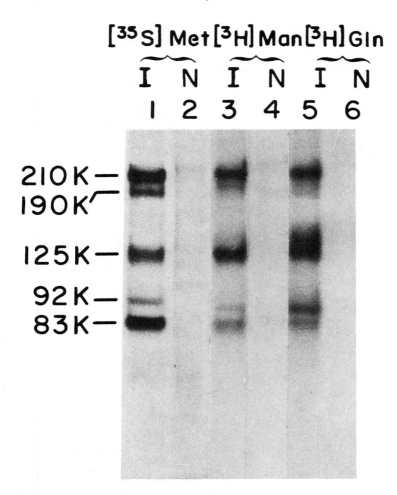

Figure 7 Autoradiograms of SDS-polyacrylamide gels of immunoprecipitated insulin receptor polypeptides from 3T3-L1 adipocytes labeled for 1 hr with [^{35}S]methionine (lanes 1 and 2), [^{3}H]mannose (lanes 3 and 4), or [^{3}H]glucosamine (lanes 5 and 6). In lanes 2, 3, and 5 anti-insulin receptor antiserum and in lanes 2, 4 and 6 nonimmune serum were used. From Ronnett et al. (10).

Pulse, min 15 15 15 15 15 15
Chase, min 0 15 30 60 90 120

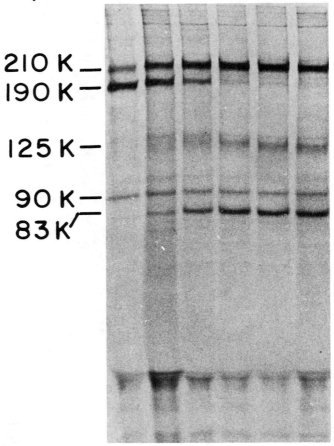

210 K
190 K
125 K
90 K
83 K

Figure 8 Autoradiograms of SDS-polyacrylamide gels of immunoprecipitated insulin receptor precursors from 3T3-L1 adipocytes labeled
for 15 min with [35S]methionine and then chased with medium containing excess unlabeled methionine. Immunoprecipitation with anti-
insulin receptor antibody and SDS-PAGE were performed at each time
indicated. From Ronnett et al. (10).

this time. The 190 K polypeptide is more heavily labeled than the 210 K polypeptide immediately following the pulse. However, after a short period of chase, ^{35}S-label in the 190 K polypeptide is rapidly lost, and by 60 min the label has disappeared completely. The 190 K polypeptide will, henceforth, be referred to as the insulin "proreceptor". There is a concomitant increase in ^{35}S labeling of the 210 K polypeptide, suggesting a precursor-product relationship between the 190 K and 210 K polypeptides.

It is also evident that as the ^{35}S label in the 210 K species disappears, the 125 K and 83 K polypeptides become labeled suggesting a precursor-product relationship. It should be noted that up to 2 hr after the initial labeling of the 190 K proreceptor, ^{35}S labeling of the mature α- and β subunits 135 K and 95 K polypeptides does not occur. To determine at what time after the [^{35}S]methionine pulse the mature α and β subunits are formed, longer pulse-chase experiments were performed. The results of these experiments, taken together with those described above, support the pathway of insulin proreceptor processing outlined in Figure 9.

To further characterize the intermediates in the proreceptor processing pathway in 3T3-L1 adipocytes, four additional types of analysis were performed (10): (a) the presence of the intermediate (or subunit) at the cell surface was assessed by determining the susceptibility of each intermediate in [^{35}S]methionine-labeled intact cells to proteolysis by trypsin, (b) the presence of terminal *N*-acetylglucosamine or sialic acid was assessed by determining whether the solubilized labeled polypeptide binds to wheat germ lectin, (c) the nature of the oligosaccharide chain (whether high mannose or complex) was determined by treating each intermediate with endoglycosidase H, which cleaves high mannose, but not sialylated complex oligosaccharide chains, and (d) the presence of terminal sialic acid residues on the oligosaccharide chains was assessed by observing the effect of neuraminidase, which cleaves terminal sialic acid residues, on the labeled intermediate. In addition, Kahn and his colleagues (20) working with another cell system, compared tryptic peptide maps of the 210 K precursor with those of the α and β subunits to determine whether both subunits were derived from this common precursor. They determined that the α and β

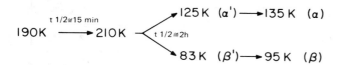

Figure 9 Proposed pathway of posttranslational processing of the 190 K proreceptor to form the α and β subunits of the mature insulin receptor in 3T3-L1 adipocytes. From Ronnett et al. (10).

subunits possess tryptic peptides in common with the 210 K polypeptide. This supports the view that the α and β subunits are derived
from the 210 K polypeptide.

The only trypsin-sensitive species detected was the 135 K α subunit, suggesting that only the mature α and β subunits (presumed to
be covalently bound to the β subunit in the plasma membrane, but which
must face the cytoplasmic compartment) have reached the plasma membrane
during a 4-hr pulse-chase experiment. This suggests that only the
mature receptor‚ reaches the plasma membrane. With the exception of
the 190 K proreceptor, all other intermediates and subunits are capable
of binding to wheat germ lectin. This indicates that intermediates beyond the 190 K species in the pathway (Fig. 9) possess oligosaccharide
chains that terminate either in N-acetylglucosamine or sialic acid. It
is evident that the 190 K proreceptor must contain a high mannose
oligosaccharide core (added contranslationally), since this polypeptide is sensitive to endoglycosidase H. Its product, the 210 K species
that binds to wheat germ lectin, is also sensitive to endoglycosidase H.
Neither of these species contain sialic acid as indicated by their sensitivity to endoglycosidase H and lack of susceptibility to neuraminidase.
These results indicate that the 190 K proreceptor does not contain
terminal N-acetylglucosamine residues, whereas the 210 K species must.
Likewise, the 125 K (α') and 83 K (β') subunits do not contain terminal
sialic acid residues, since they too are susceptible to endoglycosidase
H cleavage, but are not cleaved by neuraminidase. Only the mature
135 K (α) and 95 K (β) subunits contain terminal sialic acid residues,
since they exhibit a decreased mobility when treated with neuraminidase
and show minimal decreases in mobility when treated with endoglycosidase H. In kinetic experiments, it is evident that the sialic acid residues are added about 3 hr after the 190 K proreceptor is synthesized,
an event known to take place in the Golgi apparatus. Thus sialylation
may be the terminal event of processing, which is the signal for translocation of the mature receptor to the plasma membrane for insertion.

Taken together, our results (10) and those from Kahn's laboratory
(20) support the posttranslational processing pathway for the insulin
proreceptor shown in Fig. 10. The primary proreceptor translation
product appears to contain a 180 K polypeptide chain to which N-linked
core high mannose oligosaccharides are added cotranslationally. Therefore, the first identifiable labeled intermediate is the 190 K proreceptor.
The 190 K proreceptor leads only a transient existence, being rapidly
converted ($t_{1/2}$ = 15 min) to the 210 K intermediate precursor. The
basis for the 20 K increase in the apparent size, that occurs during
190 K to 210 K conversion, is not entirely clear. However, our results
suggest that the 210 K species contains terminal N-acetylglucosamine,
while the 190 K species does not. Since this property alone would not
account for the large (20 K) apparent size difference between the two
species, it is likely that there is an additional structural difference between the two species, i.e., 190 K and 210 K, such as a difference in
the state of sugar phosphorylation of their oligosaccharide chains.

Minutes 0——5——————20——————45———————————180

-190K   -210K   -125K +83K   -135K +95K

-Translation   -Further sugar -Peptide   -Capping sugar
               addition   cleavage   addition

-Core oligosaccharide   -Oligomerization   -Insertion
addition   (-S-S-)

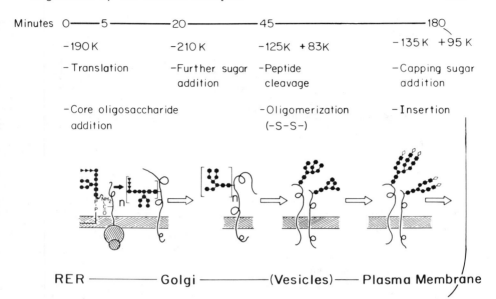

RER —————— Golgi ————————(Vesicles)—— Plasma Membrane

Figure 10   Proposed sequence of events and intracellular sites of their occurrence during the processing and maturation of the insulin proreceptor. From Lane et al. (5).

The 210 K intermediate is slowly converted ($t_{1/2}$ = 2 hr), apparently by proteolytic processing, to the previously not recognized 125 K α' and 83 K β' precursors of the α and β subunits. Importantly, the oligosaccharide side chains of these receptor precursors have not yet acquired terminal sialic (above). The time after translation at which the receptor is inserted into the plasma membrane, i.e., about 3 hr, corresponds to the time at which the receptor, particularly the 125 K α polypeptide, acquires sialic acid, thus giving rise to the mature α receptor subunit. Just preceding their translocation to the cell surface, the α' and β' receptor precursors acquire sialic acid in the Golgi apparatus and then are quickly translocated to the plasma membrane. Once inserted into the plasma membrane, the insulin receptor appears to be fully functional.

Preliminary evidence in our laboratory indicates that the disulfide bond(s) that covalently links the α' subunit to the β' subunit is formed before the 210 K precursor is proteolytically cleaved to form the α' and β' subunit precursors (see Fig. 11). The formation of this α'-β' disulfide linkage(s) prior to proteolytic cleavage of the proreceptor guarantees the firm attachment of the external α-subunit to the membrane-bound β-subunit (see Fig. 2) during processing the transit to the plasma membrane. However, the disulfide bond that links each α'-β' pair through an α'-α' linkage) to produce the oligomeric $\alpha'_2\beta'_2$ structure

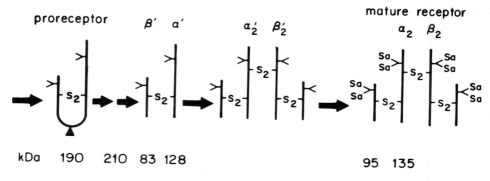

Figure 11 Postulated sequence of disulfide bond formation during the posttranslational processing of the insulin proreceptor. S_2, disulfide bond; Sa, sialic acid.

appears to be formed much later, i.e., about 1.5 hr after transla-tion of the 190 K proreceptor precursor. The formation of the $\alpha'-\alpha'$ disulfide bond occurs at approximately the same time as "acti-vation" (acquisition of insulin-binding capacity; see Section III), some 1.5 hr before the mature $\alpha_2\beta_2$ receptor appears at the cell surface. It is possible that formation of this disulfide bond(s) perfects the conformation of the insulin-binding sites of the α sub-units, enabling them to bind insulin.

VI. DEPENDENCE OF THE FORMATION OF ACTIVE RECEPTOR UPON N-GLYCOSYLATION

Glycosylation of the insulin receptor has been shown to be essential for the formation of functional insulin receptor (8,21). In the experi-ments in which it was established that N-glycosylation of the insulin proreceptor is essential for its maturation, 3T3-L1 adipocytes were treated with tunicamycin and its affect on cellular insulin binding activity was determined (21). Tunicamycin specifically blocks the initial step in the formation of the oligosaccharide-dolichol intermedi-ate, which serves as the en bloc donor of oligosaccharide to asparagine-N of nascent chains during their translation in the rough endoplasmic re-ticulum. Treatment of 3T3-L1 adipocytes with tunicamycin for 3 days led to a >95% loss of functional insulin receptor (21). Upon withdrawal of tunicamycin from the cell culture medium, insulin-binding activity was regained, even when protein synthesis was blocked by cyclo-heximide. This suggested that an inactive aglycoproreceptor, formed when tunicamycin was present, could be "rescued" to form active re-ceptor. This hypothesis was proved correct by heavy isotope

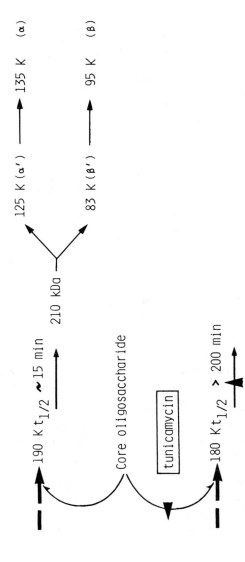

Figure 12 Effect of blocking core oligosaccharide addition with tunicamycin on pro-receptor formation and processing.

density-shift experiments (21) in which 3T3-L1 adipocytes were first
exposed to tunicamycin, then tunicamycin was withdrawn and the cells
were shifted to medium containing heavy (>95% ^{15}N, ^{13}C, ^{2}H-containing)
amino acids with or without cycloheximide. Following the withdrawal of
tunicamycin, "active" light receptor was formed along with a small
amount of newly synthesized heavy receptor (in the absence, but not
in the presence, of cycloheximide). Substantial recovery of active
light receptor also occurred after tunicamycin withdrawal, even though
protein synthesis had been inhibited by cycloheximide.

Taken together these results indicate that (a) N-linked glycosylation of the insulin proreceptor is required for formation of active insulin receptor, and (b) that aglyco-proreceptor formed in the presence
of tunicamycin can be rescued as active receptor following the withdrawal of tunicamycin.

To identify and characterize the inactive aglyco-precursor of the
receptor, 3T3-L1 adipocytes were preincubated for 24 hr with tunicamycin and then were labeled with [^{35}S]methionine or [^{3}H]mannose (10).
Tunicamycin treatment led to the accumulation of a 180 K polypeptide
that we believe is the primary proreceptor translation product, but
which lacks N-linked core oligosaccharide. This is supported by the
fact that treatment of either 190 K or 210 K precursors with endoglycosidase H yields a 180 K polypeptide that is identical to the 180 K
intermediate that accumulates in the presence of tunicamycin (Fig. 12).
The 180 K aglyco-proreceptor does not reach the plasma membrane
even upon extended incubation, as evidenced by its resistance to
cleavage by trypsin (10). Moreover, pulse-chase experiments with
[^{35}S]methionine reveal that the 180 K aglyco-proreceptor, although
rapidly formed, does not turnover (or decay) during an extended
chase with unlabeled methionine. This is in contrast to its 190 K glycosylated counterpart that turns over with a half-life of 15 min (Fig. 12).

These results underscore the importance of glycosylation to further processing and maturation of the insulin receptor. It is concluded
that N-linked oligosaccharide chains on the proreceptor are either required for its intracellular translocation to the site of proteolytic cleavage or for its identification as a target of the proteolytic cleavage enzyme. Regardless of the mechanism, it is clear the the glycosylated
insulin proreceptor is not further processed into functional insulin receptor (see Fig. 12).

VII. FATE OF INTERNALIZED INSULIN RECEPTOR:
INACTIVATION—DEGRADATION VERSUS
RECYCLING TO THE PLASMA MEMBRANE

Once the mature insulin receptor is inserted into the plasma membrane,
it can participate in transmembrane signaling in response to binding

insulin. The receptor, however, has a finite lifetime on the plasma membrane and periodically undergoes endocytosis with or without bound insulin. A large body of evidence indicates that insulin, bound to the receptor, undergoes endocytosis and is degraded (broken down by proteolysis) in the lysosome. The endocytotic process by which insulin enters the cell appears to be mediated by the insulin receptor. It has been shown (22), for example, that in the presence of chloroquine, an agent which blocks lysosomal proteolysis, [^{125}I]insulin accumulates intracellularly and is not proteolytically degraded to [^{125}I]tryosine. Thus, the pathway traversed by insulin after binding to its cell sur-face receptor and exerting its signal leads to endocytosis and ultimate degradation in the lysosomal system. This process, of course, ter-minates the signal by destroying the ligand.

Several lines of evidence indicate that the insulin receptor, which undergoes endocytosis with its bound ligand, separates from the li-gand and recycles back to the cell surface (Fig. 1, step 8). It can be calculated (22) from the rate of receptor degradation that 7% of the cellular receptors of the hepatocyte are degraded per hour, which is about 1/200 the rate of insulin degradation. If it is assumed that an insulin receptor is internalized with each insulin molecule internalized and degraded, it follows that most receptors escape degradation and are recycled about 200 times before they themselves are degraded. Experiments with mouse fibroblasts (17) have provided additional evi-dence for recycling of insulin receptors following endocytosis. Thus, upon addition of insulin to fibroblasts, cell surface insulin receptors are rapidly translocated to an intracellular, i.e., a trypsin-resistant, compartment. This translocation occurs rapidly, reaching steady-state distribution within 10 min after the addition of insulin (see Fig. 13). The translocation process is rapidly reversed ($t_{1/2}$ = 20 min) when insulin is removed, i.e., upon removal of insulin, the receptor again becomes sensitive to trypsin indicating its return to the plasma membrane. Compelling evidence with several other receptors (23) in-dicates that upon endocytosis, the endosome with its ligand-receptor

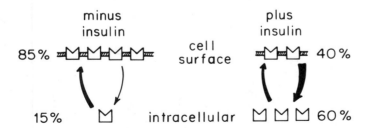

Figure 13 Effect of insulin addition (down-regulation) on the distribu-tion of insulin receptors between the cell surface and intracellular com-partments of mouse 3T3-C2 fibroblasts. See Reference 17.

complexes become acidic. Acidification of the endosome is believed (23) to cause dissociation of ligand from its receptor allowing these two components to enter different pathways, i.e., the receptor entering a recycling pathway and free ligand entering the lysosomal degradative pathway. Recent evidence from my laboratory (17 and unpublished results) with fibroblasts suggests that these pathways also operate with the insulin receptor and insulin.

Chloroquine, which prevents acidification of both endosomes and lysosomes, blocks the proteolytic degradation of insulin (17,22). Of importance is the fact that chloroquine, which has no effect on the insulin-induced internalization of insulin receptor, blocks the return, i.e., recycling, of the insulin receptor to the plasma membrane when insulin is withdrawn from the culture medium (17 and unpublished results). Thus, it appears that when the insulin receptor with bound insulin undergoes endocytosis, acidification is the driving force for the separation of ligand from receptor, allowing them to traverse their separate pathways. When acidification of the endosome is blocked by chloroquine, this separation cannot occur, leaving the receptor-insulin complex at a metabolic dead end. These results, and others using receptor labeled with photoaffinity labeled [^{125}I]insulin (24), strongly suggest that after undergoing endocytosis, the insulin receptor can return to the plasma membrane via a recycling pathway.

There is also compelling evidence which shows that a fraction of the internalized insulin receptor intracellularly undergoes inactivation and degradation (17), as illustrated in Fig. 14. One line of evidence indicates that receptor inactivation precedes and is independent of lysosomal proteolytic degradation; hence, chloroquine, which prevents lysosomal proteolysis, has no effect on the rate of insulin receptor

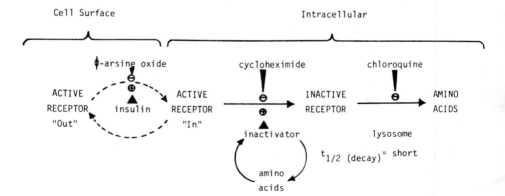

Figure 14 Postulated pathway of cell surface insulin receptors of mouse 3T3-C2 fibroblasts during insulin-induced down-regulation.

inactivation precedes and is independent of lysosomal proteolytic degradation; hence, chloroquine, which prevents lysosomal proteolysis, has no effect on the rate of insulin receptor inactivation as measured by the heavy isotope density-shift technique (17,22). This is in contrast to the lysosomal degradation of insulin, which is blocked by chloroquine (17,22). Conversely, insulin receptor inactivation is rapidly and nearly completely blocked by inhibitors of protein synthesis (e.g., cycloheximide or puromycin), but lysosomal degradation of insulin is unaffected (Fig. 14).

Moreover, when insulin is added to mouse fibroblasts, causing a rapid internalization of receptors ($t_{1/2}$ = <10 min) such that the distribution of receptor shifts from the 85% cell surface—15% intracellular to 40% cell surface—60% intracellular, as illustrated in Fig. 13, the rate of receptor inactivation is markedly increased ($t_{1/2}$ for receptor degradation shifting from 15 to about 7 hr) (17). These results show that insulin-induced translocation of its receptor into an intracellular compartment precedes its inactivation, strongly suggesting that receptor inactivation occurs intracellularly. Therefore, the rate of inactivation of cellular receptors will depend upon the fraction of the receptors that is located within the intracellular compartment. Partitioning of receptors between the cell surface and intracellular compartments in the short term will be determined by the relative rates of receptor internalization and externalization (recycling), the former being accelerated by insulin.

VIII. REGULATION OF FUNCTIONAL RECEPTOR LEVEL

Most cells have the capacity to alter their responsiveness to specific hormones as changes in the physiological state of the animal occur. There is now considerable evidence that one of the major mechanisms by which cells regulate their hormonal responsiveness is through alterations in the level of surface receptors they possess. The total number of receptors a cell possesses depends both upon the relative rates of receptor synthesis and receptor degradation (see Fig. 3). Not all cellular receptors may be functional at a given time. An intracellular pool of active or inactive receptors may exist that becomes functional upon activation and/or recruitment to the plasma membrane. Recruitment of such internal or reserve receptors could be regulated. Since receptors can recycle, returning to the cell surface following internalization, either internalization or exocytosis may be controlled. Thus, there are many points in the life cycle of the receptor at which regulation could be exerted.

Three types of regulation of functional insulin receptors have been studied extensively. These include (a) insulin-induced "down-regulation" of receptor level, (b) differentiation-induced "up-regulation" of receptor level, and (c) glucocorticoid-induced alterations of receptor level. The regulatory processes involved in these types of receptor alteration are described below.

A. Insulin-Induced Down-Regulation of Receptor Level

Like many other receptors for polypeptide hormones, insulin itself is an important modulator of the cellular level of its own receptor. Gavin et al. (25) were the first to show that chronic exposure of lymphocytes to insulin in vitro caused a decrease or down-regulation in the level of cell surface insulin receptors. This inverse relationship between ambient insulin concentration and surface insulin receptor level extends to other cell types studied in culture or in vivo.

It appears that the common feature of insulin-induced receptor down-regulation is the rapid redistribution of cellular receptors such that an increased percentage is found within the intracellular compartment after the addition of insulin. This redistribution is rapid and with some cell types, e.g., skin fibroblasts, preadipocytes, adipocytes, and lymphocytes (14,25,25), leads to an accelerated rate of receptor degradation. This not only lowers the number of receptors at the cell surface, but also lowers the total number of cellular receptors in the new steady state. The half-time for achieving this new steady state is far longer than the half-time, i.e., half-time < 10 min, for insulin-induced redistribution of receptors between the cell surface and the intracellular compartment (see Fig. 13). In certain other cell types, e.g., the hepatocyte, only the first phase (i.e. the insulin-induced redistribution of receptors toward the intracellular compartment) occurs. However, this does not lead to a decrease in the total number of cellular receptors per cell in the new steady state 12−24 hr after insulin addition (19).

The mechanism by which insulin causes down-regulation of total cellular receptor level in adipocytes and fibroblasts was investigated by the heavy isotope density-shift approach described above (see Section III). Since the number of receptors that a cell possesses in the steady state is determined by the relative rates of synthesis and decay of active receptor, ligand-induced changes in the rates of either of these processes could cause receptor down-regulation. We have shown that, for 3T3-C2 fibroblasts (15), 3T3-L1 preadipocytes (14), and 3T3-L1 adipocytes (14), insulin-induced down-regulation of total receptor number is the consequence of an increased rate of receptor inactivation. As illustrated in Table 1A for 3T3-L1 adipocytes, the rates of insulin receptor synthesis for control, i.e., up-regulated 3T3-L1 adipocytes and down-regulated adipocytes, were virtually identical—about 11,000 sites of receptor per hour per 10^6 cells. In contrast, a significant difference in the degradative rates of insulin receptors was observed in control and down-regulated cells. Control

Table 1 Effect of Insulin, Preadipocyte Differentiation, and Glucocorticoid on Receptor Level Synthesis and Inactivation[a]

Cell type and physiological state	Receptor sites/cell	K_d (nM)	Rate of receptor		
			Synthesis[b] (sites/cell/hr)	Inactivation[b] (hr^{-1})	Half-life[b] (hr)
A. Down-regulation (3T3-L1 adipocytes)					
Control (no insulin)	240,000	1–2	10,800	0.045	15
+ Insulin	120,000	1–2	11,400	0.095	7
B. Differentiation (3T3-L1 cells)					
Preadipocyte[c]	8,400	1–2	800	0.095	7
Adipocyte[c]	162,000	1–2	15,400	0.095	7
C. Up-regulation (3T3-C2 fibroblasts)					
Control[d]	59,000	1–2	4,100	0.070	10
+ Dexamethasone	110,000	1–2	4,200	0.038	20

[a]Results from References 11 and 13–15.
[b]Determined by the heavy isotope density-shift method (12).
[c]Down-regulated state (insulin present).
[d]No insulin present.

cells, maintained in the absence of insulin, exhibited a k_D for receptor decay of 0.045 hr^{-1} (half-life of 15 hr). Within 12 hr after the addition of insulin to induce down-regulation, the degradative rate increased to k_D of 0.095 hr^{-1} (half-life of 7 hr).

The effect of down-regulation on the rate of transit of newly synthesized receptors to the cell surface (from their site of synthesis in the rough endoplasmic reticulum) and the net rate of inactivation of cell surface receptors was also investigated (16). It was found that down-regulation had no effect on the time required (i.e., about 3 hr) for newly synthesized insulin receptor to reach the plasma membrane. On the other hand, down-regulation increased the first-order rate constant for inactivation of cell surface insulin receptors from 0.046 to 0.10 hr^{-1}. This indicates that either the rate of inactivation of insulin receptors (which is increased in the down-regulated state) is limited by the rate of receptor internalization or that insulin rapidly induces the redistribution of total cellular receptors raising the fraction of cellular receptors in the intracellular compartment and thereby increasing the rate of intracellular receptor inactivation. Since we know (see Section VII) that the insulin-induced redistribution of receptors to the intracellular compartment is very rapid relative to down-regulation, it is evident that redistribution is the primary cause of down-regulation, but is not the rate-limiting step in the process.

Taken together, our results indicate that the events of insulin-induced down-regulation (see Figs. 13 and 14) involve the following steps: (a) exposure of cells to insulin increases the rate of insulin receptor internalization; (b) receptor redistribution occurs rapidly ($t_{1/2} < 10$ min) changing from 85%/15% (surface/intracellular) to 40%/60%; (c) redistribution of insulin receptors to the intracellular compartment increases the rate of receptor inactivation—degradation by an, as yet, unidentified system; (d) the accelerated rate of insulin receptor decay slowly ($t_{1/2} = 3$ hr) leads to a lower steady-state level of insulin receptor.

B. Differentiation Induced Up-Regulation of Receptor Level

The 3T3-L1 preadipocyte cell line differentiates in culture into a cell type that exhibits the morphological and biochemical characteristics of an adipocyte. Expression of the adipocyte phenotype is closely correlated with the coordinate rise in the activities of the enzymes of de novo fatty acid and triglyceride synthesis. Another characteristic of the adipocyte conversion process is the acquisition of an increased sensitivity to certain hormones, in particular, the lipogenic hormone, insulin (26). Prior to differentiation, acute exposure of the preadipocyte to insulin has virtually no effect upon hexose uptake (transport across the plasma membrane). After differentiation, however, 3T3-L1 adipocytes acquire the capacity to respond acutely to insulin (26). Thus, brief exposure of 3T3-L1 adipocytes to insulin activates hexose uptake 15 to 20-fold. Undifferentiated 3T3-L1 preadipocytes exhibit no significant stimulation of hexose uptake upon exposure to insulin.

One possible cause of this increased responsiveness to insulin is an increase in the number of cell surface insulin receptors. It was found (11,13) that during differentiation of 3T3-L1 preadipocytes into adipocytes the cells exhibit a 20-fold rise in insulin receptor level, fully differentiated 3T3-L1 adipocytes possessing about 200,000 receptors per cell. The possibility that the increased insulin-binding capacity of differentiated cells might be due to a change in the affinity of the receptor for insulin was ruled out by Scatchard analysis. Rather, it was observed that the increased insulin-binding capacity of differentiated cells was the result of an increased number of receptors per cell. That this effect was specific for insulin receptors was indicated by the fact that the receptors for several other polypeptide hormones, including the receptor for EGF, remained at a constant level during preadipocyte differentiation.

Two general mechanisms could account for the rise in the level of cell surface insulin receptors during differentiation. Either the rate of insulin receptor synthesis might be increased or the rate of insulin receptor inactivation—degradation might be decreased. By applying the heavy isotope density-shift technique (see Section III), it was possible to determine which of these two processes was responsible for the rather dramatic differentation-induced rise in receptor level. Density-labeling of the receptor provided an unambiguous basis for distinguishing between "old" and newly synthesized receptor without resorting to the use of inhibitors of protein synthesis that can impair other cellular processes, including the rate at which receptor is inactivated (8).

The results of the heavy isotope density-shift experiments with 3T3-L1 undifferentiated preadipocytes and fully differentiated adipocytes are summarized in Table 1B. It was found that an increased rate of insulin receptor synthesis accounted entirely for the increased number of receptors per cell caused by differentiation. No change in the rate at which insulin receptors were inactivated was caused by differentiation. It can be concluded, therefore, that during differentiation the rate of insulin receptor synthesis increases, leading to an elevated level of functional receptors. This is likely to be due to an increase in the rate of transcription of the insulin receptor gene leading to an increased level of insulin receptor mRNA. This is inferred from results with a number of other enzyme proteins where it has been established that increased expression during the differentiation of 3T3-L1 preadipocytes is the result of an increased rate of specific gene transcription (27,28). It will be of great interest to learn how expression of the insulin receptor gene is activated.

C. Glucocorticoid–Induced Alteration of Receptor Level

The responsiveness of cells to insulin caused by changes in the
cellular level of insulin receptors is also under the control of hetero-
logous hormones. For example, it has been demonstrated that the
exposure of cells to glucocorticoids, e.g., dexamethasone, can lead
to an increase or decrease in insulin receptor level depending upon
the cell type involved. We have observed that exposure of 3T3-C2
fibroblasts to dexamethasone leads to a slow 2.5- to 3-fold increase
in cell surface and total insulin receptor level (15). Approximately
2 days are required for this change in steady-state insulin receptor
level.

The mechanism by which dexamethasone induces "up-regulation"
of insulin receptor level was investigated using the heavy isotope
density-shift technique (15). The results of these experiments (see
Table 1C) revealed that the rise in receptor level was due entirely
to changes in the rate of receptor inactivation; the first-order rate
of receptor inactivation was decreased from about 0.07 to 0.03 h^{-1}
by dexamethasone treatment. Under these conditions there was no
significant change in the rate of receptor synthesis.

IX. SUMMARY

The mature insulin receptor is an intrinsic membrane glycoprotein
composed of two types of subunits arranged in an $\alpha_2\beta_2$ oligomeric
structure in which the subunits are linked through $\alpha-\beta$ and $\alpha-\alpha$
disulfide bonds. The α subunit contains the insulin binding domain,
and the β subunit contains a tryosine protein kinase catalytic site.
Both the α and β subunits are derived form a common precursor
proreceptor, a 190 K polypeptide that contains N-linked high mannose oligosaccharide chains that are added cotranslationally. The
pathway by which the proreceptor is processed into mature receptor
is complex, involving proteolytic cleavage of the large proreceptor
polypeptide, intersubunit disulfide bond formation, and capping sugar
addition prior to insertion into the plasma membrane.

Newly synthesized insulin receptors have a finite lifetime on the
plasma membrane and undergo insulin-induced internalization into an
endosomal compartment. Upon acidification of the endosome and dissociation of the ligand-receptor complex, the receptor and its ligand
(insulin) can undergo separate pathways. The ligand enters the
lysosomal pathway where it is ultimately degraded by proteolysis.
In contrast, the receptor has two metabolic options: recycling back
to the plasma membrane that occurs about once every 7−10 min or
inactivation-degradation that occurs at a much lower rate.

The number of functional receptors a cell expresses on its plasma
membrane is rigorously controlled and determines the responsiveness

of that cell to insulin. Three mechanisms by which the level of cell surface insulin receptors are regulated have been observed; these include an alteration in the rate of receptor synthesis, alterations in the rate of receptor inactivation-degradation, and the more rapid alteration of the distribution of receptors between the plasma membrane and the intracellular compartment.

ACKNOWLEDGMENTS

The research described that was conducted in the author's laboratory was supported by research grants from the National Institutes of Health (AM-14574) and the Juvenile Diabetes Foundation.

I wish to thank Mrs. Norma Mitchell for her expert assistance in the preparation of this article.

REFERENCES

1. Krupp, M. N. and Lane, M. D. (1982). In *Membranes and Transport: A Critical Review*, A. M. Martonosi, ed., Plenum, New York, pp. 541–549.
2. Jacobs, S., Hazum, E., Schechter, Y., and Cuatrecasas, P. (1979). *Proc. Natl. Acad. Sci. USA*, 76:4918–4921.
3. Pilch, P. F. and Czech, M. P. (1980). *J. Biol. Chem. 255*: 1722–1731.
4. Kohanski, R. A. and Lane, M. D. (1985). *J. Biol. Chem. 260*:5014–5025.
5. Lane. M. D., Ronnett, G. V., Kohanski, R. A., and Simpson, T. L. (1985). *UCLA Symposium on Membrane Receptors and Cellular Regulation*, Alan R. Liss, New York, pp. 397–412.
6. Kasuga, M., Karlsson, . A., and Kahn, C. R. (1982). *Science*, 215:185–187.
7. Kasuga, M., Zick, Y., Blithe, D. L., Karlsson, F. A., Haring, H. U., and Kahn, C. R. (1982). *J. Biol. Chem.* 257:9891–9894.
8. Reed, B. C., Ronnett, G. V., and Lane, M. D. (1981). *Proc. Natl. Acad. Sci. USA* 78:2908–2912.
9. Hedo, J. A., Kasuga, M., Van Obberghen, E., Roth, J., and Kahn, C. R. (1981). *Proc. Natl. Acad. Sci. USA* 78:4791–4795.
10. Ronnett, G. V., Knutson, V. P., Kohanski, R. A., Simpson, T. L., and Lane, M. D. (1984). *J. Biol. Chem.* 259:4566–4575.
11. Reed, B. C. and Lane, M. D. (1980). *Proc. Natl. Acad. Sci. USA* 77:285–289.
12. Krupp, M. N., Knutson, V. P., Ronnett, G. V., and Lane, M. D. (1983). *Methods in Enzymology, Vol. 96, Biomembranes Part J.* Academic Press, New York, pp. 423–433.

13. Reed, B. C., Ronnett, G. V., Clements, P. R., and Lane, M. D. (1981). *J. Biol. Chem. 256*:3917—3925.

14. Ronnett, G. V., Knutson, V. P., and Lane, M. D. (1982). *J. Biol. Chem. 257*:4285—4291.

15. Knutson, V. P., Ronnett, G. V., and Lane, M. D. (1982). *Proc. Natl. Acad. Sci. USA, 79*:2822—2826.

16. Ronnett, G. V., Tennekoon, G., Knutson, V. P., and Lane, M. D. (1983). *J. Biol. Chem. 258*:283—290.

17. Knutson, V. P., Ronnett, G. V., and Lane, M. D. (1983). *J. Biol. Chem. 258*:12139—12142.

18. Lane, M. D., Reed, B. C. and Clements, P. R. (1981). *ICN-UCLA Symposium on Control of Cellular Division and Development*, Part A: Alan R. Liss, Inc., New York, pp. 523—542.

19. Krupp, M. N. and Lane, M. D. (1981). *J. Biol. Chem. 256*: 1689—1694.

20. Kasuga, M., Hedo, J. A., Yamada, K. M., and Kahn, C. R. (1982). *J Biol. Chem. 257*:10392—10399.

21. Ronnett, G. V. and Lane, M. D. (1981). *J. Biol. Chem. 256*: 4704—4707.

22. Krupp, M. N. and Lane, M. D. (1982). *J. Biol. Chem. 257*: 1372—1377.

23. Yamashiro, D. J., Tycko, B., Fluss, S. R., and Maxfield, F. R. (1984). *Cell, 37*:789—800.

24. Fehlman, M., Carpentier, J. L., Van Obberghen, E., Freychet, P., Thamm, P., Saunders, D., Brandenburg, D., and Orci, L. (1982). *Proc. Natl. Acad. Sci. USA 79*:5921—5925.

25. Gavin, J. R., Roth, J., Neville, D. M., Jr., DeMeyts, P., and Buel., D. N. (1974). *Proc. Natl. Acad. Sci., USA 71*:84—88.

26. Frost, S. C. and Lane, M. D. (1985). *J. Biol. Chem. 260*: 2646—2652.

27. Bernlohr, D. A., Angus, C. W., Lane, M. D., Bolanowski, M. S., and Kelly, Jr., T. J. (1984). *Proc. Natl. Acad. Sci. USA 81*:5468—5472.

28. Bernlohr, D. A., Bolanowski, M. A., Kelly, T. J., Jr., and Lane, M. D. (1985). *J. Biol. Chem. 260*:5563-5567.

29. Ullrich, A., Bell, J. R., Chen, E. Y., Herrera, R., Petruzzelli, L. M., Dull, T. J., Gray, A., Coussens, L., Liao, Y.-C., Tsubokawa, M., Mason, A., Seeburg, P. H., Grunfeld, C., Rosen, O. M., and Ramachandran, J. (1985). *Nature 313*:756—761.

30. Ebina, Y., Ellis, L., Jarnagin, K., Edery, M., Graf, L., Clauser, E., Ou, J.-H., Masiarz, F., Kan, Y. W., Goldfine, I. D., Roth, R. A. and Rutter, W. J. (1985). *Cell 40*: 747—758.

13

Insulin Receptor: Relationship to Obesity and Diabetes Mellitus

PAULOS BERHANU   *University of Colorado Health Sciences Center, Denver, Colorado*

JERROLD M. OLEFSKY   *University of California School of Medicine, San Diego, La Jolla, California*

I. INTRODUCTION

Diabetes mellitus is a complex disorder characterized by alterations in carbohydrate, lipid, and protein metabolism resulting from a deficiency of insulin or its cellular metabolic effects. As a function of time, these metabolic derangements lead to the development of chronic degenerative changes in the eyes, kidneys, nerves, and blood vessels, and often result in the well-known chronic clinical complications of diabetes including blindness, renal failure, peripheral and autonomic neuropathy, and occlusive peripheral vascular and coronary artery disease. Although diabetes mellitus has been recognized for several centuries, our concepts regarding its etiology and pathogenesis continue to undergo major changes. The role of the pancreas in regulating blood sugar and carbohydrate metabolism was first recognized from the work of von Mering and Minkowski, who in 1889 demonstrated that total pancreatectomy in dogs led to a syndrome of hyperglycemia, glycosuria, ketosis, and death. The similarity between this syndrome and clinical diabetes mellitus suggested that diabetes was due to pancreatic disease. Consequently, over the ensuing three decades, several investigators attempted to extract and identify the pancreatic factor responsible for blood glucose regulation. In 1921, Banting and Best succeeded in obtaining pancreatic extracts that contained biologically active insulin and then demonstrated its effectiveness in treating diabetes (Refs. 1, 2; see Chap. 2). This major discovery sparked numerous other investigations that subsequently led to the crystallization, purification, structural determination, and commercial preparation of insulin for clinical use. The availability of insulin has had an enormous impact on the treatment of diabetes and has resulted in saving the lives of

untold numbers of diabetics who used to die from the acute complications of their disease. However, despite the earlier view that all
diabetes mellitus resulted from insulin deficiency and the optimism
that all of the manifestations of the disease could potentially be corrected by insulin replacement, it later became evident that diabetes
is a heterogeneous disorder with more diverse etiologies than simple
insulin deficiency. One of the first to recognize the heterogeneity of
the disease was Himsworth, who pointed out that diabetes could be
differentiated into "insulin-sensitive" and "insulin-insensitive" types
on the basis of the blood glucose response to insulin administered immediately after an oral glucose load (3). Based on this and other lines
of evidence, he later suggested that insulin insensitivity, and not insulin deficiency, was present in many of the diabetics who tended to
be middle aged and nonketotic. This notion was further supported
following the introduction of insulin radioimmunoassay by Yalow and
Berson (4), when it was found that endogenous insulin was measurable
in the plasma of diabetics, and that on the average higher levels were
found in patients with the adult onset form of the disease, thus suggesting that resistance to insulin contributed to this form of diabetes.

The most current classification of diabetes (5) divides the disease
into two major types. Approximately 10% of all diabetics have type I
or insulin-dependent diabetes mellitus (IDDM). This form of the disease is characterized by insulinopenia, a more or less abrupt onset of
symptoms, susceptibility to ketoacidosis and dependence on exogenous
insulin to prevent ketoacidosis and to sustain life. In most instances,
this form of the disease has its onset in the young; hence, the term,
juvenile onset diabetes. Type I diabetes is due to insulin deficiency
resulting from pancreatic beta cell damage. Thus, in this form of the
disease target tissue insulin resistance is not a major feature and insulin resistance, when it occurs, is most likely due to the metabolic
derangements resulting from the diabetic state itself rather than from
intrinsic target tissue defects in insulin action. For this reason, IDDM
will not be discussed in the remainder of this chapter.

Type II or non-insulin-dependent diabetes mellitus (NIDDM) comprises approximately 90% of the diabetic population. Subjects with this
form of diabetes in whom the disease is usually diagnosed in adulthood
(hence, the term adult-onset diabetes mellitus) are not ketosis prone
and are not dependent on exogenous insulin to sustain life, although
insulin may be used to treat persistent hyperglycemia that does not
respond to diet or oral hypoglycemic agents. Target tissue insulin
resistance is a characteristic feature of NIDDM. Furthermore, the
majority (60—90%) of patients with NIDDM have obesity, which by itself is characterized by hyperinsulinemia and insulin resistance. For
these reasons, the major portion of this chapter will be devoted to
discussing the role of insulin receptor and postreceptor defects in the

overall target tissue insulin resistance in obesity and non-insulin-dependent diabetes mellitus. To facilitate a systematic discussion of insulin resistance in these disorders, we will begin this chapter with an overview of normal insulin-receptor interaction and some of the general mechanisms of cellular insulin resistance.

II. GENERAL ASPECTS OF INSULIN-RECEPTOR INTERACTION AND INSULIN ACTION

Insulin plays a central role in the control of a number of cellular metabolic processes. Its diverse biological actions include: stimulation of membrane transport of glucose, amino acids, nucleotide precursors, and certain ions; increased storage of glycogen and triglycerides; inhibition of lipolysis and hepatic gluconeogenesis; and stimulation of protein, RNA, and DNA synthesis. Although the basic mechanisms by which insulin exerts such diverse cellular effects remain largely unknown, important advances have been made in understanding the characteristics of insulin's interactions with its target cells, and also in identifying some of the alterations of these interactions in pathophysiological states such as obesity and type II diabetes mellitus. Figure 1 depicts a schematic representation of insulin action on a target cell in which the integrated sequence of physiological processes from insulin synthesis, secretion, and transport to its action on a target cell have been conveniently divided into three phases—prereceptor, receptor binding, and postreceptor phases.

A. Prereceptor Phase

The prereceptor phase, which is the most characterized in the overall insulin action scheme, encompases the series of events from insulin synthesis and secretion to its transport to the target tissue site of action. In the pancreatic β-cell, insulin is produced as the primary biosynthetic product, preproinsulin, that is rapidly converted to proinsulin (M.W. ~ 9000). Proinsulin is in turn converted to insulin (M.W. ~ 6000) and connecting peptide (C-peptide, M.W. ~ 3000) by specific proteolytic steps within the β-cell secretory granule. Therefore, the normal secretory products from the β-cell are insulin, an equimolar amount of C-peptide, and a small amount ($\sim 5\%$) of unconverted proinsulin. After a brief circulation time in the vascular compartment ($t_{1/2} \sim 6-10$ min), insulin interacts with the cells of its target tissues and exerts its biological effects. The major mammalian target tissues of insulin action are liver, muscle, and fat.

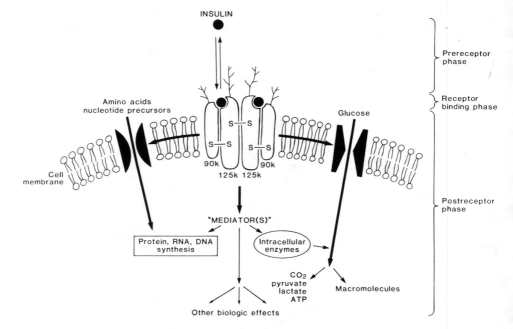

Figure 1 Schematic representation of insulin receptor structure and overall insulin action (see text for details).

B. Receptor Binding Phase

The multiple biological actions of insulin at the cellular level are initiated by binding of the hormone to its specific high-affinity glyco-protein receptors on the surface of target cells (Fig. 1). From the considerations outlined in Chapter 6, it is evident that the magnitudes of the biological responses to insulin can be regulated not only by the concentrations of circulating insulin, but also by the number and affinity of cell surface insulin receptors as well as by the complex series of postreceptor events which, at the present time, are poorly understood. The insulin-receptor interaction has been extensively studied in intact cells and in membrane preparations (6,7), and it is now well established that receptor number and/or affinity are altered in a variety of physiological and pathological conditions (8,9). As will be discussed later, these changes in the receptor are in turn reflected by concomitant changes in cellular sensitivity or responsiveness to insulin. As indicated in Chapters 3 and 4, the insulin receptor has been characterized using biochemical purification, affinity cross-linking, photo-affinity labeling, and biosynthetic labeling procedures (see also

Refs. 6,7,10−12). From such studies the emerging concept is that the receptor is a glycoprotein macromolecule composed of disulfide linked subunits of M_r 125,000−135,000 (α subunit) and M_r 90,000−95,000 (β subunit). As summarized in Chapter 4, one model of the receptor suggests subunit stoichiometry of $\alpha_2\beta_2$ (Fig. 1). An alternative receptor model, also involving the α and β subunits is described in Chapter 3. Essentially all of the insulin binding activity is believed to reside in the α subunit, in view of the results of the affinity cross-linking and photoaffinity labeling studies. While the β subunit (M_r 90,000−95,000) does not appear to participate in insulin binding to any major extent, it has been suggested that this subunit is involved in modulation of insulin action as discussed further below.

C. Postreceptor Phase

This phase in insulin action encompasses all of the complex series of steps distal to insulin binding by which the interaction of insulin with its receptor is transformed into specific cellular biological responses. Unfortunately, the nature of these steps are not well understood, although there have been some important recent developments. One of insulin's major biological effects is to stimulate the transport of substrates (glucose, amino acids, ions, fatty acids, and nucleic acid precursors) across the cell membrane of target cells. Of these, the effect of insulin on glucose transport is the most extensively studied (13). |Recent evidence indicates that insulin stimulates glucose transport by increasing the number of transport units on the plasma membrane through a rapid and reversible translocation of the transporters from an intracellular pool, possibly located in the Golgi apparatus (14, 15).| However, the precise mechanisms by which the insulin-receptor interaction is coupled to the transport stimulation is not known.| Besides its effects on membrane transport, insulin also modulates a number of important intracellular processes, including stimulation (or inhibition) of several intracellular enzymes; stimulation of protein, RNA, and DNA synthesis; and effects on cell growth and differentiation. Although much remains to be learned about the biochemical mechanisms by which insulin exerts such diverse biological effects, several new developments have significantly contributed to research in this area. One of these is the demonstration that insulin generates "chemical mediator(s)" that modulate the activities of certain key insulin-sensitive enzymes (see Chap. 9 for detailed discussion). The exact chemical structure of these substances and their role (if any) in mediating insulin's physiological actions remain to be determined. \Another recent development is the demonstration that the insulin receptor exhibits tyrosine-specific kinase activity localized to the β subunit and that binding of insulin to the receptor stimulates this kinase activity (16−20). This receptor kinase activity results in autophosphorylation of the β subunit of the insulin receptor and is also capable of phosphorylating other proteins. Since the kinase activity actually resides in the M_r 90,000–95,000 (β) subunit, which itself does not participate in the insulin binding to any major extent, it appears that the binding of insulin to the M_r 125,000–135,000 (α) subunit of its receptor triggers enhanced phosphorylation of the β subunit as an early postbinding event. However, the specific endogenous cellular substrates for the receptor kinase activity and the functional significance of insulin receptor phosphorylation in mediating insulin's physiological actions remain to be demonstrated.

An important physiological process that occurs following the binding of insulin to cell surface receptors is the internalization of the bound insulin and its receptor by adsorptive endocytosis. Earlier morphological and biochemical studies demonstrated that following initial binding to the cell surface receptors, a portion of the bound insulin is internalized and degraded intracellularly, most probably within lysosomes (21,22). In insulin target cells, such as adipocytes and hepatocytes, recent findings show that the insulin receptor is also internalized along with the bound insulin (23–26) and is then degraded at chloroquine-sensitive intracellular sites (23,24,26), suggesting lysosomal involvement in the degradation of internalized insulin receptors. In contrast, in cultured IM-9 human lymphocytes, a transformed cell line in which no glucoregulatory effects of insulin are demonstrable, insulin receptors are lost primarily by shedding into the incubation media (27). Thus, the available data indicate that in insulin target cells, both ligand and receptor are internalized as insulin-receptor complexes and are then degraded at similar, if not the same, intracellular sites. While all of the internalized insulin may be committed to eventual degradation, there is evidence indicating that a proportion of the internalized receptors may be recycled back to the plasma membrane (28). Figure 2 shows a schematic representation of the cellular fate of insulin and insulin receptors following binding on the cell surface. Also schematically shown is the pathway of receptor biosynthesis and incorporation into the plasma membrane. Thus, the homeostatic maintenance of the net number of insulin receptors on the plasma membrane of target cells represents a balance between receptor biosynthesis and membrane insertion and its removal by internalization and degradation. Internalization of insulin-receptor complexes may play an inportant physiological role in mediating the well-known process of insulin-induced receptor loss or "down-regulation" first demonstrated by Gavin et al. (29) in cultured human lymphocytes and subsequently also observed in various other cell types. The internalization process may also be important in the termination of insulin action by removing it from the cell surface and transporting it to intracellular degradation sites. The demonstration of insulin binding sites in various intracellular organelles (30,31) had led to the speculation that the intracellular

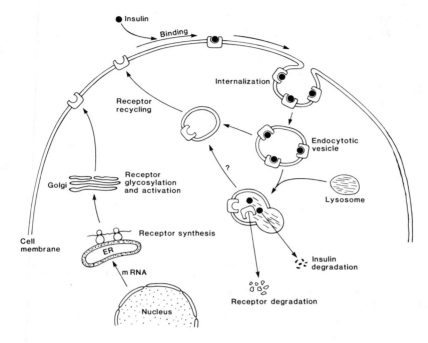

Figure 2 Schematic representation of insulin receptor turnover in insulin target cell (see text for details).

effects of insulin may be mediated through the interaction of these binding sites with internalized insulin. However, there is no experimental evidence to support this view, and it seems more likely that the intracellular binding sites represent newly synthesized receptors en route to the plasma membrane or internalized receptors en route to degradation sites.

This overview of the prereceptor, receptor, and postreceptor phases in insulin action points out the complexity of the overall process and also indicates that insulin action and cellular response can potentially be regulated at several points in the overall insulin action scheme.

III. INSULIN RESISTANCE: MECHANISMS AND CAUSES

Insulin resistance is a metabolic state in which a normal concentration of insulin produces a less than normal biological response. This resistance can involve any of the multiple metabolic effects of insulin. However, from the standpoint of relevance to diabetes mellitus and

obesity, resistance to insulin's effect on glucose metabolism has been
the most extensively studied. Consideration of normal insulin action,
as discussed in the preceding section, makes it apparent that insulin
resistance can potentially result from abnormalities at any point in the
integrated sequence of steps from insulin synthesis and secretion to
its transport and action at target tissue level. Table 1 lists the
causes of insulin resistance in which the different abnormalities have
been grouped under prereceptor, receptor, and postreceptor causes.
Receptor and postreceptor abnormalities together constitute target
tissue resistance to insulin action and, as will be discussed further,
these play a major role in the pathophysiology of obesity and diabetes
mellitus.

A. Prereceptor Causes of Insulin Resistance

Abnormal β-Cell Secretory Product

   Synthesis of abnormal insulin molecule due to mutation in the
structural gene for insulin: Although it had been postulated for
several years that in some patients diabetes may result from the synthesis and secretion of a structurally abnormal insulin molecule, the
actual documentation of such a case was made only recently (32). The
patient studied displayed fasting hyperglycemia ($\sim$200 mg/100 ml) and

Table 1   Causes of Insulin Resistance

   I. Prereceptor Phase

      1. Abnormal β-cell secretory product
         a. Synthesis of abnormal insulin molecule
         b. Incomplete conversion of proinsulin to insulin

      2. Circulating insulin antagonists
         a. Elevated levels of counterregulatory hormones, e.g.,
            growth hormone, cortisol, glucagon, catecholamines
         b. Anti-insulin antibodies
         c. Anti-insulin receptor antibodies

  II. Receptor Phase

      1. Decreased number of insulin receptors
      2. Decreased binding affinity of insulin receptors

 III. Postreceptor Phase

      Post receptor defects in insulin action

---

fasting hyperinsulinemia ($\sim$100 μU/ml), but responded normally to exogenously administered insulin. Isolation and biochemical charac-terization of the patient's insulin revealed that it contained a single amino acid substitution (leucine for phenylalanine) at position 25 of the insulin B chain (33). Since this substitution was within the bio-logically active site of the insulin molecule, the mutated insulin species displayed markedly reduced receptor binding and biological potency, thus accounting for the patient's diabetic state. The key clinical fea-tures that lead to the suspicion of this abnormality are the presence of hyperglycemia and hyperinsulinemia in a patient who responds nor-mally to exogenous insulin. It is likely that more patients with this syndrome will be discovered.

Incomplete conversion of proinsulin to insulin: Proinsulin is normally converted to insulin by proteolytic action within the β-cell secretory granule. This conversion is usually largely complete, and in normal subjects only about 5% of the β-cell secretory product con-sists of proinsulin. When the conversion of proinsulin to insulin is incomplete, excess amounts of proinsulin are secreted into the cir-culation. Since proinsulin has reduced biological activity compared to insulin, β-cell secretory activity is increased to maintain glucose homeostasis. Thus, elevated circulating proinsulin levels occur, and since proinsulin cross-reacts with insulin in the radioimmunoassay for insulin, an apparent hyperinsulinemic state exists. Two families with this disease, termed familial hyperproinsulinemia, have been reported (34,35). The defect is in the structural gene for proinsulin, and the proinsulin molecule produced by these patients has an amino acid sub-stitution at the C-peptide cleavage point, thus preventing normal pro-teolytic conversion of proinsulin to insulin and C-peptide. These pa-tients do not necessarily display abnormal glucose tolerance and can apparently compensate for their defect by secreting sufficient amounts of proinsulin and insulin to maintain adequate glucose homeostasis. Since these patients respond normally to exogenously administered in-sulin, and since their apparent hyperinsulinemia is due to elevated levels of proinsulin rather than insulin, in a strict sense they are not insulin resistant.

Circulating Insulin Antagonists

Elevated levels of counterregulatory hormones: Circulating hor-monal antagonists of insulin action include the counterregulatory hor-mones, such as cortisol, growth hormone, glucagon, and catecholamines. Although in the usual case of obesity or type II diabetes mellitus ex-cessive levels of these hormones do not play a major contributory role in the insulin resistance, clinically significant glucose intolerance or a frank diabetic state can be observed in Cushing's syndrome, acromeg-aly, or pheochromocytoma due to the excessive levels of cortisol, growth hormone, or catecholamines, respectively.

Glucocorticoids: It is well known that excess endogenous or exogenous glucocorticoids (such as in Cushing's syndrome or during pharmacological glucocorticoid therapy) antagonize the actions of insulin. Intolerance to administered glucose load can be demonstrated in up to 80--90% of patients with Cushing's syndrome, while overt diabetes occurs in about 15--20% of the patients. Thus, a spectrum of glucocorticoid-induced insulin resistance exists, and the mechanisms by which this occurs are also varied. For example, in the liver, insulin inhibits glucose production, whereas glucocorticoids increase gluconeogenesis. This effect of glucocorticoids involves multiple loci in the overall gluconeogenic pathway, including increase in the availability of gluconeogenic substrates (amino acids, lactate) and increase in the intrinsic hepatic capacity to produce glucose (36-38). Glucocorticoids also stimulate glucagon secretion (37), which in turn auguments hepatic glucose production. At the level of peripheral tissues, glucocorticoids antagonize insulin's effect to stimulate glucose utilization; this occurs by several mechanisms (39-41). These include a decrease in the activity of the plasma membrane glucose transport system by decreasing the transport V_{max}, a decrease in insulin binding to receptors resulting from decrease in receptor number or affinity, and a defect at the postreceptor level. Thus, the overall effect of glucocorticoids to antagonize insulin action and thereby decrease glucose utilization results from a combination of their multiple effects.

Growth hormone: Chronic excessive secretion of growth hormone as occurs in acromegaly can be associated with hyperinsulinemia, glucose intolerance, and decreased effectiveness of exogenous insulin. Although mild abnormalities of glucose tolerance may commonly be seen in acromegaly, less than 15% of the patients develop clinical diabetes with fasting hyperglycemia. The mechanism underlying the anti-insulin effects of growth hormone have not been clearly eludicated, and this is in part due to the multiplicity of cellular effects of growth hormone, including its induction of the production of somatomedins and the heterogeneity of circulating forms of the hormone. However, decreased number of insulin receptors on circulating monocytes and an inverse correlation of receptor number with plasma insulin level in acromegaly have been reported (42).

Glucagon: Glucagon influences glucose metabolism by augmenting hepatic glycogenolysis and gluconeogenesis, and in this sense, glucagon can counteract some of insulin's effects. However, glucagon has no influence on insulin's ability to promote peripheral glucose metabolism and does not lead to a true state of insulin resistance.

Catecholamines: Excessive levels of circulating catecholamines can also antagonize the effects of insulin. Several mechanisms are involved. Catecholamines can stimulate glucagon secretion (β effect) and increase hepatic glucose production by direct stimulation of glycogenolysis and gluconeogenesis ($\alpha + \beta$ effect). In combination, these effects will tend to cause hyperglycemia and are opposite to the actions of insulin.

Additionally, catecholamines directly inhibit peripheral glucose uptake (β effect), and this is at least partly mediated by suppression of glucose transport activity (43). Furthermore, since it has also been shown that α-adrenergic stimulation (or β-adrenergic blockade) inhibits basal insulin secretion, it is possible that excessive levels of cathecholamines may cause impaired glucose tolerance partly through their effect on inhibition of insulin secretion. It is also possible that the β-adrenergic-induced augmentation of lipolysis may lead to secondary fatty acid-induced decrease in glucose uptake. Thus, in patients with pheochromocytoma, glucose intolerance can result from the multiplicity of the effects of excess endogenous catecholamines on carbohydrate homeostasis.

Placental lactogen: This is a placental-derived hormone that may be causally involved in the insulin resistance that develops during normal pregnancy. Obviously, this hormone would have little relevance to obesity or non-insulin-dependent diabetes mellitus. The mechanisms of action of this hormone are not understood.

Anti-insulin antibodies: Essentially all patients who receive exogenous insulin for long enough periods eventually develop anti-insulin antibodies, although the titers of these antibodies and their clinical significance are quite variable among individuals. Commercial insulin preparations are commonly a mixture of pork and beef insulin, which differ from human insulin by one and three amino acid residues, respectively. Thus, the antigenicity of these insulin preparations has been related both to the differences in the primary structures of the beef and pork insulins from human insulin as well as to the impurities within the commercial preparations. In recent years, highly purified insulins have been made available, and with the use of these newer preparations, the development of anti-insulin antibodies is much less of a problem than in the past. One theoretical advantage in using human insulin (made by transpeptidation from porcine insulin or by biosynthesis using recombinant DNA technology) has been the hope that the development of anti-insulin antibodies would not occur because of the structural identity with endogenous human insulin. Nevertheless, the development of anti-insulin antibodies have been reported with the use of these insulin preparations in clinical trials, although the immunogenicity of these preparations (possibly as a result of subtle structural alterations during preparation) is significantly less than that of highly purified monocomponent procine insulin (44). Although anti-insulin antibodies do not usually lead to a clinically significant insulin-resistant state, the presence of these antibodies can alter the pharmacokinetics of insulin (45). High titers of high-affinity antibodies can act as a reservoir for insulin by binding the hormone when it initially enters the circulation with later release. Thus, patients with clinically significant anti-insulin antibodies may manifest apparent resistance to administered insulin.

Anti-insulin receptor antibodies: Insulin resistance due to circulating autoantibodies directed against the insulin receptor has been
described in recent years (46). Although this syndrome is a rare
cause of insulin resistance, its study has provided important information regarding the role of insulin receptor in insulin resistance and
the availability of the naturally occurring anti-insulin receptor antibodies has been very useful in studies of insulin receptor dynamics
and action. Most of the patients with this syndrome have acanthosis
nigricans and also have other features suggestive of immunological disease. The characteristic finding is the presence in the serum of
these patients of antibodies directed against the insulin receptor as
detected by their ability to inhibit insulin binding or to immunopre-
cipitate solubilized insulin receptors on target tissues, and, by acting
as competitive antagonists for endogenous or exogenous insulin, cause
insulin resistance. Thus, depending on the severity of the syndrome,
patients would have carbohydrate intolerance ranging from mild abnormalities of glucose tolerance test to severe hyperglycemia requiring large amounts of exogenous insulin administration.

B. Receptor and Postreceptor Causes of Insulin Resistance

As depicted in Figure 1 and discussed earlier in this chapter, following its synthesis and transport to target tissues, insulin exerts its
biological effects by binding initially to its specific cell surface receptors. It is apparent that abnormalities at either the receptor binding
step or at any step distal to binding can result in target tissue de-
fect(s) in insulin action. Thus, for convenience, overall target tissue
insulin resistance can be subdivided into receptor and postreceptor
defects and these are further discussed.

Receptor Defects in Insulin Action

Since the binding of insulin to its cell surface receptors is a key first
step in its action, it becomes apparent, as outlined in Section VI of
Chapter 6, that the magnitude of the specific insulin-mediated cellular
biological response will be proportional to the number of insulin-receptor
complexes formed. Thus, a decrease in insulin binding resulting from
either reduced receptor numbers or decreased binding affinity of the
receptors could lead to insulin resistance. However, since target cells
possess "spare receptors" (47,48) for most of insulin's biological effects, the relationship between a change in receptor number and insulin
action is not straightforward.

The spare receptor concept is based on the observation that a
maximal insulin effect is achieved at an insulin concentration that
occupies less than the total number of cell surface receptors. For
example, it has been shown that in isolated adipocytes, maximal insulin
stimulation of glucose transport and oxidation occurs when only about

10% of the cell surface receptors are occupied (47,49). This degree
of receptor occupancy occurs at physiological concentrations of insulin.
Thus, under normal circumstances, 90% of the full complement of receptors are "spare." These spare receptors are all potentially fully
functional, and it is only a random statistical chance that determines
which receptors are occupied at any given point in time. Thus, any
group of occupied receptors amounting to 10% of the total would lead
to the same maximal insulin-stimulated metabolic response, such as
glucose transport, glucose oxidation, or lipogenesis. Therefore, the
cellular response to increasing insulin concentrations is a continuous
increase in receptor occupancy and biological action until the critical
number of receptors needed to generate a maximal response is occupied.
Further increases in the ambient insulin concentration beyond this
point leads to a continued increase in receptor occupancy with no further increase in biological response, since a step(s) distal to the receptor would now be the rare limiting event.

Given this relationship between insulin binding and insulin action,
the predicted functional consequence of a progressive decrease in the
number of receptors would be a concomitant decrease in insulin action
only at insulin levels that occupy less than the absolute number of
receptors required for a maximal effect, with a normal response occurring in the presence of maximally effective hormone levels (50,51).
As shown in Figure 3, this results in a rightward shift in the insulin
biological function dose-response curve with decreased responses at
all submaximal insulin concentrations and normal insulin action at maximally effective hormone concentrations. As receptor loss becomes
more pronounced, the insulin biological function dose-response curve
shifts further to the right, and the degree of rightward shift becomes
proportional to the decrease in receptors. When the decrease in insulin receptors becomes great enough so that less than 10% (in the
example in Fig. 3) of the normal complement of receptors are left, then
a decrease in maximal insulin effect occurs even at very high insulin
concentrations. The precise proportion of spare receptors varies
among different target cell types and is also dependent upon which
particular metabolic action of insulin is being measured.

Postreceptor Defects in Insulin Action

In the overall insulin action scheme, any abnormality distal to the
initial receptor-binding event constitutes a postreceptor defect and
can cause or contribute to cellular insulin resistance. Such defects
may involve abnormalities in postbinding functions of the receptor
such as phosphorylation or other covalent modifications, the coupling
of insulin-receptor complexes to cell membrane or intracellular effector
systems, or any of the many insulin-modified intracellular biochemical
steps. Since alterations of insulin receptor function (e.g., phosphorylation) are possible and may lead to insulin resistance, a more proper

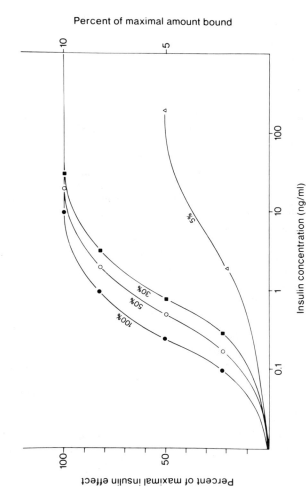

Figure 3 Predicted functional consequence of a progressive loss of insulin receptors on insulin biological function dose-response curve. Shown are the theoretical dose-response curves in which percent of maximal insulin effect (left
axis) and percent of normal maximal amount bound (right axis) are plotted as
a function of insulin concentration for conditions in which 100% (●), 50% (○),
30% (■), or 5% (△) of the normal complement of cell surface receptors are
present.

term for this type of abnormality would be postbinding rather than postreceptor defect. Although the precise biochemical nature of this type of abnormality is not presently known, its functional consequence can be predicted. In the simplest situation, if decreased insulin action exists in the presence of normal insulin binding, then clearly the abnormality is at the post receptor level. However, in the usual case of the insulin resistance of obesity and type II diabetes mellitus, this is not the typical findings, since receptor abnormalities also exist (52). In the usual forms of postreceptor defects, one sees a proportionate decrease in insulin action at all insulin concentrations, including maximally effective hormone levels (51,52). Thus, a decrease in the capacity of a rate-limiting step in the insulin action-glucose metabolism scheme leads to a reduction in the maximal insulin response, and this defect cannot be overcome by the addition of more insulin.

The insulin resistance of obesity and type II diabetes mellitus is a heterogeneous disorder with both receptor and postreceptor defects contributing to the overall insulin resistance (52). On the basis of our understanding of normal insulin action and the spare receptor concept, the predicted effects of receptor versus postreceptor defects on the in vivo insulin biological function dose-response curve can be established. Based on this formulation, reasonable distinctions can then be made regarding the role of receptor, postreceptor, or combined defects in the overall insulin resistance. This is summarized in Figure 4. A decrease or defect in insulin receptors leads to a rightward shift in the insulin dose-response curve with no change in maximal insulin action that is attained at the cost of higher insulin concentrations, and this is termed a decrease in insulin sensitivity. A postreceptor defect in insulin action leads to a proprotionate reduction in cellular biological response, and a less than normal maximal response is attained at all insulin concentrations. This is termed decreased responsiveness to insulin action. It should be noted, however, that since the biochemical steps that follow insulin binding to receptors are not known, it is possible that certain kinds of postreceptor defects invovling the coupling mechanisms could lead to rightward-shifted dose-response curves. In combined receptor and postreceptor defect, both a rightward shift in the dose-response curve and a decrease in maximal insulin responsiveness are seen.

In the usual forms of exogenous obesity and type II diabetes mellitus, the available evidence indicates that resistance to insulin action occurs at target tissue levels, and the other (prereceptor) causes of insulin resistance listed in Table 1 can only rarely be implicated in these common disease states. Therefore, in the following sections the concepts depicted in Figure 4 will be used in discussing the role of receptor, postreceptor, and combined defects in the insulin resistance of obesity and type II diabetes mellitus.

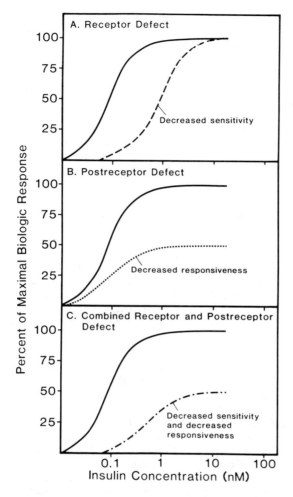

Figure 4 Theoretical insulin dose-response curves showing the predicted results of isolated defects at (A) receptor level, (B) postreceptor level, and (C) combined receptor and postreceptor defects.

IV. INSULIN RESISTANCE IN OBESITY

Insulin resistance has been widely described in human obesity; the cause of this decrease in insulin action has received considerable attention. The notion that chronic hyperinsulinemia in obesity somehow leads to adaptive insulin resistance has been suggested over the years, but Gavin et al. (29) were the first to report positive evidence to support this hypothesis. These workers found that high media insulin concentrations in vitro led to decreased insulin receptors on cultured human lymphocytes. This suggested further that in vivo the plasma insulin concentration inversely regulates the number of cellular insulin receptors and that in obesity the hyperinsulinemia causes the decreased insulin binding. In other studies, an inverse relationship has been found between the plasma insulin concentration and insulin receptors in obese humans (50,53-55). These data support the concept that it is the hyperinsulinemia that leads to decreased insulin receptors.

Insulin binding to receptors has been extensively studied in obesity. Significant decreases in insulin receptors have been demonstrated in a variety of tissues from obese human subjects and animals (8,9,52—56). As a first approximation, this decrease in insulin receptors would appear to be a reasonable etiology for this insulin-resistant state. However, the relationship between insulin binding and insulin action is complex, and examination of the biological activity of insulin in obesity is necessary. To evaluate the mechanisms of insulin resistance in human obesity, the overall in vivo insulin dose-response curve has been evaluated by means of the euglycemic glucose clamp technique developed by Andres and colleagues (57,58).

With this technique, insulin is infused at varying rates to achieve different steady-state plasma insulin levels. Plasma glucose is maintained at euglycemic levels (80—90 mg/100 ml) by monitoring the glucose level at 5-min intervals and adjusting the infusion rate of a 20% glucose solution using a servocontrol negative-feedback principle (59). Under these conditions, steady-state euglycemia is maintained, and all of the glucose infused is metabolized by peripheral tissues. Thus, the total amount of glucose metabolized serves as a measure of the sensitivity of the subject to the prevailing steady-state serum insulin concentration. Studies were done at insulin infusion rates of 40, 120, 240, or 1200 mU/m^2/min to define the shape of the in vivo insulin dose-response curve. In this manner, the rate of overall glucose disposal can be determined under euglycemic conditions at a variety of steady-state serum insulin levels. This allows one to construct the classic dose-response curve in which the rate of the reaction (V, overall glucose disposal) is measured as a function of the insulin concentration at a constant substrate (S) level, i.e., euglycemia.

The mean in vivo insulin dose-response curves for seven normal subjects and a group of thirteen obese subjects is shown in Figure 5A. In all of the study subjects, increasing the steady-state serum insulin level led to a dose-dependent increase in their glucose disposal rates. However, it is evident that the shapes of the dose-response curves for the obese subjects are shifted to the right and are different from those of the normal controls. Furthermore, the obese subjects displayed two kinds of response patterns and have been divided into two separate groups for the purpose of further analysis. The first group, hereafter referred to as group I obese, consists of the four obese subjects who exhibited a rightward shift in the dose-response curve but achieved normal maximal rates of insulin-stimulated glucose disposal

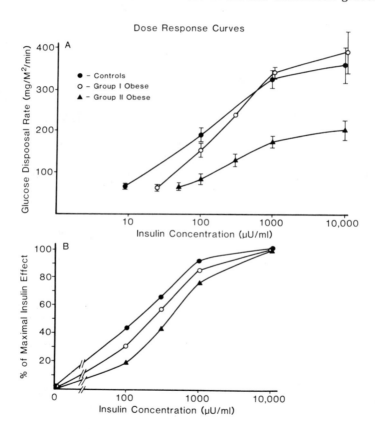

Figure 5 (A) Mean dose-response curves of insulin stimulated glucose disposal rates for normal subjects (●) and for the obese subjects separated into two groups: group I (○) and group II (▲) (see text for details). (B) Dose-response curves plotted as percent of maximal effect.

at high insulin concentrations. The second group (group II obese) is composed of the remaining nine obese subjects who demonstrated both a rightward shift in their dose-response curve plus markedly decreased maximal glucose disposal rates. It should be emphasized that this division of the obese subjects into two groups is done simply to demonstrate and contrast the different response patterns that can be seen in human obesity. The individual response curves of the 13 obese subjects comprise a spectrum and do not imply that these arbitrarily defined groups represent distinctly different populations of obese patients.

The data in Figure 5A indicate that the insulin resistance associated with the obese state in human beings appears to be heterogeneous; some patients (group I obese) display a dose-response relationship consistent with decreased insulin receptors as the sole abnormality (decreased insulin sensitivity), whereas the results in other (group II obese) are most consistent with both a decrease in cellular insulin receptors and a postreceptor defect (decreased insulin sensitivity and responsiveness). To analyze more accurately the functional form of the dose-response curves, the absolute values for glucose disposal were converted to percentage terms (Fig. 5B). For each group, the maximal glucose disposal rate was taken as 100%, and the glucose disposal rate at each submaximal insulin level is plotted as a percent of this value. For purposes of this analysis, 70% of the absolute basal glucose disposal rate is initially subtracted from all values because it represents non-insulin-mediated glucose uptake (60−62). With this approach, potential influences of differences in postreceptor effector systems are eliminated because all maximal rates are taken as 100%, and the proportion of the total possible insulin effect elicited at any hormone level can be seen. Figure 5B clearly shows that the dose-response curves are shifted to the right in obesity, and the magnitude of this effect is greatest in the patients with the most severe receptor reduction. Thus, the half-maximally effective insulin levels are 130, 210, and 370 μU/ml in the normal, group I, and group II obese objects, respectively.

It is apparent that the patients with normal maximal rates of glucose disposal (group I obese) are less insulin resistant than those with reduced maximal insulin responsiveness (group II obese). Furthermore, fasting serum insulin levels were found to be generally higher in the group II obese subjects as compared to the group I obese subjects. Thus, the less insulin-resistant patients tended to be less hyperinsulinemic. Additionally, studies of insulin binding by isolated adipocytes from the different study subjects (Fig. 6) also demonstrated that the reduction in insulin receptors (decreased binding) was more pronounced in the more insulin-resistant group II obese subjects as compared to the group I obese subjects who were less insulin resistant.

Hepatic glucose output was measured during all of the studies, and the effect of insulin to suppress basal hepatic glucose output was determined. The results are shown in Figure 7. It can be seen that hepatic

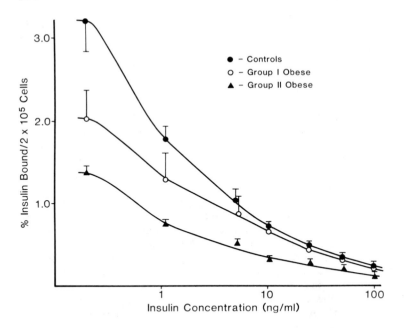

Figure 6 Insulin binding by isolated adipocytes from control (●), group I obese (○), and broup II obese (▲) subjects. All data are corrected for nonspecific binding and represent mean (± SE) percentage of tracer [^{125}I]insulin specifically bound/2 × 10^5 cells.

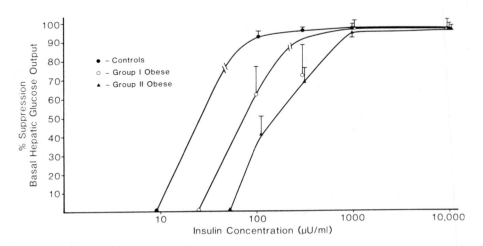

Figure 7 Mean dose-response curves for insulin-mediated suppression of basal hepatic glucose output for control (●), group I obese (○), and group II obese (▲) subjects.

glucose production can be totally suppressed in all subjects, provided that high enough insulin concentrations are employed. Thus, in contrast to the effects of insulin on peripheral glucose disposal, livers of obese subjects do not exhibit decreased responsiveness (postreceptor defect) in this insulin effect. It is also clear that the dose-response curves for hepatic glucose output are shifted to the right in the obese groups, and the half-maximally effective insulin levels were 33, 75, and 130 µU/ml in normal, group I, and group II obese subjects, respectively. This parallels the results for peripheral glucose disposal and reflects the magnitude of the decrease in insulin receptors in the two obese groups. Finally, it should also be noted that lower insulin levels are required to suppress hepatic glucose output than are required to stimulate glucose disposal. During the glucose clamp studies, portal and peripheral insulin levels are similar, and the half-maximal plasma insulin levels are about 3.5- to 4.0-fold greater for glucose disposal. Thus, the proportion of spare receptors is greater for suppression by insulin of hepatic glucose output than it is for stimulation of peripheral glucose uptake. This finding plus the fact that under physiological conditions portal insulin levels are two- to three-fold greater than peripheral levels (63) demonstrate the sensitivity of hepatic glucose production to insulin and indicate that this process should be suppressed under physiological conditions in which stimulated insulin levels exist. The differences in sensitivity between the ability of insulin to suppress hepatic glucose output or stimulate peripheral glucose uptake are striking when one compares the dose-response curves for the group II obese patients in Figures 5A and 7. For example, at an insulin concentration of 100 µU/ml, stimulation of glucose disposal was negligible, whereas hepatic glucose production was about half-maximally inhibited. Thus, at a high physiological insulin level, glucose uptake is only marginally stimulated, indicating that in these kinds of insulin-resistant patients, insulin regulates glucose metabolism predominantly by modulating hepatic glucose balance.

As shown in Figure 6, the obese subjects exhibited decreased cellular insulin receptors. The dose-response data (Fig. 5) indicate that this is physiologically significant in both obese groups, since all of the curves are displaced to the right. To assess the absolute effectiveness of bound insulin, the relationship between the actual amount of insulin bound at a given insulin concentration and the in vivo biological effect of insulin at the concentration was examined. The amount of insulin bound was determined from the curves shown in Figure 6 at the insulin concentrations indicated in Figure 5. This analysis assumes that insulin binding to adipocytes accurately reflects insulin binding to other target tissues in vivo. In view of the heterogeneity demonstrated in obese subjects, one would expect to see different relationships for the two obese groups. As can be seen in Figure 8A, this is the case. It is apparent that, for any given amount of insulin bound, in vivo insulin effectiveness is comparable in the control and group I obese subjects;

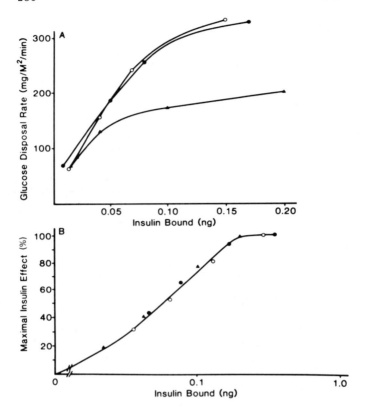

Figure 8 (A) Mean glucose disposal rates plotted as a function of
amount of insulin bound for control (●), group I obese (○), and
group II obese (▲) subjects. Amount of insulin bound was calculated
by multiplying insulin concentrations plotted in Figure 5 by percentage
of insulin bound at that concentration (as calculated from competition
binding curves in Fig. 6). (B) Percentage of maximal insulin effect
plotted as a function of amount of insulin bound.

this again demonstrates that the abnormality in the in vivo dose-
response curve (Fig. 5) in these subjects was the result of a decrease
in cellular insulin receptors. On the other hand, in vivo insulin action
is less at any given amount of insulin bound in the group II obese
group (Fig. 8A), and this suggests "uncoupling" between insulin-
receptor complexes and the biological function measured, i.e., overall
glucose disposal. This is the predicted consequence of a postreceptor
defect, and the uncoupling can be the result of any abnormality in the
insulin action-glucose metabolism sequence after the initial binding event.

To evaluate the site of this postbinding defect and to evaluate more accurately coupling between insulin-receptor complexes and glucose disposal, the relationship between percent of maximal insulin effect and the actual amount bound was also analyzed (Fig. 8B). As can be seen, the results in all three groups are comparable, indicating that when differences in postreceptor effector units are taken into account, insulin-receptor complexes are equally functional in all situations. Thus, actual coupling of insulin receptors to the biological effect is intact in obesity, and the reduction in glucose disposal in the group II obese subjects is the result of a defect distal to this step.

The close relationship between the decrease in insulin binding and the rightward shift in the dose-response curve in individual obese subjects plus the results of the analyses presented in Fig. 8 indicate that the receptor defect accounts for the decrease in insulin sensitivity (rightward shifted dose-response curve) and that the postreceptor defect lies distal to the coupling step. Thus, the possibility that a unique kind of postreceptor defect could cause a decrease in insulin action at submaximal insulin levels with normal response at maximal insulin levels can be excluded in this condition.

To elucidate the possible site of the postreceptor defect in obesity, an important effector unit, i.e., the glucose transport system, was evaluated in isolated adipocytes (64). The in vitro insulin dose-response curves for adipocyte 3-O-methylglucose transport in normals, group I obese, and group II obese are shown in Figure 9. In group I, decreased glucose transport is seen at submaximal insulin concentrations, whereas the maximal rates of insulin-stimulated glucose transport are normal. Thus, insulin sensitivity is decreased, but the maximum responsiveness to insulin is normal. This result is consistent with a decrease in insulin receptors and no postreceptor defect (51,52). In the group II obese patients, not only are the dose-response curves shifted to the right, but there is also a marked decrease in both the basal and maximal insulin-stimulated rates of glucose transport.

The data in Figure 9 demonstrate that the in vitro adipocyte glucose transport data are consistent with the in vivo glucose disposal rates as measured by the glucose clamp technique (Fig. 5). Furthermore, when the maximal in vitro glucose transport rates in individual patients are plotted as a function of the in vivo maximal glucose disposal rates in these patients, a statistically significant positive correlation is observed between these two variables (64). This indicates that the measurement of the adipocyte glucose transport rate provides an accurate estimate of the overall capacity of target tissues to dispose of glucose in vivo. Because adipocytes are a known peripheral target tissue for insulin action and because physiological and pathophysiological changes in adipocyte glucose transport are reflected by similar changes in the glucose transport system of skeletal muscle in animals (65), it seems reasonable to postulate that the findings in human

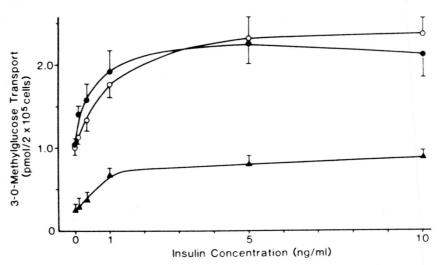

Figure 9 Dose-response curves for insulin stimulated 3-O-methylglucose transport in isolated adipocytes from normal (●), group I obese (○) and group II obese (▲) subjects. Isolated fat cells were incubated for 60 min at 37°C with the indicated concentrations of insulin and initial rates of 3-O-methylglucose transport were then measured and the values corrected for diffusion and extracellular trapping of substrate (by simultaneous measurement of L-glucose uptake). Transport values shown are per 10-sec periods.

adipocytes are representative of the other peripheral insulin target tissues in general. This conclusion is supported by the strong correlation observed between maximal insulin-stimulated overall glucose disposal observed in vivo and the adipocyte glucose transport rates observed in vitro (64). From these results, one can infer that the postreceptor defect demonstrated in many obese patients is due to a defect in the activity of the plasma membrane glucose transport carrier. Whether this is due to a decrease in the number of glucose carriers or a decrease in the accessibility of the carriers to the cell surface (14, 15) remains to be determined. In addition, it should be noted that although these results indicate that the rate-limiting step of the postreceptor defect in human obesity is localized to the glucose transport system, this does not exclude other more distal intracellular postreceptor defects in insulin action.

The results of these in vitro and in vivo studies in human obesity demonstrate that the cause of insulin resistance in this condition is heterogeneous. A likely explanation for this apparent heterogeneity is that the greater the hyperinsulinemia the more severe the insulin resistance; those patients with mild insulin resistance display only a defect in insulin receptors, whereas those obese patients with more severe hyperinsulinemia and insulin resistance also develop a post-receptor defect. The site of this postreceptor defect is distal to the coupling step and appears to involve a decrease in glucose transport system activity. Other more distal intracellular defects in glucose metabolism may also coexist.

V. INSULIN RESISTANCE IN TYPE II DIABETES MELLITUS

Insulin resistance is a characteristic feature of patients with impaired glucose tolerance and patients with type II or non-insulin-dependent diabetes mellitus (NIDDM) (52,66–69). Patients with impaired glucose tolerance have relatively mild insulin resistance, whereas patients with non-insulin-dependent type II diabetes mellitus have more severe insulin resistance. Furthermore, as the degree of carbohydrate intolerance worsens, the frequency of insulin resistance increases (68, 69). Thus, although not all patients with impaired glucose tolerance are insulin resistant, the great majority of type II diabetics with significant fasting hyperglycemia display this abnormality.

As discussed in the preceding section, obesity leads to the development of insulin resistance. Because the great majority of adult type II diabetic patients are overweight, obesity-induced insulin resistance is frequently a contributing factor in the hyperglycemia of these patients. However, obesity cannot account for all of the insulin resistance in this type of diabetic patient because the insulin resistance is greater than can be accounted for on the basis of the obesity alone. Furthermore, many nonobese non-insulin-dependent diabetic patients are also insulin resistant (52,66).

The euglycemic glucose clamp technique has been used to provide direct quantitative evidence for insulin resistance in patients with impaired glucose tolerance (chemical diabetes) and in overt type II diabetic patients (67). The patients with "chemical diabetes" consistently have normal fasting glucose levels (<115 mg/100/ml) but have abnormal oral glucose tolerance tests. The type II diabetic patients have fasting hyperglycemia (>140 mg/100 ml); the mean fasting glucose level in this group of patients is 255/mg/100 ml. These patients were divided into two groups consisting of thirteen nonobese (rel wt, <1.10; mean, 0.96) and ten obese (rel wt, >1.15; mean, 1.31) subjects. Figure 10 presents the mean steady-state plasma insulin levels and peripheral glucose disposal rates during euglycemic glucose clamp studies performed at an insulin infusion rate of 120 mU/m^2/min. As can be seen, despite comparable steady-state insulin levels, the glucose disposal rates are decreased in the diabetic groups, and the magnitude of this defect is

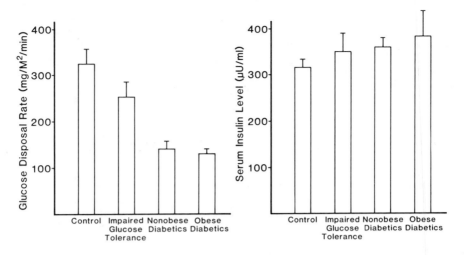

Figure 10 Mean steady-state glucose disposal rates (left panel) and serum insulin levels (right panel) for control subjects, subjects with impaired glucose tolerance, and nonobese and obese type II diabetics during euglycemic glucose clamp studies performed at an insulin infusion rate of 120 mU/m^2/min. The data shown are mean ± SE values.

greatest in the most carbohydrate-intolerant patients. Thus, the mean was reduced by 24% in the subjects with impaired glucose tolerance and by 56 and 60% in the nonobese and obese type II diabetic groups, respectively.

Since prereceptor causes of insulin resistance, such as abnormal β-cell secretory products or circulating insulin antagonists (Table 1), can only rarely be implicated in the pathogenesis of the insulin resistance in impaired glucose tolerance and type II diabetes, the most likely site of the insulin resistance in these disorders is at the level of target tissues (at receptor and postreceptor phases in insulin action). To assess the contribution of abnormalities at the receptor level to the overall insulin resistance, studies of insulin binding have been performed. Figure 11A summarizes measurements of insulin binding to receptors on circulating monocytes from normal and type II diabetic patients with fasting hyperglycemia. It is clear that the ability of cells from the diabetic patients to bind insulin is reduced due to a reduced number of cellular insulin receptors. When similar studies were performed in a group of patients with impaired glucose tolerance, analogous results were obtained (Fig. 11B). Thus, taken as a group, insulin binding to circulating monocytes is reduced in these patients, and the overall magnitude of this decrease in insulin binding is about the same for both diabetic groups. Because circulating monocytes are not a major target tissue for insulin, similar studies were performed using a known target tissue, i.e., isolated adipocytes. Figure 11C demonstrates that analogous results were found in this cell type. Scatchard analysis and average affinity profile analysis revealed that the decrease in insulin binding seen in Figure 11A−C are due to decreases in receptor number with no change in binding affinity (67).

As discussed earlier, the simple demonstration of decreased insulin receptors in the setting of insulin resistance does not necessarily imply cause and effect. To clarify the role of this cellular abnormality in the pathogenesis of the in vivo insulin rsistance of diabetes, the in vivo dose-response relationship was examined by performing additional euglycemic glucose clamp studies at insulin infusion rates of 40, 240, 1200, or 1800 mU$/$m$^2/$min (67).

As can been seen in Figure 12A, the curve for the subjects with impaired glucose tolerance lies to the right of the curve for the control subjects. Thus, the mean glucose disposal rates at insulin levels of 100, 300, and 1000 µU$/$ml are significantly less (P < 0.01) than those of controls. However, the subjects with impaired glucose tolerance achieve a maximal rate of glucose disposal not significantly different from that of the control subjects. Therefore, the insulin-resistant state associated with impaired glucose tolerance appears to result from a decrease in cellular insulin receptors with no evidence of a post-receptor defect in insulin action. The type II diabetic subjects exhibit both a rightward shift in their dose-response curve and a marked decrease in the maximal rate of glucose disposal, and there appears to be a tendency for these changes to be more pronounced in the obese diabetic subjects. Clearly, the predominant abnormality responsible for the insulin-resistant state in the patients with fasting hyperglycemia appears to be a postreceptor defect in insulin action leading to a marked decrease in maximal insulin responsiveness; this abnormality is present in both nonobese and obese type II diabetics. This demonstrates that in subjects with impaired glucose tolerance, the insulin resistance is due to decreased insulin receptors leading to decreased insulin sensitivity; in the patients with significant fasting hyperglycemia, decreased insulin receptors and a postreceptor defect in insulin action exist, leading both to decreased insulin sensitivity and decreased insulin responsiveness.

The functional form of the dose-response curves for the normals and the subjects with impaired glucose tolerance can be better appreciated by plotting the data as a percent of the maximal insulin effect (Fig. 12B). This analysis could not be done accurately for the type II diabetic subjects because their dose-response curves were so flat. The results show that the half-maximally effective insulin level is 135 µU$/$ml for the control subjects compared to 240 µU$/$ml for the subjects with impaired glucose tolerance (note the log scale on the abscissa).

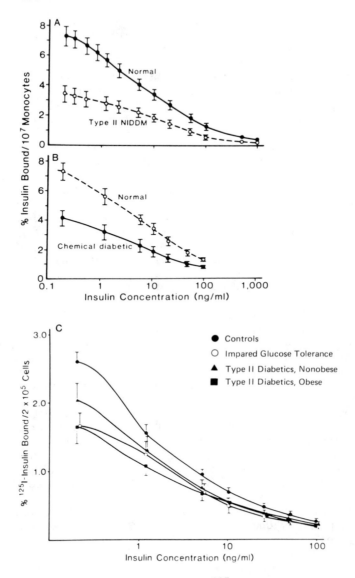

Figure 11   (A) Comparison of [^{125}I]insulin binding to isolated monocytes obtained from 40 normal subjects (●) and 31 type II diabetic patients (○).   (B) Comparison of [^{125}I]insulin binding to isolated monocytes obtained from 24 normal subjects (○) and from 14 patients with
chemical diabetes (●).   Mononuclear leukocytes (50 × 10^6/ml containing
6.5 × 10^6 monocytes/ml) were incubated with [^{125}I]insulin (0.2 ng/ml)

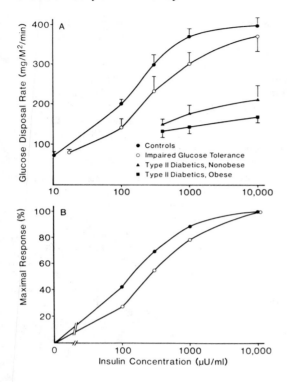

Figure 12 (A) Mean dose-response curves for insulin-stimulated glucose disposal rates in control subjects (●), subjects with impaired
glucose tolerance (○), and nonobese (▲) and obese (■) type II diabetics. (B) Mean dose-response curves for control subjects (●) and
subjects with impaired glucose tolerance (○) plotted as percent of
maximal response.

at 15°C for 100 min in the absence (initial point) or in the presence of
increasing unlabeled insulin concentrations. The binding data are corrected for nonspecific binding, and the percent of [125I]insulin specifically bound at the indicated total insulin concentrations are shown on
the ordinate. Each point represents the mean ± SE. (C) Insulin binding by isolated adipocytes from control subjects (●), subjects with impaired glucose tolerance (○), and nonobese (▲) and obese (■) type II
diabetics. All data are corrected for nonspecific binding and represent means ± SE of percentage [125I]insulin specifically bound by
2×10^5 cells.

Therefore, this form of analysis quantitates the rightward shift in the
dose-response curve for the subjects with impaired glucose tolerance,
thus demonstrating decreased insulin sentivitiy.

Hepatic glucose output was also measured during these studies,
and the results are presented in Figure 13. It is apparent that the
dose-response curves for hepatic glucose output are shifted to the
right in the patients with impaired glucose tolerance and in type II
diabetic subjects, and this is consistent with a decrease in insulin
sensitivity secondary to decreased insulin receptors. On the other
hand, it is also apparent that hepatic glucose production can be totally
suppressed in all patients, provided that high enough insulin concentrations are used. This is analogous to the situation seen in obesity
(see Fig. 7) and demonstrates that for this important insulin action no
postreceptor defect exists in livers of diabetic patients.

The biochemical nature of the postreceptor defect in the patients
with significant fasting hyperglycemia remains to be elucidated. However, because no postreceptor defect exists in the ability of insulin to
inhibit hepatic glucose production or in its antilipolytic effect (70), it
seems likely that the postreceptor abnormality is specific for one or
more aspects of cellular glucose uptake and metabolism. To pursue this
idea, studies of adipocyte glucose transport in diabetic subjects have
been completed recently (71).

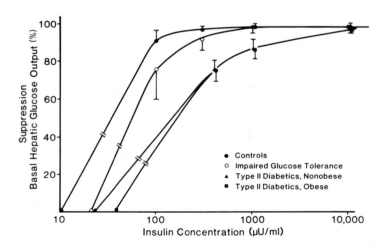

Figure 13 Mean dose-response curves for insulin-mediated suppression
of hepatic glucose output for control subjects (●), subjects with impaired glucose tolerance (○), nonobese type II diabetics (▲), and obese
type II diabetics (■).

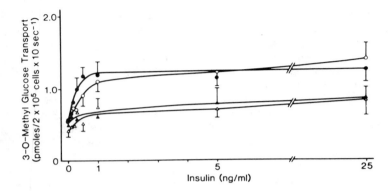

Figure 14 Dose-response curves for insulin stimulated 3-O-methyl-glucose transport in normal subjects (●), subjects with impaired glucose tolerance (○), lean type II diabetic (▲), and obese type II diabetic (△) subjects. Adipocytes are preincubated for 60 min at 37°C with the indicated concentrations of insulin and initial rates of 3-O-methylglucose transport then measured.

The in vitro insulin dose-response curves for adipocyte 3-O-methylglucose transport in normals, subjects with impaired glucose tolerance, and lean and obese patients with NIDDM are seen in Figure 14. In the subjects with imapired glucose tolerance, both basally (in the absence of insulin) and maximally (25 ng/ml) insulin-stimulated glucose transport rates are normal, while decreased glucose transport is seen at submaximal insulin concentrations. Thus, insulin sensitivity is decreased and insulin responsiveness is normal, consistent with a decrease in insulin receptors and no postreceptor defect. In both lean and obese NIDDM groups, not only are the dose-response curves shifted to the right, but there is also a decrease in both basally and maximally insulin-stimulated rates of glucose transport. Thus, both decreased insulin sensitivity and decreased insulin responsiveness are demonstrated, consistent with both receptor and postreceptor defects. These findings are consistent with what was observed in the in vivo multiple glucose clamp studies in these same patients (Fig. 12).

From the preceding data on insulin resistance in type II diabetes mellitus, a number of conclusions and generalizations can be made. In most patients with impaired glucose tolerance who are insulin resistant and relatively hyperinsulinemic, the pathogenesis of the carbohydrate intolerance seems to be due to decreased insulin receptors. This leads to decreased insulin sensitivity; and if adequate hyperinsulinemia cannot be generated to overcome this defect in insulin action, then carbohydrate intolerance develops. The relationship between insulin resistance and the diabetic state in type II diabetic patients with fasting hyperglycemia is more complex. Essentially all patients with severe fasting hyperglycemia are insulin resistant, and the degree of insulin resistance is much greater than that found in patients with impaired glucose intolerance. The available evidence indicates that the insulin resistance is largely related to a postreceptor defect in insulin action. It is possible that this postreceptor defect may be secondary to the diabetic state and that the defect may mirror the severity and chronicity of the disease. At least one locus for this postreceptor defect is the glucose transport system, since in vitro studies have demonstrated decreased glucose transport activity in freshly isolated adipocytes from type II diabetic patients. Although patients with fasting hyperglycemia can have normal or elevated basal insulin levels, they are uniformly hypoinsulinemic in response to a glucose challenge. This could indicate that the insulin resistance in these patients is secondary to the insulin deficiency. A possible corollary to this idea is that most of the insulin resistance of the diabetic patients with severe hyperglycemia could be reversed if the diabetic state were corrected with insulin therapy.

In this regard, recent evidence indicates that, when non-insulin-dependent type II diabetic patients are treated with frequent insulin injections to achieve near-normal blood glucose levels, the postreceptor defect can be substantially reversed (72). This is seen in Figure 15, which compares the in vivo dose-response curves in six patients before and after a 2-week period of intensive insulin treatment (the dose-response curves of normals are also shown for comparison).

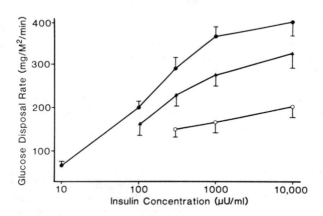

Figure 15 Mean dose-response curves for in vivo insulin-stimulated glucose disposal under euglycemic conditions (mean day long blood glucose level of ∿125 mg/100 ml) in normal subjects (●) and in six non-insulin-dependent type II diabetic subjects before (○) and after (▲) 2 weeks of intensive insulin therapy.

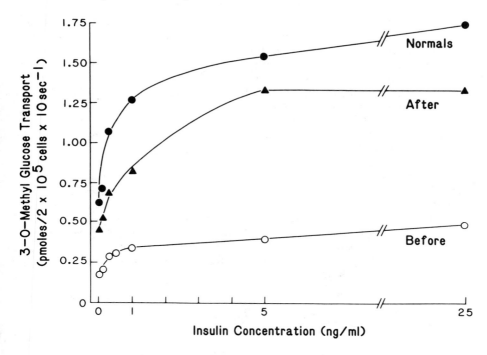

Figure 16 Mean in vitro dose-response curves for insulin stimulated 3-O-methylglucose transport in normal subjects (●), and in type II diabetic subjects before (○) and after (▲) intensive insulin treatment.

The period of intensive insulin treatment, which markedly improved glycemic control, did not change insulin binding to cells from these patients, demonstrating that the treatment-induced increase in glucose disposal rates seen in Figure 15 is due to amelioration of a postreceptor defect in insulin action. These results also confirm the interpretation that the cause of the decrease in maximally insulin-stimulated glucose disposal rates in the untreated type II patients was a postreceptor defect.

Since at least one locus for the postreceptor defect in type II diabetes is at the level of the glucose transport system (Fig. 14), it was of interest to examine if this defect can be reversed or improved by the intensive insulin treatment regimen. Figure 16 shows the in vitro insulin dose response curves for adipocyte 3-O-methylglucose transport in the diabetic subjects before and after treatment and in seven normal subjects. In the diabetic subjects prior to treatment, transport activity was significantly lower than the normal subjects' values in the basal state and at all insulin concentrations studied. After 14 days of insulin therapy, glucose transport activity increased significantly in the basal state as well as at all insulin concentrations. Although the diabetics' maximal glucose transport activity after treatment was still 24% decreased compared to the normal values, this difference was not statistically significant.

From these in vivo and in vitro studies, it can be concluded that the postreceptor defect in type II diabetes is acquired and reversible and, therefore, is secondary to some aspect of the chronic diabetic state, possibly the insulin deficiency. After the insulin treatment period, the patients are still quite insulin resistant, but now the resistance is primarily due to decreased insulin sensitivity resulting from the decreased insulin receptors with only a small residual contributory postreceptor defect. From a pathophysiological point of view, the result of the intensive insulin therapy is the conversion of the dose-response curves from a pattern indicative of combined lesions with the postreceptor defect predominant to a pattern in which the persisting receptor defect now predominates. It seems likely that if insulin treatment were carried out for longer periods or if euglycemic control were more tightly maintained, the postreceptor defect in the type II diabetic patients might be completely reversed.

VI. CONCLUDING REMARKS AND FUTURE PERSPECTIVES

In this chapter, we have presented a synopsis of our current understanding of overall insulin action, the general mechanisms subserving insulin resistance, and the role of receptor and postreceptor defects in target tissue resistance to insulin action, a phenomenon characteristically observed in obesity and non-insulin-dependent (type II) diabetes mellitus. While much progress has been made in these areas in recent years, our basic understanding of the primary pathogenetic mechanisms involved in obesity and type II diabetes mellitus remains incomplete. Although target tissue insulin resistance is a characteristic finding in type II diabetes mellitus, it is not yet established that this plays the primary pathogentic role in this disorder. This is because, in addition to insulin resistance, hypoinsulinemia, particularly in response to glucose challenge, is also commonly found in type II diabetics. This has led to the hypothesis that insulin deficiency resulting from either reduced β-cell mass or from a defect in glucose-stimulated insulin secretion may be a primary abnormality in type II diabetes mellitus. While according to this hypothesis the postreceptor defect of type II diabetes may be explained on the basis of impairment of insulin-dependent metabolic pathways resulting from the insulin deficiency, it becomes difficult to explain the receptor defect characteristically observed in type II diabetics. Furthermore, since some nonobese type II diabetics are also found to have basal hyperinsulinemia, a primary β-cell abnormality cannot explain such findings. If, on the other hand, type II diabetes mellitus results from a primary defect in target tissue insulin action, then the following sequence of events could be constructed to explain the various findings in this disorder: receptor or postreceptor defect → insulin resistance → compensatory hyperinsulinemia → further receptor reduction by down-regulation → worsening insulin resistance → more demand on β-cells leading to their exhaustion → hypoinsulinemia → more severe postreceptor defect(s). It is, however, unlikely that this sequence entirely explains all the pathophysiological findings of NIDDM. Thus, the exact interplay between insulin resistance and insulin deficiency in mediating the metabolic abnormalities in NIDDM remains to be unraveled. Furthermore, since the majority of patients with NIDDM are obese, any proposed pathogenetic mechanism should incorporate the contribution of the insulin resistance of obesity as an additional important variable. Finally, it should also be noted that even if target tissue insulin resistance is the primary lesion in type II diabetes, it appears that this abnormality is an acquired rather than an intrinsic (genetic) cellular defect. This is because in studies of cultured fibroblasts from type II diabetics, experimental conditions in which the in vivo metabolic and hormonal influences of the donors are eliminated, normal insulin binding (73) and insulin-stimulated glucose transport and metabolism (74,75) have been demonstrated. However, such results have to be interpreted with caution since fibroblasts are not major insulin target cells.

Regardless of whether target tissue insulin resistance plays a primary or secondary pathogenetic role, this abnormality is an important and consistent finding in type II diabetes. Thus, in future studies it will be important to elucidate further the precise biochemical abnormalities that lead to the receptor and postreceptor defects in this disorder. Clearly, further understanding of the cellular mechanisms involved in insulin receptor regulation (see Fig. 2) should help in defining if abnormalities in one or more of the various regulatory steps give rise to the observed reduction in insulin receptors in type II diabetes or obesity. In this regard, it should be noted that, recently, important results have appeared from different laboratories describing the pathways of insulin receptor biosynthesis. The findings indicate that the receptor is synthesized as a single chain polypeptide (proreceptor) that is subsequently glycosylated, cleaved into its constituent α and β subunits, and then expressed on the plasma membrane (see Chap. 12 and 76–78). Since the removal of the receptors from the plasma membrane by endocytosis and internalization is another major component of overall homeostatic control of receptor concentration on the cell surface, the precise mechanism by which this process occurs and is regulated also need to be further elucidated. In this regard, we have recently studied the internalization and processing of insulin receptors in isolated

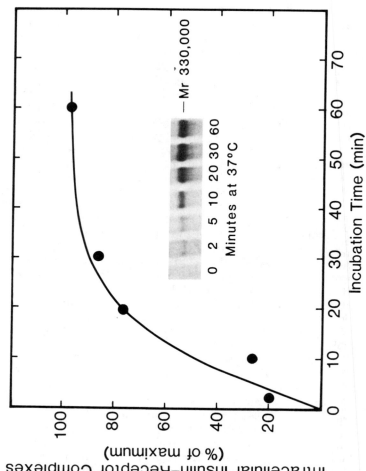

Figure 17 Time course of intracellular translocation of insulin-receptor complexes in human adipocytes. Insulin receptors were photolabeled on viable isolated human adipocytes at 16°C (a temperature at which the receptors remain on the cell surface) using a biologically active photosensitive insulin derivative (79). Under these conditions, the major specifically labeled non-reduced insulin receptor is a protein of M_r 330,000. The adipocytes photolabeled at 16°C were further incubated at 37°C to allow internalization of the receptors to occur, and, at the times shown, they were exposed to trypsin to remove labeled receptors still remaining on the cell surface; the internalized receptors remain inaccessible to trypsin. The cells were then washed, solubilized, and subjected to polyacrylamide gel electrophoresis (under nonreducing conditions) and autoradiography. The areas of the dried gel containing the trypsin-insensitive (intracellular) M_r 330,000 receptor forms were cut out, and the radioactivity was measured in a gamma counter. The results are expressed as percent of the maximal amount of intracellular labeled insulin-receptor complexes. The inset shows an autoradiogram depicting a time-dependent increase in the intensity of the intracellular M_r 330,000 receptor band.

human adipocytes using photoaffinity labeling techniques (79). With this technique, a biologically active photosensitive insulin analogue is radiolabeled and then is covalently linked to insulin receptors on the surface of viable cells through a photolytic reaction. The cellular fate of the insulin-receptor complexes is then studied at physiologic temperatures. In the example shown in Figure 17, it can be seen that in isolated human adipocytes insulin-receptor complexes are rapidly (within 2 min) internalized at 37°C. In further studies, we have also shown that a proportion of the internalized complexes are degraded intracellularly and that this process can be partially blocked by the lysosomotropic agent, chloroquine (79).

Thus, further detailed studies of the overall integrated mechanisms of insulin receptor regulation (biosynthesis, processing, internalization, recycling, degradation, etc.) should help in identifying the process(es) by which the receptor defects in obesity or type II diabetes develop. Similarly, in studies aimed at identifying the mechanisms of the postreceptor defect in obesity or type II diabetes, possible abnormalities in the insulin-induced translocation of glucose transporters, in receptor kinase activity, or in the generation or function of insulin mediator substances should all be considered.

ACKNOWLEDGMENTS

This work was supported by Grants AM 31072 and AM 32880 (to P.B.) and AM 25241 and AM 25242 (to J.M.O.) from the National Institute of Arthritis, Diabetes, and Digestive and Kidney Diseases, and in part by Grant BRSG-05357 from the Biomedical Research Grant Program, Division of Research Resources, National Institutes of Health.

The authors wish to thank Ms. Sally Frye for her expert secretarial assistance in the preparation of this manuscript.

REFERENCES

1. Banting, F. G. and Best, C. H. (1922). The internal secretion of the pancreas. *J. Lab. Clin. Med.* 7:251–266.
2. Banting, F. G. and Best, C. H. (1922). Pancreatic extracts. *J. Lab. Clin. Med.* 7:464–472.
3. Himsworth, H. (1949). The syndrome of diabetes mellitus and its cause. *Lancet 1*:465–472.
4. Yalow, R. S. and Berson, S. A. (1960). Immunoassay of endogenous plasma insulin in man. *J. Clin. Invest. 39*:1157–1175.
5. National Diabetes Data Group. (1979). Classification and diagnosis of diabetes mellitus and other categories of glucose intolerance. *Diabetes 28*:1039–1057.

6. Jacobs, S. and Cuatrecasas, P. (1981). Insulin receptor structure and function. *Endocrine Rev.* 2:251–263.
7. Czech, M. P. (1981). Insulin action. *Am. J. Med.* 70:142–150.
8. Bar, R. S., Harrison, L. C., Muggeo, M., Gorden, P., Kahn, C. R., and Roth, J. (1979). Regulation of insulin receptors in normal and abnormal physiology in humans. *Advan. Int. Med.* 24:23–52.
9. Kahn, C. R. (1980). Role of insulin receptors in insulin-resistant states. *Metabolism* 29:455–466.
10. Siegel, T. W., Ganguly, S., Jacobs, S., Rosen, O. M., and Rubin, C. S. (1981). Purification and properties of the human placental insulin receptor. *J. Biol. Chem.* 256:9266–9273.
11. Yip, C. C., Moule, M. L., and Yeung, C. W. T. (1980). Characterization of insulin receptor subunits in brain and other tissues by photoaffinity labeling. *Biochem. Biophys. Res. Commun.* 96:1671–1678.
12. Van Obberghen, E., Kasuga, M., Le Cam, A., Hedo, J. A., Itin, A., and Harrison, L. C. (1981). Biosynthetic labeling of insulin receptor: Studies of subunits in cultured human IM-9 lymphocytes. *Proc. Natl. Acad. Sci. USA* 78:1052–1056.
13. Czech, M. P. (1980). Insulin action and the regulation of hexose transport. *Diabetes* 29:399–408.
14. Suzuki, K. and Kono, T. (1980). Evidence that insulin causes translocation of glucose transport activity to the plasma membrane from intracellular storage site. *Proc. Natl. Acad. Sci. USA* 77:2542–2545.
15. Cushman, S. W. and Wardzala, L. J. (1980). Potential mechanism of insulin action on glucose transport in the isolated adipose cell. *J. Biol. Chem.* 255:4758–4762.
16. Kasuga, M., Karlsson, F. A., and Kahn, C. R. (1982). Insulin stimulates the phosphorylation of the 95,000-dalton subunit of its own receptor. *Science* 215:185–187.
17. Kasuga, M., Zick, Y., Blithe, D. L., Crettaz, M., and Kahn, C. R. (1982). Insulin stimulates tryosine phosphorylation of the insulin receptor in a cell-free system. *Nature (London)* 298:667–669.
18. Avruch, J., Nemenoff, R. A., Blackshear, P. J., Pierce, N. W., and Osathanondh, R. (1982). Insulin-stimulated tyrosine phosphorylation of the insulin receptor in detergent extracts of human placenta membranes: Comparison to epidermal growth factor-stimulated phosphorylation. *J. Biol. Chem.* 257:15162–15166.
19. Petruzzelli, L., Ganguly, S., Smith, C. J., Cobb, M. H., Rubin, C. S., and Rosen, O. M. (1982). Insulin activates a tyrosine-specific protein kinase in extracts of 3T3-L1 adipocytes and human placenta. *Proc. Natl. Acad. Sci. USA* 79:6792–6796.

20. Roth, R. A. and Cassel, D. J. (1983). Insulin receptor: Evidence that it is a protein kinase. *Science* 219:299–301.
21. Gorden, P., Carpentier, J.-L., Freychet, P., and Orci, L. (1980). Internalization of polypeptide hormones. *Diabetologia* 18:263–274.
22. Posner, B. I., Khan, M. N., and Bergeron, J. J. M. (1982). Endocytosis of peptide hormones and other ligands. *Endocrine Rev.* 3:280–298.
23. Berhanu, P., Olefsky, J. M., Tsai, P., Thamm, P., Saunders, D., and Brandenburg, D. (1982). Internalization and molecular processing of insulin receptors in isolated rat adipocytes. *Proc. Natl. Acad. Sci. USA* 79:4069–4073.
24. Green, A. and Olefsky, J. M. (1982). Evidence for insulin-induced internalization and degradation of insulin receptors in rat adipocytes. *Proc. Natl. Acad. Sci. USA* 79:427–431.
25. Fehlmann, M., Carpentier, J.-L., LeCam, A., Thamm, P., Saunders, D., Brandenburg, D., Orci, L., and Freychet, P. (1982). Biochemical and morphological evidence that the insulin receptor is internalized with insulin in hepatocytes. *J. Cell Biol.* 93:82–87.
26. Olefsky, J. M., Marshall, S., Berhanu, P., Saekow, M., Heidenreich, K., and Green, A. (1982). Internalization and intracellular processing of insulin and insulin receptors in adipocytes. *Metabolism* 31:670–690.
27. Berhanu, P. and Olefsky, J. M. (1982). Photoaffinity labeling of insulin receptors in viable cultured human lymphocytes: Demonstration of receptor shedding and degradation. *Diabetes* 31:410–417.
28. Marshall, S., Green, A., and Olefsky, J. M. (1981). Evidence for recycling of insulin receptors in isolated rat adipocytes. *J. Biol. Chem.* 256:11464–11470.
29. Gavin, J. R. III, Roth, J., Neville, D. M., Jr., DeMeyts, P., and Buell, D. N. (1974). Insulin-dependent regulation of insulin receptor concentrations: A direct demonstration in cell culture. *Proc. Natl. Acad. Sci. USA* 71:84–88.
30. Goldfine, I. D. (1981). Interaction of insulin, polypeptide hormones, and growth factors with intracellular membranes. *Biochim. Biophys. Acta* 650:53–67.
31. Posner, B. I., Bergeron, J. J. M., Josefsberg, Z., Khan, M. N., Khan, R. J., Patel, B. A., Sikstrom, R. A., and Verma, A. K. (1981). Polypeptide hormones: Intracellular receptors and internalization. *Recent Prog. Hormone Res.* 37:539–582.
32. Olefsky, J. M., Saekow, M., Tager, H., and Rubenstein, A. H. (1980). Characterization of a mutant human insulin species. *J. Biol. Chem.* 255:6098–6105.

33. Tager, H., Given, B., Baldwin, D., Mako, M., Markese, J., Rubenstein, A., Olefsky, J., Kobayashi, M., Kolterman, O., and Poucher, R. (1979). A structurally abnormal insulin causing human diabetes. *Nature (London)* 281:122—125.

34. Gabbay, K. H., De Luca, K., Fisher, Jr., J. N., Mako, M. E. and Rubenstein, A. H. (1976). Familial hyperproinsuline-mia: An autosomal dominant defect. *N. Engl. J. Med.* 294: 911—915.

35. Kanazawa, H., Hayashi, M., Ikeuchi, M., Hirmatsu, K., and Kosaka, K. (1978). Familial proinsulinemia: A possible cause of abnormal glucose tolerance. *Eur. J. Clin. Invest.* 8:327.

36. Wicks, W. D., Barnett, C. A., and McKibbin, J. B. (1974). Interaction between hormones and cyclic AMP in regulating specific hepatic enzyme synthesis. *Fed. Proc.* 33:1105.

37. Wise, J. K., Hendler, R., and Felig, P. (1973). Influence of glucocorticoids on glucagon secretion and plasma amino acid concentrations in man. *J. Clin. Invest.* 52:2774—2782.

38. Issekutz, B. and Allen, M. (1972). Effect of catecholamines and methylprednisolone on carbohydrate metabolism of dogs. *Metabolism* 21:48—59.

39. Olefsky, J. M. (1975). Effect of dexamethasone on insulin binding glucose transport, and glucose oxidation of isolated rat adipocytes. *J. Clin. Invest.* 56:1499—1508.

40. Bratusch-Marrain, P. R. (1983). Insulin-counteracting hormones: Their impact on glucose metabolism. *Diabetologia* 24: 74—79.

41. Kahn, C. R. Goldfine, I. D., Neville, D. M., Jr., and De Meyts, P., (1978). Alterations in insulin binding induced by changes in vivo in the levels of glucocorticoids and growth hormone. *Endocrinology* 103:1054—1066.

42. Muggeo, M., Bar, R. S., Roth, J., Kahn, C. R., and Gorden, P. (1979). The insulin resistance of acromegaly: Evidence for two alterations in the insulin receptor on circulating monocytes. *J. Clin. Endocrinol. Metab.* 48:17—25.

43. Sacca, L., Eigler, N., Cryer, P. E., and Sherwin, R. S. (1979). Insulin antagonistic effects of epinephrine and glucagon in the dog. *Am. J. Physiol.* 237:E487—E492.

44. Schernthaner, G., Borkenstein, M., Fink, M., Mayr, W. R., Menzel, J., and Schober, E. (1983). Immunogenicity of human insulin (Novo) or pork monocomponent insulin in HLA-DR-typed insulin-dependent diabetic individuals. *Diabetes Care* 6:43—48.

45. Kurtz, A. B. and Nabarro, J. D. N. (1980). Circulating insulin-binding antibodies. *Diabetologia* 19:329—334.

46. Kahn, C. R., Baird, K. L., Flier, J. S., Grunfeld, C., Harmon, J. T., Harrison, L. C., Karlsson, F. A., Kasuga, M., King, G. L., Lang, U. C., Podskalny, J. M., and Van

Obberghen, E. (1981). Insulin receptors, receptor antibodies and mechanism of insulin action. *Recent Prog. Hormone Res.* 37:447–538.

47. Kono, T. and Barham, F. W. (1971). The relationship between the insulin-binding capacity of fat cells and the cellular response to insulin: Studies with intact and trypsin-treated fat cells. *J. Biol. Chem.* 246:6210–6216.

48. Gliemann, J., Gammeltoft, S., and Vinten, J. (1975). Time course of insulin-receptor binding and insulin-induced lipogenesis in isolated rat fat cells. *J. Biol. Chem.* 250:3368–3374.

49. Olefsky, J. M. (1976). Effects of fasting on insulin binding, glucose transport, and glucose oxidation in isolated rat adipocytes. Relationships between insulin receptors and insulin action. *J. Clin. Invest.* 58:1450–1460.

50. Olefsky, J. M. (1976). The insulin receptor: Its role in insulin resistance in obesity and diabetes. *Diabetes* 25:1154–1165.

51. Kahn, C. R. (1978). Insulin resistance, insulin insensitivity and insulin unresponsiveness: A necessary distinction. *Metabolism* 27:1893–1902.

52. Olefsky, J. M. (1980). Insulin resistance and insulin action: An in vitro and in vivo perspective. *Diabetes* 30:148–162.

53. Bar, R. S., Gorden, P., Roth, J., Kahn, C. R., and De Meyts, P. (1976). Fluctuations in the affinity and concentration of insulin receptors on circulating monocytes of obese patients: Effects of starvation, refeeding and dieting. *J. Clin. Invest.* 58:1123–1135.

54. Olefsky, J. M. (1976). Decreased insulin binding to adipocytes and circulating monocytes from obese subjects. *J. Clin. Invest.* 57:1165–1172.

55. Roth, J., Kahn, C. R., Lesniak, M. A., Gorden, P., De Meyts, P., Megyesi, K., Neville, D. M., Jr., Gavin, J. R. III, Soll, A. H., Freychet, P., Goldfine, I. D., Bar, R. S., and Archer, J. A. (1976). Receptors for insulin, NSILA-s and growth hormone: Applications to disease states in man. *Recent Prog. Hormone Res.* 31:95–126.

56. Kahn, C. R. Neville, D. M., Jr., and Roth, J. (1973). Insulin-receptor interaction in the obese hyperglycemic mouse. A model of insulin resistance. *J. Biol. Chem.* 248:244–250.

57. Insel, P. A., Liljenquist, J. E., Tobin, J. D., Sherwin, R. S., Watkins, P., Andres, R., and Berman, M. (1975). Insulin control of glucose metabolism in man. *J. Clin. Invest.* 55:1057–1066.

58. Sherwin, R. S., Kramer, K. J., Tobin, J. D., Insel, P. A., Liljenquist, J. E., Berman, M., and Andres, R. (1974). A model of the kinetics of insulin in man. *J. Clin. Invest.* 53:1481–1492.

59. Kolterman, O. G., Insel, J., Saekow, M., and Olefsky, J. M. (1980). Mechanisms of insulin resistance in human obesity— evidence for receptor and post receptor defects. *J. Clin. Invest.* 65:1273–1284.

60. Cahill, G. F., Jr. (1970). Starvation in man. *N. Engl. J. Med.* 282:668–675.

61. Cherrington, A. D., Lacy, W. W., and Chiasson, J. L. (1978). Effect of glucagon on glucose production during insulin deficiency in the dog. *J. Clin. Invest.* 62:664–677.

62. Vranic, M. and Wrenshall, G. A. (1968). Matched rates of insulin infusion and secretion and concurrent tracer-determined rates of glucose appearance and disappearance in fasting dogs. *Can. J. Physiol.* 46:383–390.

63. Blackard, W. G. and Nelson, N. C. (1970). Portal and peripheral vein immunoreactive insulin concentrations before and after glucose infusion. *Diabetes* 19:302–306.

64. Ciaraldi, T. P., Kolterman, O. G., and Olefsky, J. M. (1981). Mechansim of the post receptor defect in insulin action in human obesity. A decrease in glucose transport system activity. *J. Clin. Invest.* 68:875–880.

65. Le Marchand-Brustel, Y., Jeanrenaud, B., and Freychet, P. (1978). Insulin binding and effects in isolated soleus muscle of lean and obese mice. *Am. J. Physiol.* 234:E348–E358.

66. Reaven, G. M. and Olefsky, J. M. (1978). Role of insulin resistance in the pathogenesis of diabetes mellitus. *Advan. Metab. Res.* 9:313–331.

67. Kolterman, O. G., Gray, R. S., Griffin, J. Burstein, P., Insel, J., Scarlett, J. A., and Olefsky, J. M. (1981). Receptor and post-receptor defects contribute to the insulin resistance in non-insulin-dependent diabetes mellitus. *J. Clin. Invest.* 68:957–969.

68. Olefsky, J. M. and Reaven, G. M. (1977). Insulin binding in diabetes: Relationship with plasma insulin levels and insulin sensitivity. *Diabetes* 26:680–688.

69. Reaven, G. M., Bernstein, R., Davis, B., and Olefsky, J. M. (1976). Non-ketotic diabetes mellitus: Insulin deficiency or insulin resistance? *Am. J. Med.* 60:80–88.

70. Ginsberg, H., Kimmerling, G., Olefsky, J. M., and Reaven, G. M. (1975). Demonstration of insulin resistance in maturity onset diabetic patients with fasting hyperglycemia. *J. Clin. Invest.* 55:454–460.

71. Ciaraldi, T. P., Kolterman, O. G., Scarlett, J. A., Kao, M., and Olefsky, J. M. (1982). Role of the glucose transport system in the post-receptor defect of non-insulin-dependent diabetes mellitus. *Diabetes* 31:1016–1022.

72. Scarlett, J. A., Gray, R. S., Griffin, J., Olefsky, J. M., and Kolterman, O. G. (1982). Insulin treatment reverses the insulin resistance of type II diabetes mellitus. *Diabetes Care* 5:353—363.
73. Prince, M. J., Tsai, P., and Olefsky, J. M. (1981). Insulin binding internalization, and insulin receptor regulation in fibroblasts from type II, non-insulin-dependent diabetic subjects. *Diabetes* 30:596—600.
74. Howard, B. V., Hidaka, H., Ishibashi, F., Fields, R. M., and Bennett, P. H. (1981). Type II diabetes and insulin resistance. Evidence for lack of inherent cellular defects in insulin sensitivity. *Diabetes* 30:562—567.
75. Berhanu, P., Tsai, P., and Olefsky, J. M. (1982). Insulin-stimulated glucose transport in cultured fibroblasts from normal and non-insulin-dependent (type II) diabetic human subjects. *J. Clin. Endocrinol. Metab.* 55:1226—1230.
76. Kasauga, M., Hedo, J. A., Yamada, K. M., and Kahn, C. R. (1983). The structure of insulin receptor and its subunits. Evidence for multiple nonreduced forms and a 210,000 dalton possible proreceptor. *J. Biol. Chem.* 257:10392—10399.
77. Deutsch, P. J., Wan, C. F., Rosen, O. M., and Rubin C. S. (1983). Latent insulin receptors and possible prereceptors in 3T3-L1 adipocytes. *Proc. Natl. Acad. Sci. USA* 80:133—136.
78. Jacobs, S., Kull, F. C., Jr., and Cuatrecasas, P. (1983). Monensin blocks the maturation of receptors for insulin and somatomedin C: Identification of receptor precursors. *Proc. Natl. Acad. Sci. USA* 80:1228—1231.
79. Berhanu, P., Kolterman, O. G., Baron, A., Tsai, P., Olefsky, J. M., and Brandenburg, D. (1983). Insulin receptors in isolated human adipocytes: Characterization by photoaffinity labeling and evidence for internalization and cellular processing. *J. Clin. Invest.* 72:1958—1970.

BIBLIOGRAPHY

Baxter, J. D. and Funder, J. W. (1979). Hormone receptors. *N. Engl. J. Med.* 301:1149—1161.
Catt, K. J., Harwood, J. P., Aguilera, G. and Dufau, M. L. (1979). Hormonal regulation of peptide receptors and target cell responses. *Nature (London)* 280:109—116.
Flier, J. S. (1983). Insulin receptors and insulin resistance. *Ann. Rev. Med.* 34:145—160.
Kahn, C. R., Megyesi, K., Bar, R. S., Eastman, R. C. and Flier, J. S. (1977). Receptors for peptide hormones. New insights into the pathophysiology of disease states in man. *Ann. Intern. Med.* 86:205—219.

Pollet, R. J. and Levey, G. S. (1980). Principles of membrane receptor physiology and their application to clinical medicine. *Ann. Intern Med.* 92:663—680.

Roth, J. and Grunfeld, C. (1981). Endocrine systems. Mechanisms of disease, target cells, and receptors. In *Textbook of Endocrinology*, Sixth ed. (R. H. Williams, ed), W. B. Saunders Co., Philadelphia, pp. 15—72.

Index

A

Acetyl-CoA carboxylase, 192—195
Acromegaly, 273
ATPase, Na^+-K^+-activated, 150
Adipocyte(s), 30—35, 78, 109—118, 127—132, 284, 295, 297
   receptor distribution, 112
   receptor mobility, 111—113
   receptors, 30—35, 109—118
3T3-L1, 243—244
Allen, 16
α-Amanitin, 227
Antidiuretic hormone, 63
Antireceptor antibodies, 39, 91—95, 276, 288, 291
   monoclonal, 93—94
   polyclonal, 92—93
   receptor down-regulation, 95
Aryl azide, 29
4-Azidobenzoate, 29

B

Banting, 7—17
Best, 7—17
β-D-Galactosidase, 197
Bifunctional cross-linking reagent, 244

C

Chloroquine, 131, 133, 255
Chromatography, affinity, 39—40
Circumventricular organs, 206—216
   and diabetes, 214—215
   functional topography of receptors, 212—214
   hormone receptors, 207—208
   localization, 206—207
   neuronal circuitry, 208—212
   role in health and disease, 214—216